Migration, Health and Survival

Migration, Health and Survival

International Perspectives

Edited by

Frank Trovato

Department of Sociology, University of Alberta, Canada

Edward Elgar
PUBLISHING

Cheltenham, UK • Northampton, MA, USA

Published by
Edward Elgar Publishing Limited
The Lypiatts
15 Lansdown Road
Cheltenham
Glos GL50 2JA
UK

Edward Elgar Publishing, Inc.
William Pratt House
9 Dewey Court
Northampton
Massachusetts 01060
USA

A catalogue record for this book
is available from the British Library

Library of Congress Control Number: 2017947085

This book is available electronically in the **Elgar**online
Social and Political Science subject collection
DOI 10.4337/9781785365973

MIX
Paper from responsible sources
FSC® C013056
FSC www.fsc.org

ISBN 978 1 78536 596 6 (cased)
ISBN 978 1 78536 597 3 (eBook)

Typeset by Servis Filmsetting Ltd, Stockport, Cheshire
Printed and bound in Great Britain by TJ International Ltd, Padstow

Contents

Contributors

Olga Anikeeva is a postdoctoral research fellow at the Torrens Resilience Institute at Flinders University in Adelaide, Australia. Her key research interests include migrant mortality and morbidity trends, the health indicators of vulnerability, and disaster preparedness and resilience. Some of her recent publications in the field of migrant health appear in *Asia-Pacific Journal of Public Health*, *Cancer Epidemiology* and *Ethnicity and Health*.

Peng Bi is Professor of Public Health Medicine, The University of Adelaide, Australia. His main research areas include environmental epidemiology, infectious disease epidemiology and international health including migrant health. Among his recent works is a study of the impact of climate change on the health of migrants, mainly focusing on risk assessment and risk communication among the culturally and linguistically diverse (CALD) communities in Australia. Some of his recent publications appear in the journals *Ethnicity and Health* and *Science Communication*.

Nicholas Biddle is an Associate Professor and Senior Fellow at the Centre for Aboriginal Economic Policy Research (CAEPR) at the Australian National University (ANU) and Deputy Director of the ANU Centre for Social Research and Methods. He has a Bachelor of Economics (Hons.) from the University of Sydney and a Master of Education from Monash University. He also has a PhD in Public Policy from the ANU where he wrote his thesis on the benefits of and participation in education of Indigenous Australians. He previously held a Senior Research Officer and Assistant Director position in the Methodology Division of the Australian Bureau of Statistics. Associate Professor Biddle has written extensively on the demographic and socioeconomic characteristics of the Indigenous Australian population and also co-authored the first major comparative study of immigrant health profiles across four large English speaking countries.

Patrick Brzoska, DrPH, MSc, EMPH, is Junior Professor of Epidemiology at the Faculty of Behavioural and Social Sciences at Chemnitz University of Technology, Germany. His research interests comprise social and health services epidemiology, the health and health care of migrants, illness perceptions and coping with chronic diseases, rehabilitative and nursing care, international public health and the development of epidemiological research methods. Some of his most recent research appears in *BMJ Open Health Services Research* and *International Journal of Public Health*.

Graziella Caselli is Honorary Professor of Sapienza University of Rome. She is a IUSSP Laureate (2012) and Honorary President of the European Association for Population Studies – EAPS, and Editor in Chief of *GENUS – Journal of Population Sciences*. She is a co-editor of the four-volume *Demography, Analysis and Synthesis – A Treatise in Population Studies*. Many of her papers have been published in international journals, including *Population Studies* and *Demography*. Her main fields of research are population longevity and ageing; analysis of the role of socio-demographic factors on the welfare state; elderly health and survival; projections and forecast models for mortality by cause of death; devising demographic models for longitudinal analyses, and population heterogeneity.

Patrick Deboosere is Professor of Demography at the Vrije Universiteit Brussel, Belgium, where he is also director of Interface Demography. Among his recent publications, his works appear in the *Journal of Epidemiology and Community Health*, *European Journal of Public Health*, the *International Journal of Tuberculosis and Lung Disease*, *BMC Public Health*, *PLoS Medicine*, *Ethnicity and Health* and the *International Migration Review*.

Michel Guillot is Professor of Sociology at the University of Pennsylvania and Research Associate at the French Institute for Demographic Studies (INED). His research is organized primarily around two main areas: formal demography and understanding health disparities across and within populations. In the area of formal demography Dr Guillot has designed new methodologies for better understanding mortality levels and trends, and for studying their impact on population growth and ageing, and has made contributions in the area of model age patterns of mortality and indirect estimation methods. In the area of health disparities, his research has examined the burden of disease among the global poor. He has also studied the health of vulnerable ethnic, religious, and migrant groups in a range of populations, including India. Among his other research interests is the analysis of the health crisis in the former Soviet Union, with a special focus on the Central Asia region. Among his many publications is his book, *Demography: Modeling Population Processes*, co-authored with Samuel H. Preston and Patrick Heuveline.

Myriam Khlat is Senior Researcher at the Institut National d'Etudes Démographiques (INED) in Paris. Her main research interests are in the social determinants of health and differential mortality. Dr Khlat served as

Co-Editor of the *European Journal of Population* and as deputy director of INED. In the late 1980s, she was in charge of the statistical aspects of an international study on cancer among Italian migrants throughout the world at the International Agency for Research on Cancer. In the mid-1990s, with her colleague Dr Courbage, Dr Khlat undertook a study on the mortality of Moroccans in France, which remains to date the only one of its kind to have corrected their mortality data for under-registration using indirect estimation techniques. Among her many publications, her recent work appears in *Social Science & Medicine*, *International Archives for Occupational and Environmental Health*, *AIDS*, and *Journal of Epidemiology and Community Health*.

Lihua Liu, PhD, has worked as a demographer and social epidemiologist at the Los Angeles Cancer Surveillance Program for many years and currently serves as its Director for Data Utilization. She is also an Associate Professor in the Department of Preventive Medicine at Keck School of Medicine of the University of Southern California. Her research interest is in the health disparities and disease patterns in various racial/ethnic populations in the USA. She is particularly interested in understanding the changing cancer risks among immigrant populations. Among her recent publications is a chapter on cancer among Chinese Americans, appearing in the book, *Cancer Epidemiology Among Asian Americans*. Her research on cancer has been published in *Cancer Causes Control*, *Journal of the National Cancer Institute* and *International Journal of Cancer*.

Silvia Loi is a Research Scientist at the Max Planck Institute for Demographic Research in Rostock, Germany. She obtained her PhD in demography from the Department of Statistical Sciences, University of Rome, La Sapienza, with a dissertation on migrant health in Italy. Her research interests include international migration, migrant health and its socioeconomic determinants. Her current research focuses on migrant health as a driver for integration.

Doug G. Manuel, Dr Med., has a Master's in epidemiology and Royal College specialization in public health and preventive medicine. He is a Senior Scientist of Ottawa Hospital Research Institute and a Senior Medical Advisor for Statistics Canada, Professor in the Departments of Family Medicine and the School of Epidemiology, Public Health and Preventive Medicine at the University of Ottawa. He is also a Clinician Scientist at the Bruyère Research Institute. Dr Manuel's research interest is the population health impact assessment of health interventions and the assessment of population health status. He has developed performance measures and planning tools for health planning. Dr Manuel's research combines his interests in public health, health-care systems and primary care. The overarching question that spans his research is how to most effectively improve health of communities and reduce inequities. He performs two types of studies: modelling studies or 'what if' studies that examine the potential impact of interventions; and, observational or 'what is' studies that examine the actual impact of interventions that are provided routinely in our society or that are experimentally being tested. His studies typically focus on prevention such as immunization and healthy living. His laboratory also performs supporting studies that describe or predict the future health of Canadians and health care use. Dr Manuel has been a primary care physician for 25 years, serving rural, remote and underserviced populations across Canada. His current practice is with refugees at the Ottawa Newcomer Clinic.

K. Bruce Newbold is Professor of Geography at McMaster University, Hamilton, Ontario, Canada. He has held guest positions at the University of Glasgow, UK, and the University of California San Diego, USA. Trained as a population geographer, his research interests include migration, immigration, health, and human capital. He is the author or co-author of over 100 academic articles, and has also authored the population textbook *Population Geography: Tools and Issues*. He has received awards for his work and service from the Population Specialty Group of the Association of American Geographers and the North American Regional Science Council.

Edward Ng is a Senior Analyst with the Health Analysis Division at Statistics Canada, and is also an Adjunct Professor at the School of Epidemiology, Public Health and Preventive Medicine at the University of Ottawa. He obtained his PhD in social demography from the University of Western Ontario. His research interest is on the use of record linkage to study immigrant health. He has conducted analyses using national population health surveys in Canada to understand the healthy immigrant effect. Recently, he used census or immigrant landing files linked to hospital data to examine liver-related disease and vaccine-preventable diseases among immigrants, as well as on circulatory disease-related hospitalization from the generational perspective. He also provided a big picture overview on immigrant health research in Canada in the *Health Research Bulletin* published by Health Canada to chronicle the development of health data in Canada to understand immigrant health.

Brit Oppedal is a Senior Researcher in the Division of Mental Health of the Norwegian Institute of Public Health. She has a PhD in psychology from the University of Oslo. She is the Principal Investigator of the research programme 'Youth, culture and competence' (YCC), and of the various national and international subprojects under this umbrella, such as 'Social support, coping and mental health among unaccompanied minor asylum-seekers', 'Identity, adaptation and well-being among Tamil children and youth', 'Classroom psychosocial environment and well-being in multicultural schools' and 'Social integration of migrant children: uncovering family and school factors promoting resilience'. Her research focus is on predictors of the mental health of immigrant and refugee background children, and on factors promoting their positive bicultural development and psychological adjustment.

David Ponka, MD, CCFP, MSc (Int. Prim Care), is Medical Advisor to the Migration Health Branch of Immigration, Refugees and Citizenship Canada and an Associate Professor in the Faculty of Medicine at the University of Ottawa, Canada. In his work, Dr Ponka strives to combine research with clinical and educational practice.

Oliver Razum, PhD, Dr med., MSc Epidemiology, is Professor and Dean of the School of Public Health, Bielefeld University, Germany, where he also heads the Department of Epidemiology & International Public Health. His main research area is social epidemiology with a focus on the health of immigrants and refugees; and on the role of contextual factors in the production of health inequalities. Before moving into epidemiology, he worked as district medical officer in Zimbabwe. Dr Razum has published over 180 scientific papers and co-authored or co-edited numerous books and book chapters.

Claudia Sanmartin currently works at Statistics Canada as Assistant Director in the Health Analysis Division. She received her Master of Science in health administration from the University of Toronto and a PhD in health services research from the University of British Columbia. She also holds an Adjunct Research Assistant Professorship at both the University of Calgary and University of Toronto. Claudia has worked extensively on the development and use of linked data to understand the role of broader determinants of health on use of health care services.

Gopal K. Singh, PhD, is a Senior Health Equity Advisor with the Health Resources and Services Administration, US Department of Health and Human Services, Rockville, Maryland. His research interests include global health inequalities, socioeconomic determinants of health and mortality, immigrant health, obesity and physical activity, and spatial and time trends in chronic disease morbidity and mortality. He has published two books and nearly 150 peer reviewed articles in the field of health inequalities, social determinants of health, immigrant health, and cancer epidemiology. His recent papers have appeared in *American Journal of Public Health*, *American Journal of Preventive Medicine*, *Pediatrics*, *JAMA Pediatrics* and *International Journal of Epidemiology*.

Salvatore Strozza is Professor of Demography at the University of Naples Federico II. He is the coordinator of the bachelor degree programme in political science and Master's degrees in international relations, and European studies. He is President of the Italian Association for Population Studies (AISP-SIS). Dr Strozza's main fields of research are international migration, with major contributions on: sources and methods of measurement and estimates; demographic consequences of international migration; fertility of immigrants; measures and determinants of immigrant integration; and second generation and school system. Among his publications are articles appearing in *International Migration Review*, *European Journal of Population* and *Journal of Ethnic and Migration Studies*.

Frank Trovato is Professor of Sociology and Demography at the University of Alberta, Canada. He is Editor-in-Chief of *Canadian Studies in Population*. His research interests intersect diverse topics across the disciplines of sociology, demography and social epidemiology. In 2012 he was awarded the Nathan Keyfitz Book Prize for his book, *Canada's Population in a Global Context: An Introduction to Social Demography*. Some of his recent works appear in *Journal of Biosocial Science*, *Cahiers québécois de démographie* and *Review of Religious Research*.

Jack V. Tu, MD, holds a Tier 1 Canada Research Chair in Health Services Research and an Eaton Scholar Award. He is a senior scientist at the Institute for Clinical Evaluative Sciences, where he oversees the cardiovascular programme, a professor of medicine at the University of Toronto and also an attending physician in Cardiology at Sunnybrook Schulich Heart Centre. He is internationally recognized and has published over 380 peer-reviewed articles in many leading journals. He holds several million dollars in peer-reviewed grants from the Canadian Institutes of Health Research, Heart and Stroke Foundation, and other funding agencies. His research focuses on use of 'big data' for cardiovascular quality of care and outcomes research.

Hadewijch Vandenheede is Professor at the Vrije Universiteit Brussel, Belgium. She is team member of Interface Demography. Among her many publications, some of her recent works appear in the *European Journal of Public Health*, *BMC Public Health*, *PLoS One*, *Tropical Medicine & International Health*, *Health & Place* and *Ethnicity and Health*.

Matthew Wallace, PhD, is a postdoctoral researcher at the French National Institute for Demographic Studies (INED) in the Health, Mortality and Epidemiology unit. Dr Wallace was awarded his doctoral degree from the University of Liverpool (under the supervision of Professor Hill Kulu, who is the co-author of three of the four articles summarized in his chapter). From his thesis, Dr Wallace has published articles in *Social Science & Medicine*, *Population, Space and Place*, and the *Journal of Ethnic and Migration Studies*.

Samuel G. Weldeegzie is a postdoctoral researcher at the WORLD Policy Analysis Center, UCLA, USA. Samuel completed his PhD at the Australian National University. Prior to this, he received his MA degree in the economics of development from the International Institute of Social Studies of Erasmus University Rotterdam and his BA degree in economics from Jimma University, Ethiopia. Samuel is interested in the health of immigrants, the long-term effect of conflict on human capital outcomes, and applied microeconometrics.

Lori Wilkinson is Professor of Sociology and Director of Immigration Research West at the University of Manitoba, Canada. She is Editor-in-Chief of *Journal of International Migration and Integration*. Dr Wilkinson's research focuses on the integration of newcomers. Among her latest projects is an examination of how immigrants use settlement services aimed at identifying those who need but cannot access services. Her other works look at the long-term labour market trajectories of immigrants arriving in Canada as children or teens, the health outcomes of newcomer children and youth, and the labour market transitions of immigrant women. Among her recent publications some of her articles appear in *Canadian Review of Sociology*, *Canadian Ethnic Studies* and *Canadian Review of Sociology*.

Preface

The chapters comprising this volume are contributed by authors from selected Western countries that constitute important destinations for international migrants. The scholars focus on the immigrant experience in their own country with respect to immigrant health or mortality relying on a variety of data sources, from vital statistics and census to longitudinal administrative databases. The countries featured are the United States, Canada and Australia, and four Western European nations whose experience with immigration has intensified significantly following World War II, and particularly over the latter part of the twentieth century: England and Wales, France, Germany, and Belgium. Also included are Italy in Southern Europe, and Norway in Scandinavia. By bringing together in one volume the varied experiences of these selected countries, the volume forms a unique contribution to the rapidly expanding field of migrant studies.

I am thankful to the authors for their willingness to participate in the creation of this volume, which would not have been possible without their dedicated involvement and cooperation. Many thanks to Alex Pettifer and his associates at Edward Elgar Publishing for recognizing the scholarly importance of this work and for their support and assistance throughout the publication process. A special note of thanks goes to my esteemed colleague and friend, Anatole Romaniuk, for his wise counsel and encouragement.

Frank Trovato
Edmonton, Canada
2017

1. Introduction: migration, health and survival – international perspectives

Frank Trovato

MIGRANT STUDIES IN INTERNATIONAL CONTEXT

The chapters in this volume are authored by leading migrant studies scholars from the United States, Canada and Australia, England and Wales, France, Germany, Belgium, Italy and Norway. The United States, Canada and Australia comprise the leading countries of immigration. England and Wales, France, Germany and Belgium have all experienced intense immigration after World War II; Italy and Norway are relatively new countries of immigration.

The United States has the longest experience with migrant studies, dating back to the early twentieth century (for example, Dublin and Baker, 1920; Calabresi, 1945). Interest in this area of research has grown substantially after World War II (for example, Gordon, 1957; Stamler et al., 1960; Haenszel, 1961; Jacobson, 1963; Stout et al., 1964; Krueger and Moriyama, 1967; Haenszel et al., 1968, 1972; Kmet, 1970; King and Haenszel, 1973; Marmot et al., 1975; Marmot and Syme, 1976; King and Locke, 1980; Locke and King, 1980; Kestenbaum, 1986; Markides, and Coreil, 1986; Rosenwaike and Hempstead, 1990; Rosenwaike, 1991; Singh and Yu, 1996; Abraido-Lanza et al., 1999; Hummer et al., 1999; Singh and Siahpush, 2001; Jasso et al., 2004; Palloni and Arias, 2004; Antecol and Bedard, 2006; Kelleher et al., 2006; Turra and Elo, 2008; Lariscy et al., 2016).

Early Canadian works tended to focus mainly on regional and socioeconomic disparities in mortality (for example, Basavarajappa and Lindsay, 1976; Wigle and Mao, 1980; Wilkins and Adams, 1983; Nagnur, 1986; McInnis, 2000). Before the early 1980s, only a handful of works had linked nativity and/or ethnicity explicitly to differential mortality (for example, Coy et al., 1968; Choi, 1968; Choi et al., 1971; Abu-Zeid et al., 1978; Roy, 1975). Since then, the literature has expanded considerably, exploring varied aspects of migrant health and mortality variations through the use of vital statistics data and more recently, newly available health surveys (for example, Trovato, 1985; Nair et al., 1990; Sharma et al.,

1990; Valkonen et al., 1992; Trovato and Clogg, 1992; Chan et al., 1996a; 1996b; Sheth et al., 1999; Ali, 2002; Perez, 2002; Beiser, 2005; DesMeules et al., 2005; McDonald and Kennedy, 2004; Newbold, 2009; Trovato and Odynak, 2011; Health Canada, 2010; Ng, 2011; Omariba et al., 2014; Ng et al., 2016; Vang et al., 2016).

Australian studies began to appear in the early 1970s, examining group variations in suicide and other external types of mortality, as well as chronic diseases such as cancer and cardiovascular disorders (for example, Stenhouse and McCall, 1970; Whitlock, 1971; Burwill et al., 1973). Since the 1980s, this research tradition focused on immigrant populations has intensified (for example, McMichael et al., 1980; Burwill et al., 1982; Young, 1986a, 1986b, 1987, 1991; Khlat, 1993; McMichael and Giles, 1988; Kliewer, 1992; Kliewer and Smith, 1995; Burwill, 1998; Kouris-Blazos, 2002; Hajat et al., 2010; Richardson et al., 2013; Anikeeva et al., 2012, 2015; Kennedy et al., 2015).

In Europe, late in the twentieth century important works appeared based on the experiences of France and the United Kingdom (for example, Brahimi, 1980; Marmot et al., 1983, 1984a, 1984b; Vallin, 1985). Over recent years the European literature beyond these countries has been expanding rapidly. To some extent, this is a reflection of these countries' growing experience with immigration brought on by the combined forces of globalization, expansion of the European Union, and periodic refugee crises in the regions surrounding Europe (for example, Geddes et al., 1993; Balzi et al., 1994; Courbage and Khlat, 1996; Wild and McKeigue, 1997; Sundquist and Johansson, 1997a, 1997b; Razum et al., 1998; Uitenbroek and Verhoeff, 2002; Harding, 2004; Stiribu et al., 2006; Regidor et al., 2011; Agyemang, de-Graft Aikins and Bhopal, 2012; Boulogne et al., 2012; Spallek et al., 2012; Hollander, 2013; Wallace and Kulu, 2013, 2014a, 2014b; Norredam et al., 2014; Moncho et al., 2015; Ikram et al., 2015; Vandenheede et al., 2015; Juárez and Revuelta-Eugercios, 2016; Verropoluou and Tsimbos, 2016; Wallace, 2016).

COMMON THEMES

Three consistent themes emerge from the studies. First, in one form or another, authors examine the idea that immigrant populations are selected for better health and longevity, and that by virtue of this property share a health and survival advantage over their native-born host populations. Much of the empirical evidence confirms the healthy migrant explanation, as first-generation immigrants tend to be healthier and have lower mortality risk from virtually all major causes of death in relation to their host populations. Data errors do not explain away this differential. Second, some of the studies show that the migrant health advantage is not a permanent feature. With increased time in the host country, migrants experience a deterioration of their initial health advantage, and their health profile increasingly approximates that of the host society. Underlying this general phenomenon is the experience of negative acculturation – the tendency for immigrants to, on the one hand, relinquish traditions and, on the other, to incorporate the health behaviors of the host culture. Third, the health and mortality advantage in first-generation immigrants does not typically extend to the second generation.

PHYSICAL AND MENTAL HEALTH VARIATIONS

Bruce Newbold looks at physical and mental health variations among immigrants in Canada based on the Canadian Community Health Survey, the National Population Health Survey, and the Longitudinal Survey of Immigrants to Canada. With respect to changes in self-rated health status, Newbold's analysis indicates that while immigrants enjoy an initial health advantage early in their settlement experience, the advantage diminishes with time. Even though new immigrants are less likely to report having a chronic condition, the proportions with these types of health ailments rise notably with increased duration in Canada.

As indicated by Ng, Sanmartin, Tu and Manuel, while immigrants on the whole tend to have better health than the Canadian-born, variations by disease and by source country can be considerable. For instance, circulatory disease mortality risk among South Asians tends to be similar to that of the Canadian-born population, but higher than that of other immigrant or ethnic groups. Circulatory disease risk among the Chinese population is relatively low while among Canadians of South Asian descent there is an increased risk of hypertension and heart disease which rises with duration of residence in Canada. In their chapter, Ng and associates examine immigrant generations of United Kingdom, Chinese and other Asian origins with respect to all-cause and circulatory disease related hospitalization rates. Compared with third-generation and beyond descendants (that is, native-born Canadians), age-adjusted odds of all-cause hospitalization among first-generation recent immigrants (in Canada for less than ten years) were significantly lower than for longer-term immigrants (in Canada more than ten years), and also for second-generation descendants. Statistical controls for variations in socioeconomic status attenuated these differentials but the lower circulatory disease hospitalization risk among first- and second-generation immigrants of Chinese origin persisted while, among those of South Asian descent, only the first generation showed a lowered risk but not the second generation.

Biddle and Weldeegzie analyze four waves of the Household Income and Labour Dynamics survey in Australia to examine whether self-assessed health of migrants deteriorates over time. They report that for the immigrant population as a whole longer duration is associated with worsening health, even after age, gender, education, employment, and income have been taken into account statistically. However, they find some differences across migrant groups. Immigrants from English-speaking countries have higher self-assessed health than native-born Australians, while those from 'other' countries tend to show either no difference or worse health relative to the Australian born.

Oppedal gives a comprehensive overview of research on the mental health of immigrant children, youths, and young adults in Norway. Inter-group as well as intra-group variations are examined. An important point raised by Oppedal is that in multicultural contexts such as Norway, concepts such as 'the immigrant health paradox' may not be very useful because such generalizing concepts can often lead to misperceptions of the real complexities associated with the psychosocial adjustment of migrant children and youths. It is argued that a deeper understanding of the mental health of immigrant youth must be based on a clear appreciation of the dynamic interactions between macro-level policies of the host country in conjunction with the unique socio-cultural orientations and practices of the immigrant groups.

Wilkinson and Ponka turn their attention to the Canadian literature concerning the mental health of immigrants and refugees, approaching their overview from two differing perspectives – one from a sociologist (Wilkinson) and the other from a practicing physician (Ponka). They challenge many misperceptions about mental health and newcomers, including the idea that the experience of migration, particularly among refugees, is somehow psychologically and irreversibly damaging. After summarizing the state of knowledge concerning the mental health outcomes of immigrant and refugee adults, children and youth, they explore a number of interrelated dimensions, including: the complexities associated with identifying and tracking over time the mental health of refugees from the point of entry throughout their post-settlement experience; the necessity for medical practitioners to treat refugees as a special case given their pre-migration experience with trauma and for many, their post-settlement experience with post-traumatic stress disorder (PTSD); and challenges associated with ensuring proper access for refugees to the health-care system and needed systemic accommodations to better treat refugee mental health concerns in Canada.

HEALTH, MORTALITY AND SURVIVAL VARIATIONS

Trovato investigates differential mortality between immigrant and native-born populations in Canada during the period 2010 to 2012, looking at causes of death encompassing chronic and external types. The immigrant population shows lower death rates on virtually all causes examined. Acculturation (proxied by years in Canada since immigration) was found to have an eroding effect on the immigrant mortality advantage across most causes examined. The protective effect of health selection on survival probabilities is estimated to persist for 25 years or more for certain diseases, particularly ischemic heart disease in males, whereas for diseases such as diabetes the protective effect of selection lasts only between five and ten years for female migrants. Trovato's findings are consistent with the proposition that the passage of time in the host country entails varying degrees of health erosion for immigrants, and that the mortality advantage afforded by selection dissipates with time, though at varying degrees of intensity depending on the type of disease.

For the United States, Singh and Liu look at mortality and life expectancy trends and differentials among immigrant and US-born populations based on death certificate and population data from the National Vital Statistics System (NVSS) and decennial censuses, as well as prospective data from the National Longitudinal Mortality Study (NLMS). These authors also discuss differentials in health status, chronic disease morbidity, disability, injuries, mental health, health-risk behaviors, such as obesity, physical inactivity, diet, smoking, alcohol use, and hypertension, health-care access and use. The similarity of the US findings regarding mortality differentials with those reported for Canada by Trovato is striking, as in both countries immigrants share a substantial survival advantage over the native born. As argued by Singh and Liu, the migrant mortality advantage is due to a combination of factors, ranging from health selection to cultural practices that promote health and survival. These authors also recognize that the extent of negative assimilation on migrant health and survival can vary across nationality groups.

In Australia, Anikeeva and Bi study differential patterns of mortality in migrants for the most common cancers in relation to the role of diet, lifestyle factors and acculturation. In general, immigrants have lower mortality rates than do Australians. Greeks and Italians in particular enjoy a significant cancer mortality advantage. This is attributed to the predominantly Mediterranean diet adopted by Greeks and Italians, and to salutogenic effects of aggregative affiliation, as these groups are mostly clustered in the larger cities where a supportive environment exists within the ethnic community that reinforces maintenance of traditions, and in particular, traditional food preparation and consumption. On the other hand, for some cancers mortality rates are higher in immigrants. Upon arrival, East and South East Asian migrants have an approximately thirty-fold higher age-adjusted risk of dying from nasopharyngeal cancer compared with the Australian-born, which reduces to nine-fold after 30 years in Australia. Migrants from the United Kingdom, the former Yugoslavia, Greece and Italy have higher age-adjusted mortality rates from cancer of the stomach and pancreas. However, this higher death rate among the migrants tends to decrease with increasing duration of residence in Australia. It is suggested that such group differentials and patterns of cancer mortality reflect group variability in dietary and lifestyle habits linked to differential retention of Old World traditions.

Wallace examines differential mortality among migrants and their descendants living in England and Wales. It is confirmed that the healthy migrant effect cannot be explained away by data errors, nor can the 'salmon bias' (return selectivity) account for the observed migrant mortality advantage. The low mortality among migrants is mainly a function of low mortality from cancer, and in some groups also reduced death rates from cardiovascular disease. The descendants of migrants were not observed to share a mortality advantage. A succinct overview of the accelerated health transition thesis is given by Wallace. This thesis posits a mortality advantage for migrants, most especially from developing countries, as a function of reduced mortality from infectious diseases and perinatal and maternal mortality very soon after arrival to the new country. This accelerated health transition occurs because upon arrival, the newcomers benefit from a more sanitary environment and access to better health care, thereby permitting a rapid reduction in mortality from infectious diseases. However, with increased duration in the new country, the migrants are progressively exposed to western lifestyles and related risk factors for chronic diseases, and consequently, after a lag period they experience increased death rates from chronic diseases.

The evolution of migrant studies in France is the subject of Khlat and Guillot's chapter. It is observed that there has been a shift in research orientation in France, from an early period in the 1980s when the focus was mostly on cancer epidemiology concerning the foreign born, to a more recent period since 2000 focused largely on the social determinants of health and mortality inequalities. It is noted that the French literature agrees in many respects with that based on other immigrant-receiving western countries: younger migrants in the pre-labor force ages tend to show relatively high death rates, and those in the prime labor force ages enjoy a notably low mortality risk. Female migrants from sub-Saharan Africa, particularly Morocco, have unusually high rates of maternal mortality. This raises the interesting juxtaposition that within the larger immigrant population – usually found to be in better health than the native born – there are vulnerable subgroups in poor health. In fact, according to Khlat and Guillot, in France, the 'healthy migrant effect' is visible in only a subset of studies, and quite a number of other studies are more in line with a representation of migrants as 'vulnerable populations'.

According to Brzoska and Razum, one-fifth of the population of Germany are individuals with a migration background (16.4 million out of 80.9 million total population), that is, persons who may have immigrated to Germany from another country, or persons that are direct descendants of immigrants. Aside from having a lower socioeconomic status, immigrants in Germany tend to also encounter barriers in health care that limit their access to health services and that may also affect health-care quality and outcomes. It is indicated that based on the available evidence it is difficult to say definitively whether migrants have a higher or lower mortality than non-migrants, even though age standardized death rates do for the most part suggest an immigrant mortality advantage. Immigrants appear to have a higher incidence of certain infectious diseases and a higher prevalence of some chronic conditions. This is attributed to unfavorable social determinants in the immigrant population in conjunction with access barriers to, and a limited effectiveness of, health services to migrants.

As reported by Caselli, Loi and Strozza, since the late 1970s Italy has become a country of immigration after being one of the main European countries of emigration for more than a century. Currently, foreign residents in Italy are estimated to number more than 5 million. If non-residents are taken into account the total arrives at almost 6 million, or about 10 percent of the total population. The immigrants are almost all citizens of developing countries. Many others are from Central and Eastern Europe, with a significant presence of those from countries that have joined the European Union (EU) during the past decade. Notwithstanding these trends, Caselli and colleagues indicate that there is limited knowledge of the health conditions and mortality of immigrants and refugees in Italy. These authors rely on a variety of data sources, including regional-based surveys and studies, administrative records and hospital data to form a picture of the health condition of immigrants in Italy. Looking at differences in hospitalization rates, it is seen that for the foreign population the rates are lower compared with Italians, thus suggesting an immigrant health advantage, though over time the migrant advantage reduces, changing toward convergence with the host population. Specific to foreign women, there appear to be problems associated with pregnancy and perinatal complications, the most disadvantaged group being mothers from West and sub-Saharan Africa. It is suggested that in future research it would be important to consider the unique experiences of the different nationalities in Italy in order to better understand how culture and work histories interact to determine differential health and mortality risk.

The case of Belgium is investigated by Deboosere and Vandenheede. Based on their findings these authors underscore the need to move beyond mono-causal explanations of immigrant group variations in mortality rates. Notwithstanding a possible healthy migrant effect, it is argued that in reality many factors contribute over the life course to differences in life expectancy, and these factors can have negative and positive effects on mortality risk. For instance, the fact that the labor migration to Belgium was composed of healthy men has certainly contributed to lower mortality in adult migrant populations in the past and also currently. However, harsh working conditions for immigrants had negative effects on health which only became evident several decades after the time of arrival, as indicated, for example, by the higher death rates from respiratory diseases among older immigrant men. The negative impact of bad socioeconomic conditions on health can be compensated by better dietary habits, but again, some aspects of the diet can also have a negative impact on mortality risk, as illustrated by the higher stomach cancer mortality among several migrant groups in Belgium. Finally, cultural background (and religion as part of the culture of origin) plays an obvious role in containing the negative impact of some causes, as witnessed in connection with the low mortality due to alcohol-related diseases and the very low suicide figures.

Given the variety of experiences observed in this volume and in the broader migrant studies literature, an all-encompassing theory of immigrant health and mortality may be difficult, if not impossible. In the final chapter of this volume, Trovato proposes a heuristic framework to help organize empirical observations concerning immigrant mortality variations based largely on established features of the migrant studies literature.

REFERENCES

Abraido-Lanza, A.F., B.P. Dohrenwend, D.S. Ng-Mak and J.B. Turner (1999), 'The Latino mortality paradox: A test of the salmon bias and healthy migrant hypothesis', *American Journal of Public Health*, **89** (10), 1543–8.

Abu-Zeid, H.A.H., K.K. Maini, and N.W. Choi (1978), 'Ethnic differences in mortality from ischemic heart disease: a study of migrants and native populations', *Journal of Chronic Diseases*, **31** (3), 137–46.

Agyemang, C., A. de-Graft Aikins and R. Bhopal (2012), 'Ethnicity and cardiovascular health research: pushing the boundaries by including comparison populations in the countries of origin', *Ethnicity and Health*, **17** (6), 579–96.

Ali, J. (2002), 'Mental health of Canada's immigrants', *Health Reports*, **13** (supplement), Statistics Canada, Ottawa, 1–11.

Anikeeva, O., P. Bi, J.E. Hiller and G.-S. Han (2012), 'Trends in cancer mortality rates among migrants in Australia: 1981–2007', *Cancer Epidemiology*, **36** (2), E74–E82.

Anikeeva, O., P. Bi, J.E. Hiller and G.-S. Han (2015), 'Trends in migrant mortality rates in Australia 1981–2007: a focus on the National Health Priority Areas other than cancer', *Ethnicity & Health*, **20** (1), 29–48.

Antecol, H. and K. Bedard (2006), 'Unhealthy assimilation: why do immigrants converge to American health status levels?' *Demography*, **43** (2), 337–60.

Balzi, D., M. Geddes, A. Brancker and D.M. Parkin (1994), 'Cancer mortality in Italian migrants to Canada', *Tumori*, **80** (1), 19–23.

Basavarajappa, K.G. and J. Lindsay (1976), *Mortality Differences in Canada, 1960–1962 and 1970–1972*, Ottawa: Statistics Canada.

Beiser, M. (2005), 'The health of immigrants in Canada', *Canadian Review of Public Health*, **96** (Supplement 2), S30–S44.

Boulogne, R.E., E. Jougla, Y. Breem, A.E. Kunst and G. Rey (2012), 'Mortality differences between the foreign-born and locally born population in France (2004–2007)', *Social Science & Medicine*, **74**, (8), 1213–23.

Brahimi, M. (1980), 'La mortalite des estrangers en France', *Population*, **35** (3), 603–22.

Burwill, P.W. (1998), 'Migrant suicide rates in Australia and in country of birth', *Psychological Medicine*, **28** (1), 201–8.

Burwill, P.W., M.G. McCall, N.S. Stenhouse and T.A. Reid (1973), 'Deaths from suicide, motor vehicle accidents and all forms of violent deaths among migrants in Australia, 1962–66', *Acta Psychiatrica Scandinavica*, **49** (1), 28–50.

Burwill, P.W., T.L. Woodings, N.S. Stenhouse and M.G. McCall (1982), 'Suicide during 1961–70 of migrants in Australia', *Psychological Medicine*, **12** (2), 295–308.

Calabresi, M. (1945), 'The relation of country of origin to mortality from various causes in New York State', *Human Biology*, **17** (4), 340–67.

Chan, J., E. Ng and R. Wilkins (1996a), 'The health of Canada's immigrants in 1994–95', *Health Reports*, **7** (4), 33–45.

Chan, J., R. Wilkins and E. Ng (1996b), 'Health expectancy by immigrant status', *Health Reports*, **8** (3), 29–37.

Choi, N.W. (1968), 'Ethnic distribution of gastrointestinal cancer in Manitoba', *American Journal of Public Health*, **58** (11), 2067–81.

Choi, N.W., D.W. Entwistle, W. Michaluk and N. Nelson (1971), 'Gastric cancer in Icelanders in Manitoba', *Israel Journal of Medical Sciences*, **7** (11), 1500–1508.

Courbage, Y. and M. Khlat (1996), "Mortality and causes of death of Moroccans in France, 1979–91', *Population*, **8**, 59–94.

Coy, P.S., S. Grzybowski and J.F. Rowe (1968), 'Lung cancer mortality according to birthplace', *Canadian Medical Association Journal*, **99** (September), 476–83.

DesMeules, M., J. Gold, S. McDermott, Z. Cao, J. Payne and B. Lafrance et al. (2005), 'Disparities in mortality patterns among Canadian immigrants and refugees, 1980–1998: results of a national cohort study', *Journal of Immigrant Health*, **7** (4), 221–32.

Dublin, L.I. and C.W. Baker (1920), 'The mortality of race stocks in Pennsylvania and New York', *Quarterly Publications of the American Statistical Association* (*Journal of the American Statistical Association*), **17**(129), 13–44.

Geddes, M., D. Balzi, E. Bulatti, M. Khlat and D. Parkin (1993), *Cancer in Italian*

Migrant Populations, IARC Scientific Publications No. 123, Lyon: International Agency for Research on Cancer.
Gordon, T. (1957), 'Mortality experience among the Japanese in the United States, Hawaii and Japan', *Public Health Reports*, **72** (6), 543–53.
Gray, L., S. Harding and A. Reid (2007) 'Evidence of divergence with duration of residence in circulatory disease mortality in migrants to Australia', *European Journal of Public Health*, **17** (6), 550–54
Haenszel, W. (1961), 'Cancer mortality among the foreign-born in the United States', *Journal of the National Cancer Institute*, **26** (1), 37–132.
Haenszel, W. and M. Kurihara (1968), 'Studies of Japanese migrants. I. Mortality from cancer and other diseases among Japanese in the United States', *Journal of the National Cancer Institute*, **40** (1), 43–68.
Haenszel, W., M. Kurihara, M. Segi and R.K. Lee (1972), 'Stomach cancer among Japanese in Hawaii', *Journal of the National Cancer Institute*, **49** (4). 969–88.
Hajat, A., T. Blakely, S. Dayal and S. Jatrana (2010), 'Do New Zealand's immigrants have a mortality advantage? Evidence from the New Zealand Census-Mortality Study', *Ethnicity & Health*, **15** (5), 531–47.
Harding, S. (2004), 'Mortality of migrants from the Caribbean to England and Wales: effect of duration of residence', *International Journal of Epidemiology*, **33** (2), 382–6.
Health Canada (2010), *Health Policy Research Bulletin. Special issue, Migration Health: Embracing a Determinants of Health Approach*, no. 17, December, Ottawa: Minister of Health Canada.
Hollander, A.-C. (2013), 'Social inequalities in mental health and mortality among refugees and other immigrants to Sweden – epidemiological studies of register data', *Global Health Action*, **6** (1), 1–11.
Hummer, R.A., M. Biegler, P.B. De Turk, D. Forbes, W.P. Frisbie, Y. Hong and S.G. Pullum (1999), 'Race/ethnicity, nativity, and infant mortality in the United States', *Social Forces*, **77** (3), 1083–117.
Ikram, U.Z., D. Malmusi, K. Juel, G. Rey and A.E. Kunst (2015), 'Association between integration policies and immigrants' mortality: an explorative study across three European countries', *PlosOne*, **10** (6), e0129916, doi:10.1371/journal.pone.0129916.
Jacobson, P.H. (1963), 'Mortality of the native and foreign-born population in the United States', in *1961 IUSSP Conference Proceedings*, vol. 1, New York: IUSSP, pp. 667–74.
Jasso, G., S.D. Massey, M.R. Rosenzweig and J.P. Smith (2004), 'Immigrant health: selectivity and acculturation', in N.B. Anderson (ed.), *Critical Perspectives on Racial and Ethnic Differences in Health in Late Life*, Washington, DC: National Academies Press, pp. 227–66.
Juárez, S.P. and B. Revuelta-Eugercios (2016), 'Exploring the "healthy migrant paradox" in Sweden. A cross sectional study focused on perinatal outcomes', *Journal of Immigrant and Minority Health*, **18** (1), 42–50.
Kelleher, C.C., J.W. Lynch, L. Daly, S. Harper, N. Fitz-simon, Y. Bimpeh et al. (2006), 'The "Americanization" of migrants: evidence for the contribution of ethnicity, social deprivation, lifestyle and life-course processes to the mid-20th century coronary heart disease epidemic in the US', *Social Science and Medicine*, **63** (2), 465–84.
Kennedy, S., M.P. Kidd, J.T. McDonald and N. Biddle (2015), 'The healthy immigrant effect: patterns and evidence from four countries', *Journal of International Migration & Integration*, **16** (2), 317–32.

Kestenbaum, B. (1986), 'Mortality by nativity', *Demography*, **23** (1), 87–90.

Khlat, M. (1993), 'Mortalité des Levantins en Australie' ('Mortality of Levantines in Australia'), *Population*, **48** (4), 1072–81.

King, H. and W. Haenszel (1973), 'Cancer mortality among foreign- and native-born Chinese in the United States', *Journal of Chronic Diseases*, **26** (10), 623–46.

King, H. and F.B. Locke (1980), 'American white Protestant clergy as a low-risk population for mortality research', *Journal of the National Cancer Institute*, **65** (5), 1115–24.

Kliewer, E. (1992), 'Epidemiology of diseases among migrants', *International Migration*, **30** (supplement 1), 141–65.

Kliewer, E. and K.R. Smith (1995), 'Breast cancer mortality among immigrants in Australia and Canada', *Journal of the National Cancer Institute*, **87** (15), 1154–61.

Kmet, J. (1970), 'The role of migrant population in studies of selected cancer sites: a review', *Journal of Chronic Diseases*, **23** (5), 305–24.

Kouris-Blazos, A. (2002), 'Morbidity mortality paradox of 1st generation Greek Australians', *Asia Pacific Journal of Clinical Nutrition*, **11** (Supplement 3), S569–S575.

Krueger, D.E. and I.M. Moriyama (1967), 'Mortality of the foreign-born', *American Journal of Public Health*, **57** (3), 496–503.

Lariscy, J.T., C. Nau, G. Firebaugh and R.A. Hummer (2016), 'Hispanic-White differences in lifespan variability in the United States', *Demography*, **53** (1), 215–39.

Locke, F.B. and H. King (1980), 'Cancer mortality risk among Japanese in the United States', *Journal of the National Cancer Institute*, **65** (5), 1115–24.

Markides, K.S. and J. Coreil (1986), 'The health of Hispanics in the southwestern United States: an epidemiological paradox', *Public Health Reports*, **101** (3), 253–65.

Marmot, M.G. and L.S. Syme (1976), 'Acculturation and coronary heart disease in Japanese-Americans', *American Journal of Epidemiology*, **104** (3), 225–47.

Marmot, M.G., A.M. Adelstein and L. Bulusu (1983), 'Immigrant mortality in England and Wales, 1970–78', *Population Trends*, **33** (Autumn), 14–17.

Marmot, M.G., A.M. Adelstein and L. Bulusu (1984a), *Immigrant Mortality in England and Wales, 1970–78. Cause of Death by Country of Birth*, Studies on Medical and Population Subjects No. 47, London: Her Majesty's Stationery Office.

Marmot, M.G., A.M. Adelstein and L. Bulusu (1984b), 'Lessons from the study of immigrant mortality', *Lancet*, **323** (8392), 1455–7.

Marmot, M.G., S.L. Syme, A. Kagan, H. Kato, J.B. Cohen and J. Belsky (1975), 'Epidemiologic studies of coronary heart disease and stroke in Japanese men living in Japan, Hawaii and California: prevalence of coronary and hypertensive heart disease and associated risk factors', *American Journal of Epidemiology*, **102** (6), 514–24.

McDonald, J.T. and S. Kennedy (2004), 'Insights into the "healthy immigrant effect": health status and health service use of immigrants to Canada', *Social Science & Medicine*, **59** (8), 1613–27.

McInnis, M. (2000), 'The population of Canada in the twentieth century', in M.R. Haines and R. H. Steckel (eds), *A Population History of North America*, Cambridge: Cambridge University Press, pp. 529–600.

McMichael, A.J. and G.G. Giles (1988), 'Cancer in migrants to Australia: extending the descriptive epidemiological data', *Cancer Research*, **48** (3), 751–6.

McMichael, A.J., M.G. McCall, J.M. Hartshorne and T.L. Woodings (1980),

'Patterns of gastrointestinal cancer in European migrants to Australia: the role of dietary change', *International Journal of Cancer*, **25** (4), 431–7.
Moncho, J., P. Pereyra-Zamora, A. Nolasco, N. Tamayo-Fonseca, I. Melchor and L. Macia (2015), 'Trends and disparities in mortality among Spanish-born and foreign-born populations residing in Spain, 1999–2008', *Journal of Immigrant and Minority Health*, **17** (5), 1374–84.
Nagnur, D. (1986), *Longevity and Historical Life Tables 1921–1981 (Abridged), Canada and the Provinces*, Ottawa: Minister of Supply and Services, cat. no. 89-506.
Nair, C., M. Nargundkar, H. Johansen and J. Strachan (1990), 'Canadian cardiovascular disease mortality: first generation immigrants versus Canadian born', *Health Reports*, **2** (3), 203–28.
Newbold, B. (2009), 'The short-term health of Canada's new immigrant arrivals: evidence from LSIC', *Ethnicity & Health*, **14** (3), 315–36.
Ng, E. (2011), 'The healthy immigrant effect and mortality rates', *Health Reports*, **22** (37), 25–9.
Ng, E., C. Sanmartin, D.E. Massenat and D.G. Manuel (2016), 'Vaccine-preventable disease-related hospitalization among immigrants and refugees to Canada: study of linked population-based databases', *Vaccine*, **34** (37), 4437–42.
Norredam, M., C. Agyemang, O.K.H. Hansen, J.H. Petersen, S. Byberg, A. Krasnik and A.E. Kunst (2014), 'Duration of residence and disease occurrence among refugees and family reunited immigrants: test of the "healthy migrant effect" hypothesis', *Tropical Medicine and International Health*, **19** (8), 958–67.
Omariba, W.R., E. Ng and B. Vissandjée (2014), 'Differences between immigrants at various durations of residence and host population in all-cause mortality, Canada 1991–2006', *Population Studies*, **68** (3), 339–58.
Palloni, A. and E. Arias (2004), 'Paradox lost: explaining the Hispanic adult mortality advantage', *Demography*, **41** (3), 385–415.
Perez, C.E. (2002), 'Health status and health behaviour among immigrants', *Health Reports*, **13**, supplement, Ottawa: Statistics Canada.
Razum, O., H. Zeeb, H.S. Akgun and S. Yilmaz (1998), 'Low overall mortality of Turkish residents in Germany persists and extends into a second generation: merely a healthy migrant effect?', *Tropical Medicine and International Health*, **3** (4), 297–303.
Regidor, E., P. Astasio, P. Ortega, D. Marinez, M.E. Calle and L de la Fuente (2011), 'Healthy and unhealthy migrant effect on the mortality of immigrants from wealthy countries residing in Spain', *European Journal of Epidemiology*, **26** (4), 265–73.
Richardson, K., S. Jatrana, M. Tobias and T. Blakely (2013), 'Migration and Pacific mortality: estimating migration effects on Pacific mortality rates using Bayesian models', *Demography*, **50**, (6), 2053–73.
Rosensweike, I. (1991), *Mortality of Hispanic Populations in the United States*, New York: Greenwood Press.
Rosenwaike, I. and K. Hempstead (1990), 'Differential mortality by ethnicity and nativity: foreign-and native-born Irish, Italians, and Jews in New York City, 1979–1981', *Social Biology*, **37** (1–2), 11–25.
Roy, L. (1975), *La Mortalite Selon la Cause de Deces et L'Origine Ethnique au Quebec, 1951, 1961, 1971*, Quebec: Division de Etudes Demographiques, Ministeres des Affaires Sociales.
Sharma, R.D., M. Mikalowski and R.B.P. Verma (1990), 'Mortality differentials

among immigrant populations in Canada', *International Migration*, **28** (4), 443–50.

Sheth, T., C. Nair, M. Nargundkar, S. Anand and S. Yusuf (1999), 'Cardiovascular and cancer mortality among Canadians of European, south Asian and Chinese origin from 1979 to 1993: an analysis of 1.2 million deaths', *Canadian Medical Association Journal*, **161** (2), 132–8.

Singh, G.K. and S.M. Yu (1996), 'Adverse pregnancy outcomes: differences between US- and foreign-born women in major racial and ethnic groups', *American Journal of Public Health*, **86** (6), 837–43.

Singh, G.K. and M. Siahpush (2001), 'All-cause and cause-specific mortality of immigrants and native born in the United States', *American Journal of Public Health*, **91** (3), 392–9.

Spallek J., M. Arnold, O. Rzaum, K. Juel, G. Rey, P. Deboosere et al. (2012), 'Cancer mortality patterns among Turkish immigrants in four European countries and in Turkey', *European Journal of Epidemiology*, **27** (12), 915–21.

Stamler, J., M. Kjelsberg, Y. Hall and N. Scotch (1960), 'Epidemiologic studies on cardiovascular-renal diseases: III. Analysis of mortality by age–sex–nationality', *Journal of Chronic Diseases*, **12** (4), 464–75.

Stenhouse, N.S. and M.G. McCall (1970), 'Differential mortality from cardiovascular disease in migrants from England and Wales, Scotland and Italy, and native-born Australians', *Journal of Chronic Diseases*, **23** (5–6), 423–31.

Stiribu, I., A. Kunst, F.A. Vlems, O. Visser, V. Bos, et al. (2006), 'Cancer mortality rates among first and second generation migrants in the Netherlands: convergence toward the rates of the native Dutch population', *International Journal of Cancer*, **119** (11), 2665–72.

Stout C., J. Morrow, E.N. Brandt and S. Wolf (1964), 'Study of an Italian-American community in PA. Unusually low incidence of death from myocardial infarction', *Journal of the American Medical Association*, **188** (1), 845–9.

Sundquist, J., and S.E. Johansson (1997a), 'The influence of country of birth on mortality from all causes and cardiovascular disease in Sweden 1979–1993', *International Journal of Epidemiology*, **26** (2), 279–87.

Sundquist, J., and S.E. Johansson (1997b), 'Self-reported poor health and low educational level predictors for mortality: A population-based follow-up study of 39 156 people in Sweden', *Journal of Epidemiology and Community Health*, **51** (1): 35–40.

Trovato, F. (1985), 'Mortality differences among Canada's indigenous and foreign-born populations, 1951–1971', *Canadian Studies in Population*, **12** (1), 49–80.

Trovato, F. and C.C. Clogg (1992), 'General and cause-specific adult mortality among immigrants in Canada, 1971 and 1981', *Canadian Studies in Population*, **19** (1), 47–80.

Trovato, F. and D. Odynak (2011), 'Sex differences in life expectancy in Canada: immigrant and native-born populations', *Journal of Biosocial Science*, **43** (3), 353–67.

Turra, C.M. and I.T. Elo (2008), 'The impact of salmon bias on the Hispanic mortality advantage: new evidence from social security data', *Population Research and Policy Review*, **27** (October), 515–30.

Uitenbroek, D.G. and A. P. Verhoeff (2002), 'Life expectancy and mortality differences between migrant groups living in Amsterdam, The Netherlands', *Social Science & Medicine*, **54** (9), 1379–88.

Valkonen, T., A. Brancker and M. Reijo (1992), 'Mortality differences between three populations – residents of Scandinavia, Scandinavian immigrants to Canada and Canadian-born residents of Canada, 1979–1985', *Health Reports*, **4** (2), 137–59.

Vallin, J. (1985), 'La mortalite des immigres en Engleterre et Galles' ('The mortality of immigrants in England and Wales'), *Population*, **40** (1), 156–61.

Vandenheede, H., D. Willaert, H. De Grande, S. Simoens, and C. Vanroelen (2015), 'Mortality in adult immigrants in the 2000s in Belgium: A test of the "healthy-migrant" and the "migration-as-rapid-health-transition" hypotheses', *Tropical Medicine and International Health*, **20** (12), 1832–1845.

Vang, Z.M., S. Jennifer, F. Astrid and A. Gagnon (2016), 'Are immigrants healthier than native-born Canadians? A systematic review of the healthy immigrant effect in Canada', *Ethnicity & Health*, **22** (3), 1–33.

Verropoluou, G. and C. Tsimbos (2016), 'Mortality by cause of death among immigrants and natives in a South European country: the case of Greece, 2011', *Journal of Immigrant and Minority Health*, **18** (2), 337–44.

Wallace, M. (2016), 'Adult mortality among the descendants of immigrants in England and Wales: does a migrant mortality advantage persist beyond the first generation?', *Journal of Ethic & Migration* Studies, **42** (9), doi:org/10.1080/1369183x.2015.1131973.

Wallace, M., and H. Kulu (2013), 'Migration and health in England and Scotland: a study of migrant selectivity and salmon bias', *Population, Space & Place*, **20** (8), 694–708, doi.org/10.1002/psp.1804.

Wallace, M. and H. Kulu (2014a), 'Low immigrant mortality in England and Wales: a data artefact?', *Social Science & Medicine*, **120** (November), 100–109.

Wallace, M., and H. Kulu (2014b), 'Mortality among immigrants in England and Wales by major causes of death, 1971: a longitudinal analysis of register-based data', *Social Science & Medicine*, **147** (December), 209–21.

Whitlock, F.A. (1971), 'Migration and suicide', *Medical Journal of Australia*, **2** (17), 840–48.

Wigle, D.T. and Y. Mao (1980), *Mortality by Income Level in Urban Canada*, Ottawa: Health Protection Branch, Health and Welfare Canada.

Wild, S. and P. McKeigue (1997), 'Cross sectional analysis of mortality by country of birth in England and Wales, 1970–92', *British Medical Journal*, **314** (7082), 705–10.

Wilkins, R. and O.B. Adams (1983), 'Health expectancy in Canada, late 1970s: demographic, regional, and social dimensions', *American Journal of Public Health*, **73** (9), 1073–80.

Wolf, S. and J.G. Bruhn (1998), *The Power of Clan: A 25-Year Prospective Study of Roseto, Pennsylvania*, New Brunswick, NJ: Transaction.

Young, C.M. (1986a), *Selection and Survival: Immigrant Mortality in Australia*, Canberra: Canberra Publishing.

Young, C.M. (1986b), 'Differential mortality of birthplace groups in Australia during 1980–82', *Journal of the Australian Population Association*, **3** (2), 144–68.

Young, C.M. (1987), 'Migration and mortality: the experience of birthplace groups in Australia', *International Migration Review*, **21** (3), 531–54.

Young, C.M. (1991), 'Changes in the demographic behaviour of migrants in Australia and the transition between generations', *Population Studies*, **45** (1), 67–89.

2. Understanding the healthy immigrant effect: evidence from Canada

K. Bruce Newbold

INTRODUCTION

With the arrival of approximately 250000 immigrants in Canada annually, immigration is set to become the primary source of Canada's population growth over the coming decades. By arriving in Canada, new immigrant arrivals have moved from one set of health risks to another, potentially impacting their health. Given high levels of immigration into Canada and the associated need to understand the health needs of new arrivals and how this changes over time, an extensive literature has developed over the past decade that explores immigrant health issues. Although Canada, like other immigrant destinations, actively screens new arrivals to protect the Canadian population by ensuring satisfactory health, such measures do not guarantee that the health of arrivals will be maintained. In fact, the health of new arrivals tends to be better than that of native-born Canadians at the time of arrival, reflecting intake policies such as Canada's point system and self-selection among immigrants. However, within a comparatively short period of time – approximately five to ten years – the health status of new arrivals declines to levels below that of the Canadian born (Newbold and Danforth, 2003; Dean and Wilson, 2009; Newbold, 2009).

Known as the 'healthy immigrant effect', the literature has consistently identified a process whereby immigrants are initially healthier (or as healthy) as the receiving population on arrival. However, with the passage of time, their health levels tend to converge or even fall below the levels of the receiving population. Much of the evidence for the healthy immigrant effect is based upon self-reported health, whereby respondents are asked to rank their health relative to their peers as 'excellent', 'very good', 'good', 'fair' or 'poor' (Dunn and Dyck, 2000; McDonald and Kennedy, 2004; Newbold, 2005; Blair and Schneeberg, 2014). Additional measures, including the Health Utilities Index (Newbold and Danforth, 2003), disability and life expectancy (Chen et al., 1996), and mental health have also captured the healthy immigrant effect (Ali, 2002; Lou and Beaujot, 2005; Smith et al., 2007). Likewise, the prevalence of chronic conditions also converges upwards toward the Canadian population (Chen et al., 1996; Dunn and Dyck, 2000).

Interestingly, the healthy immigrant effect has also been observed with respect to mortality, with overall death rates among immigrants typically lower than those observed in the receiving society (Trovato, 2003; Ng and the LHAD research team, 2011). Although Ng and the LHAD research team (2011) observed that immigrants had an advantage with respect to all-cause mortality (determined by considering age-specific mortality rates), circulatory diseases and cancer at the national level in Canada, substantial differences were noted at the sub-national scale, gender, duration of residence, and for specific immigrant origins (Ng and the LHAD research team, 2011). Moreover, the healthy immigrant phenomena has also been observed in the United States, Australia and Europe (McDonald and Kennedy, 2004; Fennelly, 2007; Setia et al., 2011; Gotsens et al., 2015; Kennedy et al., 2015) and for a variety of health outcomes (Vang et al., 2016).

This chapter provides an overview of the healthy immigrant effect from the Canadian perspective. In part, it draws upon existing work by the author to illustrate the effect, while also updating the literature with new findings. The chapter first explores the data supporting the healthy immigrant effect by considering changes to both physical and mental health among immigrants, with comparisons made with the native-born population. It then considers some of the hypothesized reasons associated with the healthy immigrant effect. The conclusion provides some insight into the evolving research agenda.

UNDERSTANDING THE HEALTHY IMMIGRANT EFFECT: PHYSICAL AND MENTAL HEALTH

Three datasets, inclusive of the Canadian Community Health Survey (CCHS), National Population Health Survey (NPHS) and the Longitudinal Survey of Immigrants to Canada (LSIC), have been widely used to look at the healthy immigrant effect in the Canadian context. All three surveys are conducted by Statistics Canada and are nationally representative, although they typically exclude individuals living on Aboriginal reserves, Canadian Forces Bases, or residents of some remote places. Ideally, we wish to capture the healthy immigrant effect through longitudinal data which traces the changes to health and health care behavior over time, a feature of

Table 2.1 Health status (%): immigrant and native-born aged 20+ years in 1994

	1994/95	1996/97	1998/99	2000/01
% fair or poor health				
Foreign-born	10.1	10.6	11.3	15.9
Arrived 1990–94	3.9	6.4	12.7	17.0
Native-born	9.1	8.7	9.5	12.6
% reporting chronic conditions				
Foreign-born	55.7	65.1	67.0	69.0
Arrived 1990–94	26.5	47.0	45.9	46.2
Native-born	55.9	62.5	63.1	65.8

Source: Reproduced from Newbold (2009) with permission from Taylor and Francis (www.tandfonline.com). Results based on NPHS 1994/95–2000/01.

the latter two surveys (NPHS and LSIC), and which underlie the analysis in the subsequent tables. The CCHS, which has also been widely used, is a cross-sectional 'snapshot' of the health of the Canadian population at the time of the survey, meaning that there is no indication of the trajectory or changes to health over time. In the case of the NPHS, a randomly selected individual is followed through a series of cycles, with detailed information including health status and other socio-demographic and socio-economic information collected. The LSIC traced a cohort of immigrants (arriving between 1 October 2000 and 30 September 2001) over a period of time following arrival, with data (similar to that collected for the NPHS but inclusive only of immigrants) collected at six months, two years, and four years after arrival.

Table 2.1 documents the change in the proportion of immigrants and native-born reporting fair or poor health over a six year period from 1994/95 to 2000/01. Overall, immigrants tended to rank their health worse than their native-born counterparts at each time point. While the observed declines in health status can be partially attributed to increasing age, declines in health are clearly noticeable when considering just those immigrants who arrived in Canada between 1990 and 1994 and capturing a comparatively recent cohort of arrivals. With only 3.9 percent reporting fair or poor health in 1994/95, the proportion reporting fair or poor health within the same arrival cohort had grown to 17.0 percent by 2000/01, a proportional increase which was far greater than observed within the native-born population, and evidence of rapidly declining health status for these new arrivals.

Declines in self-assessed health are echoed in terms of chronic conditions. For the same 1990 to 1994 arrival cohort, the proportion reporting a chronic condition increased by nearly 20 percentage points (26.5 percent to 46.2 percent). Although the proportion reporting a chronic condition increased within the immigrant and native-born populations as well, the increase was not nearly as large as within the single 1990–94 arrival cohort.

Although the healthy immigrant effect has most frequently been identified by physical and self-assessed health outcomes, it has also been identified in terms of mental health outcomes (Ali, 2002; Lou and Beaujot, 2005; Smith et al., 2007). Recent immigrants are less likely to self-report psychological distress as compared to non-immigrants (Tiwari and Wang, 2008; Bergeron et al., 2009), a finding which has not been explained by the typical social determinants of health framework which includes factors such as income, education, or social relationships. Stafford et al. (2011), however, suggested that areas with a higher density of immigrants were protective against threats to mental health. That is, the context of the settlement area is vital to ensuring mental health among newcomers (Chadwick and Collins, 2015).

However, such generalizations raise multiple questions. First, is the decline in health universal? That is, do all immigrant groups, regardless of immigrant status, life-course position, race or origin, experience declines in health? The answer is that there are important differences across these dimensions. Although the healthy immigrant effect has been observed in multiple places, Vang et al's (2016) systematic review of the literature associated with immigrant health explored the role of life-course stage, observing significant variations across the life course, noting that the healthy immigrant effect was strongest during adulthood (as well as adolescents; Kwak, 2016), but less so either in childhood or in later life.

Differences in health are also observed with respect to immigrant status, with refugees experiencing some of the largest declines in health status. Although much of the literature that has explored the healthy immigrant effect has not addressed the potentially unique health experiences of refugees, it has also generally acknowledged that refugees are more vulnerable and have greater health needs than most immigrant arrivals, with their particular health needs shaped by the refugee experience and the resettlement process (Drennan and Joseph, 2005; Lawrence and Kearns, 2005; Proctor, 2005; Wynaden et al., 2005). In addition, the need to navigate through a new and different health-care system in the receiving country, along with other barriers to health care including language, cost, transportation, lack of physicians, cultural roles and knowledge, may further constrain access and use of health care and result in increased health needs (Wynaden et al., 2005). In addition to concerns related to accessing health care, refugees may also require access to employment services, shelter, and specialized health services including mental health and counseling. As such, refugees are a particularly vulnerable population with multiple health risks (Nolin, 2002; Lawrence and Kearns, 2005).

Race, origin and/or ethnicity also influence the healthy immigrant effect (Veenstra, 2009). Ng et al. (2005), for example, found that immigrants from non-European origins were most likely to experience declining health. In part, such differences are contextual. For example, shaped by their refugee experience and based on work in the USA, South-East Asian refugees disproportionately suffer from tuberculosis (TB), malaria, hepatitis B, malnutrition, anemia, leprosy, and intestinal parasites, among other problems. In part, these health outcomes are a manifestation of the conditions refugees experienced in their origin countries or refugee camps, including inadequate health care and poor nutrition, HIV and violence (Harrison et al., 1999). Other studies have noted mental health issues among refugee arrivals owing to refugee camp conditions, separation or loss of family and friends, and lack of acceptance in the destination country (Sinnerbrink et al., 1997; Whittaker et al., 2005). Post-arrival, the need to navigate through a new and different health-care system and other barriers to health care including language, cost, transportation, and cultural roles and knowledge may further challenge their health (see, for example, Kalich et al., 2016), leading to lower levels of health relative to other immigrant groups.

Declines in health relative to immigrant arrival status are further illustrated by an analysis using Statistics Canada's Longitudinal Survey of Immigrants to Canada (Newbold, 2009). Table 2.2 reports changes to self-assessed health based on the LSIC, with the added advantage that the type of immigrant arrival (family, economic or refugee) can be discerned within the data, with the LSIC being one of the few data files that enables this disaggregation. Self-assessed health is aggregated to a three-point scale (excellent/very good, good, and fair/poor). While the majority of all immigrants (78.3 percent) reported excellent or very good health just six months after arrival, this proportion had fallen to just 60 percent four years after arrival. At the same time, the proportion reporting fair or poor self-assessed health increased from 3 percent to 8.1 percent over the same period, clearly showing declines in health over a short period consistent with the healthy immigrant effect. Further, differences in health are noted relative to immigrant status, with refugees typically more likely to report fair/poor health and less likely to report excellent or very good health as compared with other groups. Conversely, economic immigrants report some of the highest levels of health, and are the least likely to report fair or poor health.

Table 2.2 Self-assessed health status (%) by immigrant status and duration of residence in Canada

	Family	Economic	Refugee	Total
6 months post-arrival				
Excellent/very good	73.5	81.1	70.1	78.3
Good	21.8	16.9	23.7	18.7
Fair/poor	4.7	2.0	6.2	3.0
2 years post-arrival				
Excellent/very good	65.5	72.8	64.0	70.2
Good	26.0	23.1	28.8	24.3
Fair/poor	8.5	4.1	7.2	5.5
4 years post-arrival				
Excellent/very good	53.5	62.8	59.8	60.0
Good	35.2	30.8	27.8	31.9
Fair/poor	11.3	6.4	12.4	8.1

Source: Newbold (2005). Copyright 2017 by K. Bruce Newbold. Reprinted by permission of SAGE Publications, Ltd. Results based on LSIC.

Given declining health status and increased need for care after arrival, does the use of health care increase? That is, does health-care use increase as health status declines? Table 2.3 displays a series of measures that capture the use of health-care facilities, including the proportion reporting physician use, hospital use, and the mean number of nights spent in the hospital. Although the analysis does not control for age or gender, the results in Table 2.3 suggest that immigrants are more likely to report the use of a physician, as compared to the native-born. For example, 84.3 percent reported contact with a physician in 2000/01, compared with 80.9 percent of the native-born. Even among those who arrived between 1990 and 1994, their use of a physician was greater than or essentially equal to that of the native-born in both 1996/97 and 2000/01.

Although a larger proportion of immigrants reported contact with a physician, is their use of physician services consistent with increased need, as demonstrated by declining health status over time? Although there is a general sense that the proportion using a physician increases between 1994/95 and 2000/01, the difference is not large (4.8 percentage points), with a nearly similar increase (3.5 percentage points) observed for the native-born.

Patterns and differences between the native- and foreign-born in terms of hospital use are far less clear, with year-to-year variations. That is, neither the incidence of hospital use nor the mean number of nights

Table 2.3 Health-care use: immigrant and native-born aged 20+ years in 1994

	1994/95	1996/97	1998/99	2000/01
Physician use (%)				
Foreign-born	79.7	83.0	83.7	84.3
Arrived 1990–94	74.6	81.8	75.9	79.4
Native-born	77.4	77.3	79.0	80.9
Hospital use (%)				
Foreign-born	9.7	9.0	8.1	8.9
Arrived 1990–94	7.7	11.5	11.2	7.2
Native-born	9.6	8.7	7.9	9.0
Mean no. of nights in hospital				
Foreign-born	8.9	6.8	9.8	9.9
Arrived 1990–1994	5.5	3.7	11.4	5.6
Native-born	9.6	8.2	9.4	9.6

Source: Newbold (2005). Copyright 2017 by K. Bruce Newbold. Reprinted by permission of SAGE Publications, Ltd. Results based on National NPHS 1994/95–2000/01.

consistently increased over time, as might be expected. For instance, 7.7 percent of immigrants who arrived between 1990 and 1994 reported use of the hospital in 1994/95. While a larger proportion of this same arrival cohort indicated use in both 1996/97 and 1998/99, the proportion using a hospital was just 7.2 percent in 2000/01. The mean number of nights spent in a hospital for this same arrival cohort also varied, with a maximum of 11.4 nights in 1998/99, and a minimum number of nights spent in hospital observed in 1996/97 (3.7). More than likely, hospital use (both overall use and mean number of nights) reflects the role of 'gatekeepers' or individuals (typically general practitioners) who control access to related health-care services, including specialists and hospitals, rather than true variations in use.

Of course, the above analyses present only a partial picture of health status and the use of health-care facilities, given that they do not control for age, gender or other variables that are typically associated with both how individuals perceive their health and their use of health-care facilities. Despite the appearance that immigrants may have some advantage in the use of physician services, further multivariate analysis (see Newbold, 2005, 2009), including ordinary and proportional hazards regression models, revealed that there is no difference in physician use between immigrants and the native-born, after controlling for other effects. Likewise, the period of arrival was not observed to impact the use of physician services

Table 2.4 Health care not received (%), 1994/95–2000/01: foreign-born and native-born, aged 20+ in 1994

	1996/97	1998/99	2000/01
		Foreign-born	
Care not received	3.3	4.4	7.6
Reason care not received			
Difficult to access	46.3	53.2	56.7
Chose not to access	26.4	25.3	17.3
Other	27.3	11.5	26.1
		Native-born	
Care not received	5.4	6.5	8.4
Reason care not received			
Difficult to access	46.7	50.4	58.9
Chose not to access	32.8	29.6	24.3
Other	20.6	20.0	16.8

Source: Author's calculations based on the 1996/97–2000/01 NPHS. Results from the 1994/95 NPHS are not presented given changes in question/coding between 1994/95 and 1996/97 cycles.

Further, analysis of the risk of a change to poor health indicated no difference between immigrants and the native-born.

The use of hospital services potentially represents greater need for care. Again, multivariate results (Newbold, 2009) revealed that hospital use was related to health status (need for care), with individuals in fair or poor health more likely to use a hospital. However, the foreign-born were neither more nor less likely to have used a hospital as compared to the native-born. Therefore, little evidence was found to support the idea that increased need for care among immigrants resulted in increased use of health care facilities over time. More specifically, it may be that the foreign-born are actually underserved given the declines in health status and the lack of a concomitant increase in their use of health care services.

Table 2.4 explores whether the foreign- and native-born are underserved by considering the extent to which health care is not received. Results demonstrate that a smaller proportion of the foreign-born consistently report that health care was not received, as compared to the native-born. Although the proportion of both the native- and foreign-born reporting unmet needs increased over the period, the low proportion of the foreign-born reporting unmet needs may reflect their lack of awareness of the health-care system. Table 2.4 also reports the reason care was not received, with respondents allowed to identify more than one reason in each case.

In each year of the NPHS, nearly similar proportions of the foreign- and native-born reported difficulty in accessing a health service as a reason why care was not received. The foreign-born were consistently less likely to indicate that they chose not to access care, although this could reflect reasons including cost, lack of insurance coverage, or lack of awareness of services.

DETERMINANTS OF IMMIGRANT HEALTH

Despite the Canada Health Act and nationalized health care within Canada, the healthy immigrant effect identifies a divergence in the health of new immigrants and the native-born population. In large part, the good health of immigrants when they first arrive in Canada is an outcome of self-selection processes at both the individual and national levels, along with the health screening of new arrivals that is meant to restrict entry to individuals with a serious health problem that would pose an economic burden to Canada for their care. That is, immigration is typically undertaken by individuals who are young and healthy, two characteristics that are typically associated with better health. In addition, immigrant receiving countries often impose a selection process, whereby potential immigrants must satisfy a series of criteria before entry (Chiswick et al., 2006). For example, Canada's Express Entry 'points system' selects economic immigrants based on measures including education, experience, age, arranged employment in Canada, adaptability, and English and/or French language abilities. In theory, such systems select individuals in better health (see http://www.cic.gc.ca/english/immigrate/skilled/apply-factors.asp). However, the points system only applies to economic immigrants (the independent class), and does not apply to individuals who enter as family-class arrivals or refugees.

While self-selection may be important in defining good health when immigrants first arrive in Canada, it does not account for subsequent declines in health. We also know that immigrants tend to move from one set of health risks, behaviors and constraints, to an environment that is often associated with a different mix of risks impacting health. However, these explanations – self-selection and risk effects – simply identify why immigrants arrive in Canada in good health, and do not provide a reason as to why health status deteriorates after arrival in the destination country. In part, aging of the immigrant stock could account for declines in health, but the change in health status is likely too fast to account for the large declines in health that are observed. As such, four broad reasons have been put forward.

First, much of the research has focused on lifestyle change and the adoption of riskier health practices among immigrants as a primary reason for declining health. In part, the health advantage experienced by immigrants when they first arrive may be due to 'cultural buffering' effects, whereby immigrants are less likely to participate in activities such as smoking and drinking and the increased consumption of prepared foods that have negative health outcomes (Hochhausen et al., 2010). Work by Subedi and Rosenberg (2014) suggests that alcohol consumption among recent immigrants does increase after arrival, and evidence of the negative impact of dietary change on health outcomes is found in work by Sanou et al. (2014) and Popovic-Lipovac and Strasser (2015). Consequently, these studies suggest that there is some merit to explaining declines in health due to changing lifestyle habits. However, the evidence supporting the uptake of unhealthy lifestyles as a determinant of declining health is limited (Vang et al., 2016). Moreover, beyond changes to diet which can reflect the ability to buy food along with access to healthy food sources, immigrants are unlikely to suddenly adopt unhealthy behaviors simply because of the immigrant experience, and the uptake of poor lifestyles is more likely to become apparent only after decades, rather than the five to ten years typically observed in the literature.

Second, barriers to health care may result in declining health status. Despite their increased need for care (as measured by declining health status), the use of health-care facilities by immigrants does not necessarily increase (Newbold 2009; Kobayashi and Prus, 2012). The more limited use of health-care facilities by immigrants reflects barriers that have been widely noted within the literature, including language, knowledge, and social/cultural roles (that is, Pottie et al., 2008; McKeary and Newbold, 2010). In particular, access to health-care services may be limited among immigrant women whose cultural expectations and roles limit opportunities. Unease or distrust of the medical system, or a medical system that does not provide culturally sensitive and appropriate care may create additional barriers (Deinard and Dunnigan, 1987; Anderson et al., 1998). For example, recent immigrants are less likely to use health-screening services such as Pap tests or prostate examinations as compared to immigrants who have resided in Canada longer and the native-born, typically because they are not considered essential and/or are relatively low priority compared to other needs (Woltman and Newbold, 2007).

Supply-side factors will also create barriers to accessing health care, with structural explanations providing an alternative explanation for the observed declines in health (Birch and Gafni, 1999). Providers, for instance, may not be aware of the health needs of newcomers (Asanin and Wilson, 2008) and/or may not have the experience and knowledge to work with the diversity found in the immigrant population. In addition, structural changes to the Canadian health-care system during the 1990s may have decreased the accessibility among immigrants to health-care services (Birch and Gafni, 1999), particularly among low-income groups and the poorly educated, even within Canada's publicly financed system.

Third, declines in health status may reflect the broader social determinants of health literature which recognizes that the health of a population is influenced by a variety of factors beyond health care (Evans and Stoddart, 1990; Evans et al., 1994; Dunn, 1996). On its own, settlement – whether in Canada or elsewhere – along with the tasks associated with finding housing, employment, transportation, building social networks, and so on, will pose challenges that impact on health status. Included within this is the recognition that poor socioeconomic status, limited social networks, language barriers, and other systemic barriers contribute to poor and declining health status.

In addition, the actual settlement location could also affect the health trajectories of newcomers (Wang and Hu, 2013; Chadwick and Collins, 2015). For instance, work by Chadwick and Collins (2015) noted the importance of geographic scale for access to mental health services, with immigrants resident in smaller urban centers having greater access to social support services. In spite of this greater access, these same individuals were more likely to report lower self-perceived mental health. Wang and Hu (2013) noted significant differences in health within the foreign-born population across metropolitan areas. At smaller spatial scales, settlement in disadvantaged neighborhoods, characterized by poorer health facilities and services and substandard housing, potentially has negative health implications. Moreover, residents of poorer neighborhoods are more likely to be unemployed (or under-employed) and exposed to crime and violence, factors which are known to negatively impact health (Stead et al., 2001; Subedi and Rosenberg, 2014).

CONCLUSION

Although the healthy immigrant effect is not a universal phenomenon in Canada, with health status often varying by country of origin, life course stage, and other factors (for example, education, age, and immigrant status), it is also commonly observed across a range of health measures (for example, self-reported health, and mental health), immigrant status (immigrant versus refugee), and other socioeconomic and demographic variables. The implications of the healthy immigrant effect are perhaps most significant for refugees, a matter that has become more pressing given the refugee crisis of 2015.

The policy implications are significant. First, although there is some evidence of increasing use of physicians by immigrants, it remains possible that immigrants are underserved relative to their need for care, a conclusion that was reinforced by Kalich et al. (2016). That is, given declines in self-reported health, there is little evidence of a systematic increase in the use of hospital resources, and only some limited increase in the use of physicians. Notwithstanding this, other literature points to the difficulties immigrants face in finding a physician and maintaining regular contact (Asanin and Wilson, 2008). The lack of change with respect to immigrants' use of hospital services suggests the potential for gatekeeping on the part of physicians or other unseen barriers to care, including discrimination (Edge and Newbold, 2013; Nakhaie and Wijesingha, 2015), structural issues, communication difficulties, insurance or other barriers to care.

Given the intensity of research considering the healthy immigrant effect, it is likely time to move beyond consideration of whether or not the effect is observed. Instead, research agendas should focus on three related topics. First, why does the healthy immigrant effect occur? As discussed previously in this chapter, numerous hypotheses have been forwarded that provide hints as to why this decline occurs. While research has started to highlight the reasons, they are undoubtedly complex and overlapping. Related to this question is the need to better understand racial, ethnic, or origin differences in the healthy immigrant effect. Veenstra (2009) has called for more attention to this question.

Second, how can the barriers to health care be overcome? That is, what programs or policies can reduce or ameliorate the healthy immigrant effect? In particular, how can programs and policies ensure that the health advantage observed among recent arrivals is retained? Following Vang et al. (2016), policies addressing immigrant health issues need to target specific life-course stages and health outcomes where immigrants are most vulnerable. In addition, perspectives from a variety of health-care workers would be valuable, enabling understanding the various ways that health care is accessed (Kalich et al., 2016).

Third, despite the fact that native-born Canadians appear to be less healthy than new immigrant arrivals, it is surprising that no research or policy-oriented attention has been given to this deficiency. Are they really less healthy? Why? In fact, it might be argued that native-born Canadians are actually healthier, but that this is somehow hidden within the data. Additional research could address this potential paradox.

REFERENCES

Ali, J. (2002), 'Mental health of Canada's immigrants', *Health Reports*, **13** (supplement), 101–11.

Anderson, R.T., M.K. James, M.E. Miller, A.S. Worley and C.E. Longino (1998), 'The timing of change: patterns in transitions in functional status among elderly persons', *Journal of Gerontology B: Psychology*, **53** (1), S17–27.

Asanin J. and K. Wilson (2008), 'I spent nine years looking for a doctor: exploring access to health care among immigrant in Mississauga, Ontario, Canada', *Social Science & Medicine*, **66** (6), 1271–83.

Bergeron, P., N. Auger and D. Hamel (2009), 'Poids, santé générale et santé mentale: La situation de divers sous-groupes d'immigrants au Canada' ('Weight, general health and mental health: the situation of various immigrant subgroups in Canada'), *Canadian Journal of Public Health*, **100** (3), 215–220.

Birch, S. and A. Gafni (1999), 'Achievements and challenges of medicare in Canada: are we there yet? Are we on course?', paper presented at the First Australia and New Zealand Health Research Conference, Manly, NSW, 8–11 August.

Blair, A.H. and A. Schneeberg (2014), 'Changes in the "healthy migrant effect" in Canada: are recent immigrants healthier than they were a decade ago?', *Journal of Immigrant and Minority Health*, **16** (1), 136–42.

Chadwick, K.A. and P.A. Collins (2015), 'Examining the relationship between social support availability, urban center size, and self-perceived mental health of recent immigrants to Canada: a mixed-methods analysis', *Social Science & Medicine*, **128** (March), 220–30.

Chen, J., R. Wilkens and E. Ng (1996), 'Life expectancy of Canada's immigrants from 1986 to 1991', *Health Reports*, **8** (3), 29–38.

Chiswick, B.R., Y.L. Lee and P.W. Miller (2006), 'Immigrant selection systems and immigrant health', IZA Discussion Paper No. 2345.

Dean, J.A. and K. Wilson (2009), 'Education? It is irrelevant to my job now. It makes me very depressed . . .': exploring the health impacts of under/unemployment among highly skilled recent immigrants in Canada', *Ethnicity and Health*, **14** (2), 185–204.

Deinard, A.S. and T. Dunnigan (1987), 'Hmong health care – reflections on a six-year experience', *International Migration Review*, **21** (3), 857–65.

Drennan, V.M. and J. Joseph (2005), 'Health visiting and refugee families: issues in professional practice', *Journal of Advanced Nursing*, **49** (2), 155–63.

Dunn, J. (1996), 'Inequalities in health and the housing question', in G. Moon, M. Gould and R. Watt (eds), *Proceedings, 7th International Symposium in Medical Geography*, Portsmouth.

Dunn, J. and I. Dyck (2000), 'Social determinants of health in Canada's immigrant population: results from the National Population Health Survey', *Social Science & Medicine*, **51** (11), 1573–93.

Edge, S. and K.B. Newbold (2013), 'Discrimination and the health of immigrants and refugees: exploring Canada's evidence base and directions for future research in newcomer receiving countries', *Journal of Immigrant and Minority Health*, **15** (1), 141–8.

Evans, R., M.L. Barer and T.R. Marmor (1994), *Why Are Some People Healthy and Others Not? The Determinants of Health of Populations*, New York: Aldine and DeGruyter.

Evans, R. and G. Stoddart (1990), 'Producing health, consuming health care', *Social Science & Medicine*, **31** (12), 1347–63.
Fennelly, K. (2007), 'The "healthy migrant" effect', *Minnesota Medical Magazine*, **90** (3), 51–3.
Gotsens, M., D. Malmusi, N. Villarroel, C. Vives-Cases, I. Garcia-Subirats, C. Hernando and C. Borrell (2015), 'Health inequality between immigrants and natives in Spain: the loss of the healthy immigrant effect in times of economic crisis', *European Journal of Public Health*, **354** (September), 1–7, doi:http://dx.doi.org/10.1093/eurpub/ckv126.
Harrison, A., L. Calder, N. Karalus, P. Martin, M. Kennedy and C. Wong (1999), 'Tuberculosis in immigrants and visitors', *New Zealand Medical Journal*, **112** (1096), 363–5.
Hochhausen, L., D.F. Perry and H.-N. Le (2010), 'Neighborhood context and acculturation among Central American immigrants', *Journal of Immigrant & Minority Health*, **12** (5), 806–9.
Kalich, A., L. Heinemann and S. Ghahari (2016), 'A scoping review of immigrant experience of health care access barriers in Canada', *Journal of Immigrant and Minority Health*, **18** (3), 697–709.
Kennedy, S., M.P. Kidd, J.T. McDonald and N. Biddle (2015), 'The healthy immigrant effect: patterns and evidence from four countries', *International Migration & Integration*, **16** (2), 317–32.
Kobayashi, K.M. and S.G. Prus (2012), 'Examining the gender, ethnicity, and age dimensions of the healthy immigrant effect: factors in the development of equitable health', *International Journal of Equity Health*, **11** (8), 1–6.
Kwak, K. (2016), 'An evaluation of the healthy immigrant effect with adolescents in Canada: examinations of gender and length of residence', *Social Science and Medicine*, **157** (May), 87–95.
Lawrence, J. and R. Kearns (2005), 'Exploring the "fit" between people and providers: refugee health needs and health care services in Mt. Roskill, Auckland, New Zealand', *Health and Social Care in the Community*, **13** (5): 451–61.
Lou, Y. and R. Beaujot (2005), 'What happens to the "healthy immigrant effect": the mental health of immigrants to Canada', PSC Discussion Paper Series, 19 (15), art.1.
McDonald, J.T. and S. Kennedy (2004), 'Insights into the "healthy immigrant effect": health status and health service use of immigrants to Canada', *Social Science & Medicine*, **59** (8), 1613–27.
McKeary, M. and K.B. Newbold (2010), 'Barriers to care: the challenges for Canadian refugees and their health care providers', *Journal of Refugee Studies*, **23** (4), 523–45.
Nakhaie R. and R. Wijesingha (2015), 'Discrimination and health of male and female Canadian immigrants', *International Migration & Integration*, **16** (4), 1255–72.
Newbold, K.B. (2005), 'Health status and health care utilization of the foreign-born in Canada: a longitudinal analysis, 1994/95–2000/01', *Journal of Health Services Research and Policy*, **10** (2), 77–84.
Newbold, K.B. (2009), 'The short-term health of Canada's new immigrant arrivals: evidence from LSIC', *Ethnicity and Health*, **14** (3), 315–36.
Newbold, K.B. and J. Danforth (2003), 'Health status and Canada's immigrant population', *Social Science and Medicine*, **57** (10), 1981–95.
Ng, E. and the LHAD research team (2011), 'Insights into the healthy immigrant

effect: mortality by period of immigration and birthplace', Statistics Canada, Ottawa, Catalogue 82-622-X No. 008.

Ng, E., R. Wilkins, F. Gendron and J.M. Berthelot (2005), 'Dynamics of immigrants' health in Canada: evidence from the National Population Health Survey', in *Healthy Today, Healthy Tomorrow? Findings from the National Population Health Survey*, Ottawa: Statistics Canada, Catalogue 82-618.

Nolin, C.L. (2002), 'Transnational ruptures: political violence and refugee and (im)migrant experiences in Guatemala and Canada', PhD dissertation, Department of Geography, Queen's University, Kingston, Ontario.

Popovic-Lipovac, A. and B. Strasser (2015), 'A review on changes in food habits among immigrant women and implications for health', *Journal of Immigrant and Minority Health*, **17** (2), 582–90.

Pottie, K., E. Ng, D. Spitzer, A. Mohammed and R. Glazier (2008), 'Language proficiency, gender and self-reported health: an analysis of the first two waves of the Longitudinal Survey of Immigrants to Canada', *Canadian Journal of Public Health*, **99** (6), 505–10.

Proctor, N.G. (2005), 'They first killed his heart (then), he took his own life. Part 1: A review of the context and literature on mental health issues for refugees and asylum seekers', *International Journal of Nursing Practice*, **11** (6), 286–91.

Sanou, D., E. O'Reilly, I. Ngnie-Teta, M. Batal, N. Mondain, C. Andrew et al. (2014), 'Acculturation and nutritional health of immigrants in Canada: a scoping review', *Journal of Immigrant and Minority Health*, **16** (1), 24–34.

Setia, M.S., J. Lynch, M. Abrahamowicz, P. Tousignant and A. Quesnel-Vallee (2011), 'Self-rated health in Canadian immigrants: analysis of the longitudinal survey of immigrants to Canada', *Health & Place*, **17** (2), 658–70.

Sinnerbrink, I., D. Silove, A. Field, Z. Steel and V. Manicavasagar (1997), 'Compounding of premigration trauma and postmigration stress in asylum seekers', *Journal of Psychology*, **131** (5), 463–70.

Smith, K.L.W., F.I. Matheson, R. Moineddin and R.H. Glazier (2007), 'Gender, income and immigration differences in depression in Canadian urban centres', *Canadian Journal of Public Health*, **98** (2), 149–53.

Stafford, M., K.B. Newbold and N. Ross (2011), 'Psychological distress among immigrants and visible minorities in Canada', *International Journal of Social Psychiatry*, **57** (4), 428–41.

Stead, M., S. MacAskill, A.M. MacKintosh, J. Reece and D. Eadie (2001), 'It's as if you're locked in: qualitative explanations for area effects on smoking in disadvantaged communities', *Health & Place*, **7** (4), e333–e343.

Subedi, R.P. and M.W. Rosenberg (2014), 'Determinants of the variations in self-reported health status among recent and more established immigrants in Canada', *Social Science & Medicine*, **115**, 103–10.

Tiwari, S.K. and J. Wang (2008), 'Ethnic differences in mental health service use among White, Chinese, South Asian and South East Asian populations living in Canada', *Social Psychiatry and Psychiatric Epidemiology*, **43** (11), 866–71.

Trovato, F. (2003), 'Migration and survival: the mortality experience of immigrants in Canada', Prairie Centre for Research on Immigration and Integration (PCRII), University of Alberta, Edmonton.

Vang, Z., J. Sigouin, A. Flenon and A. Gagnon (2016), 'Are immigrants healthier than native-born Canadians? A systematic review of the healthy immigrant effect in Canada', *Ethnicity & Health*, **22** (3), 209–41, doi:10.1080/13557858.2016.1246518

Veenstra, G. (2009), 'Racialized identity and health in Canada: results from a nationally representative survey', *Social Science and Medicine*, **69** (4), 538–42.
Wang, L. and Hu, W. (2013), 'Immigrant health, place effect and regional disparities in Canada', *Social Science and Medicine*, **98** (December), 8–17.
Whittaker, S., G. Hardy, K. Lewis and L. Buchan (2005), 'An exploration of psychological well-being with young Somali refugee and asylum-seeker women', *Clinical Child Psychology and Psychiatry*, **10** (2), 177–96.
Woltman, K. and K.B. Newbold (2007), 'Immigrant women and cervical cancer screening uptake: a multilevel analysis', *Canadian Journal of Public Health*, **98** (6), 470–75.
Wynaden, D., R. Chapman, R., A. Orb, S. McGowan, Z. Zeeman and S.H. Yeak (2005), 'Factors that influence Asian communities' access to mental health care', *International Journal of Mental Health Nursing*, **14** (2), 88–95.

3. All-cause and circulatory disease-related hospitalization, by immigrant generation status: evidence from a Canadian census-based linked cohort with a focus on South Asian, Chinese and UK populations*

Edward Ng, Claudia Sanmartin, Jack V. Tu and Doug G. Manuel

INTRODUCTION

Since the 1970s, the origins of immigrants to Canada have shifted from the West (including the United Kingdom) toward non-European sources (such as India and China) (Chui et al., 2007). As a result, 8 percent of the total population self-identify as South Asian or Chinese, a percentage that is projected to reach about 15 percent by 2031 (Statistics Canada, 2010a). Canada's changing ethnic make-up and its long-run impact on subsequent generations have implications for health care.

While immigrants tend to have better health than the Canadian-born population, variations by disease and by source country are considerable (Ng and LHAD Research Team, 2011; Rotermann, 2011). For example, regardless of where they live, South Asians have one of the highest rates of heart or circulatory disease in the world (Bhopal, 2002; Lau, 2010; Celermajer et al., 2012). In Canada, circulatory disease mortality risk among South Asians tends to be similar to that of the Canadian-born population, but higher than that of other immigrant or ethnic groups (Sheth et al., 1999; Muennig et al., 2004; Ng and LHAD Research Team, 2011). Conversely, circulatory disease risk among the Chinese population is relatively low (Chiu et al., 2010, 2012). A recent review of immigrant health research found that Canadians of South Asian descent tend to experience increased risks of heart disease and hypertension as duration of residence in Canada lengthens, and noted a need to study the effects from a generational perspective (Hyman, 2007).

Evidence of the extent to which health advantages (or disadvantages) of first-generation immigrants are transferred to future generations is mixed (Leâo et al., 2006; Hosper et al., 2007; Almeida et al., 2012). In a 1976 study of immigrant health, Marmot and Syme found a higher prevalence of heart disease among male Japanese immigrants in California and Hawaii than among men in Japan (Marmot and Syme, 1976). However, first-generation Japanese immigrants in Hawaii had a lower prevalence of heart disease than did the second generation, whose health profiles were closer to those of non-immigrant Hawaiians. In Canada, generational analyses of health tend to focus on youth and schoolchildren, specifically risk behaviors and weight gain, with little attention to cardiac health (Hamilton et al., 2009; Maximova et al., 2011; Quon et al., 2012). A study of immigrants in Montreal reported no health advantage in obesity or self-rated health among second-generation adults, especially those in disadvantaged neighborhoods (Zunzunnegui et al., 2006).

Information about the use of health-care services by generational status is limited. A key barrier is the lack of immigration and generation status variables in administrative health data (Gagnon, 2002). Area-based studies have used the percentage of immigrants in a neighborhood as a proxy for immigrant status, but such ecological approaches are limited (Carrière et al., 2012). Alternatively, linking administrative health data to sources that contain information on immigrant and generational status opens the possibility for detailed examinations of immigrant health (Ng and LHAD Research Team, 2011).

In Canada, South Asian immigrants have a circulatory disease mortality risk similar to the Canadian-born population, but higher than other immigrant groups such as the Chinese. There is a need to determine if the relatively high circulatory disease mortality risk among South Asians is reflected in hospitalization, and if the health risks affect subsequent generations. This study used data from the 2006 Census of Population (long-form respondents) linked to administrative records to examine the intergenerational transmission of the healthy immigrant effect. Specifically, this study first determines if hospitalization patterns among first-generation immigrants persist in the second generation, and if patterns differ between South Asians and Chinese subgroups, when socioeconomic covariates are taken into account. Those immigrants from the United Kingdom (UK), a country with sociocultural and economic similarity to that of Canada, were used as a contrast to the South Asians and the Chinese. Immigrants from the UK were expected to have similar all-cause hospital rates and converge faster than for those of South Asians and Chinese descents. However, for circulatory disease-related hospitalization, the Chinese expected to have a low rate, while the South Asians, due to their historically high rate in their world source region, may converge in a way similar to those from the UK.

DATA AND METHODS

Data Source

The 2006 Census (long-form) was linked to the Canadian Institute for Health Information's Discharge Abstract Database (DAD). The long-form census data represent about 20 percent of the non-institutional population and provide information about immigrant generational status, including place of birth and period of arrival of the first generation, and socioeconomic and household characteristics.

The DAD contains annual information about inpatient hospitalizations, excluding Quebec, which does not routinely submit data to the DAD. As a result of this exclusion, immigrants living in Quebec are not reflected in this study, nor are hospitalizations of residents of other provinces that occurred in Quebec.

Approximately 4.65 million census long-form respondents (excluding Quebec) were linked to the DAD for the three fiscal years from 2006/07 to 2008/09. A hierarchical deterministic linkage using date of birth, sex, and residential postal code was conducted. Postal code information from the Historical Tax File was used to account for changes in residence. The coverage rates in the linked data after weighting were relatively high (78 percent to 80 percent). The weighting using weights derived by Statistics Canada ensure representativeness of the linked data. A validation study concluded that the linked file is suitable for health-related research and is broadly representative of immigrants in Canada. Additional information about the linkage process and results is reported elsewhere (Rotermann et al., 2014). The linkage was approved by Statistics Canada's Policy Committee (Statistics Canada, 2012) and is governed by the Directive on Record Linkage (Statistics Canada, 2011).

Study Sample

The study cohort consisted of people aged 30 or older who were living in urban communities – census metropolitan areas (CMAs) or census agglomerations (CAs) outside the territories at the time of the 2006 Census (16

May 2006) (Statistics Canada, 2010b). The majority of immigrants, especially recent arrivals, reside in these urban communities (Statistics Canada, 2013). Non-permanent residents, defined as people in Canada on employment or student authorizations, and refugee claimants were excluded. After these exclusions, the final study cohort comprised 2212755 respondents, among whom 548460 hospitalizations were recorded over the three years.

Measures

Generational status was defined based on immigrant status and parental place of birth. First-generation (G1) respondents are those who were, or had been, landed immigrants in Canada. A landed immigrant is a person who is not a Canadian citizen by birth, but who has been granted the right to live in Canada permanently (Chui et al., 2007). Immigrants were categorized by their period of arrival: long-term (before 1996) or recent (from 1996 to 2006). Second-generation (G2) respondents are non-immigrants with at least one parent born outside Canada. Third-plus-generation (G3+) respondents are non-immigrants with both parents born in Canada. Although the study focuses on immigrants from China (including Hong Kong) and South Asia (Bangladesh, Bhutan, India, Maldives, Nepal, Pakistan, and Sri Lanka) as well as those from the United Kingdom (England, Scotland, Ireland, and Wales), these subgroups are not singled out in the G3+ comparison population.

Additional covariates from the census are age group (30 to 49, 50 to 64, and 65 or older), sex, secondary school graduation (yes/no), and before-tax household low-income status (yes/no/not applicable). The low-income measure is based on the low-income cut-off threshold, determined by the average spending on food, clothing and shelter of all Canadian households depending on the size of the city. A household is identified as low-income if the percentage of its spending on food, shelter and clothing exceeds the threshold (Statistics Canada, 2010b).

The primary outcome is at least one inpatient acute-care hospitalization between 1 April 2006 and 31 March 2009. Two types of hospitalization are considered in this analysis: (1) all-cause, excluding those related to pregnancy (ICD10 codes O00 to O99) and (2) circulatory disease-related (ICD10 codes I00 to I93), which accounted for 17 percent (91821) of discharges in the linked database.

Statistical Methods

Descriptive statistics were produced to profile the study population by generational status and by the selected origins: South Asia, China, and those related to the UK. Crude and age-standardized hospitalization rates (ASHR) were derived for all-cause (excluding pregnancy) and circulatory disease-related hospitalizations using the overall cohort population as the reference population. Statistical testing for differences in age-standardized rates was conducted using logarithmic transformation to adjust for the skewness in the distribution of the standardized rates for inferential purposes in analysis of rare events (Carriere and Roos, 1997). Multivariate logistic regressions were used to estimate the odds of being hospitalized at least once, by generational status using G3+ as the reference population. Separate models were estimated by sex and by origin. Two models were estimated: (1) age-adjusted, and (2) fully adjusted, controlling for age, low-income status, and secondary school graduation status. Analysis was conducted using SAS version 9.2 (SAS Institute Inc., 2009).

RESULTS

First-generation immigrants (G1) made up 34 percent of the urban population aged 30 or older, and the second generation (G2), 19 percent (Table 3.1). The third-plus generation (G3+) accounted for the remaining 48 percent. Among G1 respondents, 23 percent were recent immigrants (1996 to 2006), and 36 percent were from the U.K, South Asia, or China (12 percent each). Approximately 31 percent of G2 respondents reported that their parent(s) were born in the UK, compared with only 3 percent from South Asia or China. G2 respondents of South Asian and Chinese descent were relatively young – 85 percent and 79 percent, respectively, were aged 30 to 49, compared with about 50 percent for G2 overall and 34 percent for those from the UK.

Distributions by education level were similar across generations overall, with about 80 percent having graduated from secondary school. However, more than 90 percent of G2 respondents of South Asian and Chinese descent were secondary school graduates, but the corresponding figure for the UK was 76 percent.

A relatively large percentage of G1 respondents lived in low-income households: 18 percent versus 10 percent of G2 and G3+. The figure was particularly high for Chinese immigrants (27 percent), and low for those from the UK (4 percent).

A rising gradient in ASHRs (excluding pregnancy) was observed across the generations (Table 3.2). All-cause ASHRs for G1, G2 and G3+ were 609, 792 and 839 per 10000, respectively; the corresponding ASHRs for circulatory disease were 119, 142 and 152 per 10000. Rates for G1 and G2 were significantly lower than those for G3+. The patterns were similar

Table 3.1 Selected characteristics by generational status with special focus on South Asian, Chinese and UK groups; population aged 30 and older, urban Canada (excluding Quebec and the territories), 2006–09*

		Canadian-born					Foreign-born			
		G3+ (All)	G2				G1			
	Overall		All	UK	S. Asia	China	All	UK	S. Asia	China
Sample size	2212755	1058309	408755	146395	4755	8460	745700	86920	88315	91290
% distribution	100	47.8	18.5	6.6	0.2	0.4	33.7	3.9	4.0	4.1
Mean age (years)	52	50	54	58	40	44	54	60	48	51
Age group (%)										
30–49	49	53	49	34	85	79	45	27	59	52
50–64	30	32	23	28	9	12	31	36	27	28
65+	21	15	28	38	7	9	24	37	14	20
% males	48	48	48	47	49	51	47	47	51	46
% recent immigrants (LT 10 years)	–	–	–	–	–	–	23	5	44	37
% long-term immigrants (GE 10 years)							77	95	56	63
% high-school graduate	77	77	79	76	93	93	77	86	79	78
% low income	13	10	10	10	8	8	18	4	21	27

Notes:
* Includes Hong Kong.
G1 means generation 1; G2 means generation 2; G3+ means third generation and beyond.

Source: 2006 Census-hospitalization linked database.

Table 3.2 Crude and age-standardized hospitalization rates[†] *by 10 000 population for all-cause (excluding pregnancies) and for circulatory disease by generational status with a special focus on South Asian, Chinese and UK groups;*[‡] *population aged 30 and older, urban Canada (excluding Quebec and the territories), 2006–07*

		All		UK		South Asia		China‡	
Hospitalization rate	G3+ (reference population)	G2	G1	G2	G1	G2	G1	G2	G1
All-cause (excluding pregnancy)									
Crude	757	897	664	1124	1072	362	466	372	332
Age-standardized	839	792*	609*	830	780*	597*	544*	578*	356*
Circulatory disease									
Crude	130	169	133	222	204	52	105	43	45
Age-standardized	152	142*	119*	148*	134*	125	129*	79*	46*

Notes:
* Results statistically significantly different from overall G3+ reference group at .05 level.
† Standardization used overall cohort population as standard; statistical testing was conducted only for age-standardized rates.
‡ Includes Hong Kong.
G1 means generation 1; G2 means generation 2.

Source: 2006 Census-hospitalization linked database.

among those of South Asian and Chinese descent. Circulatory disease-specific ASHRs were generally lowest among G1 from China (46), and highest among those G2 from the UK (148), which was still significantly lower than that for G3 (152).

The logistic regression revealed rising odds of all-cause hospitalization by generation for both men and women (Table 3.3). Compared with G3+, the age-adjusted odds of at least one hospitalization among men were 0.49 for recent G1 (CI = 0.48–0.51), 0.78 for long-term G1 (CI = 0.77–0.79), and 0.95 for G2 (CI = 0.94–0.97). The trend was similar for women. Full model adjustment for education and income reduced the differences, but they remained significant. These patterns prevailed among those of South Asian and Chinese. For those from the UK, the convergence occurred among those long-term G1 with OR of .98 (CI = 0.95–1.01 for men). The pattern was similar for women. Full adjustment changed the conclusion slightly, but the G2-UK remained converged with the G3.

Although the results for circulatory disease-related hospitalizations were similar, some notable differences emerged (Table 3.3). For men, differences between G2 and G3+ were not significantly different when adjusting for covariates. For women, the odds of hospitalization for G2 converged with G3+ even before adjustment.

The results varied by origin, with higher odds of circulatory disease-related hospitalization among those from the UK and people of South Asian descent, and lower odds among those of Chinese descent. Among men from the UK, convergence occurred by G2. Also, the hospitalization odds among G2 women from the UK were higher than those for G3+. Full adjustment changed this conclusion slightly by removing the significant difference only among long-term immigrant men. Among South Asians, the odds of at least one circulatory disease-related hospitalization did not differ from those of G3+ for G2 (men and women) and long-term G1 (men only). Among the Chinese, even after adjustment, the odds of at least one circulatory disease-related hospitalization were significantly lower for G1 and G2, compared with G3+.

DISCUSSION

Using linked census-hospital data, this study examined all-cause (excluding pregnancy) and circulatory disease-related hospitalizations among first- and second-generation immigrants, particularly South Asians and Chinese with those from the UK as contrast. Convergence in hospitalization rates over immigrant generations was apparent for both men and women. Recent immigrants were the least likely to have had at least one hospitalization

Table 3.3 Age- and fully-adjusted logistic regression odds ratios of circulatory disease-related hospitalization risk (yes or no) for males by generational status with a special focus on South Asian, Chinese† and UK groups; population aged 30 and older, urban Canada (excluding Quebec and the Territories), 2006–09

	All excluding pregnancy						Circulatory disease					
	Age-adjusted	95% lC	95% UC	Fully adjusted	95% lC	95% UC	Age-adjusted	95% lC	95% UC	Fully adjusted	95% lC	95% UC
Males												
Overall												
G3+-Overall	1.00			1.00			1.00			1.00		
G2	0.95*	0.94	0.97	0.97*	0.96	0.99	0.95*	0.93	0.98	0.97	0.94	1.00
G1-(Long term GE 10 years)	0.78*	0.77	0.79	0.79*	0.78	0.80	0.82*	0.80	0.84	0.83*	0.81	0.85
G1-(Recent LT 10 years)	0.49*	0.48	0.51	0.49*	0.48	0.51	0.55*	0.52	0.59	0.56*	0.52	0.60
UK												
G3+-Overall	1.00			1.00			1.00			1.00		
G2-British	1.01	0.99	1.04	1.04	1.01	1.07	1.00	0.96	1.04	1.02	0.98	1.06
G1-UK (Long term GE 10 years)	0.98	0.95	1.01	0.78*	0.66	0.92	0.92*	0.88	0.96	1.00	0.95	1.05
G1-UK (Recent LT 10 years)	0.74*	0.63	0.88	0.82*	0.81	0.83	0.54*	0.36	0.81	0.57*	0.39	0.85
South Asia												
G3+-Overall	1.00			1.00			1.00			1.00		
G2-South Asia	0.71*	0.60	0.84	0.74*	0.63	0.88	0.87	0.64	1.21	0.91	0.66	1.25
G1-South Asia (Long term GE 10 years)	0.74*	0.71	0.77	0.75*	0.72	0.78	0.97	0.91	1.04	1.01	0.94	1.08
G1-South Asia (Recent LT 10 years)	0.50*	0.47	0.53	0.49*	0.46	0.52	0.71*	0.64	0.79	0.71*	0.64	0.79

Table 3.3 (continued)

	All excluding pregnancy						Circulatory disease					
	Age-adjusted	95% lC	95% UC	Fully adjusted	95% lC	95% UC	Age-adjusted	95% lC	95% UC	Fully adjusted	95% lC	95% UC
China												
G3+-Overall	1.00			1.00			1.00			1.00		
G2-China	0.64*	0.56	0.72	0.67*	0.59	0.76	0.52*	0.40	0.69	0.55*	0.42	0.72
G1-China (Long term GE 10 years)	0.44*	0.42	0.46	0.43*	0.41	0.45	0.37*	0.34	0.41	0.37*	0.33	0.40
G1-China (Recent LT 10 years)	0.31*	0.28	0.34	0.30*	0.27	0.32	0.24*	0.19	0.29	0.23*	0.19	0.28
Females												
Overall												
G3+-Overall	1.00			1.00			1.00			1.00		
G2	0.96*	0.94	0.97	0.97*	0.96	0.98	0.97	0.94	1.00	0.98	0.95	1.01
G1-(Long term GE 10 yrs)	0.74*	0.73	0.75	0.74*	0.73	0.75	0.79*	0.77	0.81	0.78*	0.75	0.90
G1-(Recent LT 10 years)	0.53*	0.52	0.52	0.51*	0.50	0.53	0.52*	0.48	0.56	0.49*	0.45	0.54
UK												
G3+-Overall	1.00			1.00			1.00			1.00		
G2-UK	1.04	1.02	1.06	1.02	1.00	1.05	1.05*	1.01	1.09	1.07*	1.02	1.11
G1-UK (Long term GE 10 years)	0.99	0.96	1.02	0.78*	0.66	0.92	0.95	0.90	1.00	1.02	0.96	1.07
G1- UK (Recent LT 10 years)	0.76*	0.65	0.90	0.78*	0.77	0.79	0.63	0.39	1.02	0.65	0.40	1.06

South Asia												
G3+-Overall	1.00			1.00			1.00			1.00		
G2-South Asia	0.74*	0.62	0.85	0.76*	0.65	0.88	0.67	0.42	1.07	0.71	0.44	1.13
G1-South Asia (Long term GE 10 years)	0.67*	0.64	0.70	0.65*	0.63	0.68	0.77*	0.70	0.85	0.74*	0.67	0.82
G1-South Asia (Recent LT 10 years)	0.54*	0.51	0.57	0.50*	0.48	0.54	0.67*	0.58	0.78	0.61*	0.52	0.71
China												
G3+-Overall	1.00			1.00			1.00			1.00		
G2-China	0.72*	0.64	0.80	0.75*	0.67	0.83	0.63*	0.46	0.88	0.67*	0.48	0.92
G1-China (Long term GE 10 years)	0.43*	0.41	0.45	0.41*	0.39	0.42	0.34*	0.30	0.38	0.31*	0.27	0.34
G1-China (Recent LT 10 years)	0.36*	0.34	0.39	0.34*	0.31	0.36	0.25*	0.20	0.32	0.23*	0.18	0.29

Notes:
Full-adjustment was done for age, high school graduation, and low income status.
* Results statistically significantly different from overall G3+ reference group at .05 level.
† Includes Hong Kong.
G1 means generation 1; G2 means generation 2; G3+ means third generation and beyond. lC means lower confidence limit; UC means upper confidence limit.

Source: 2006 Census-hospitalization linked database.

during the 2006/07-to-2008/09 period, followed by long-term first-generation and second-generation Canadians. All three groups were less likely to have been hospitalized, compared with the third-plus generation. While a trend toward convergence emerged for circulatory disease-related hospitalizations, second-generation Canadians overall were no different from the third-plus generation. This was more pronounced especially among those from the UK as well as those with South Asian descent than among those of Chinese descent.

Convergence of hospitalization rates in successive generations is consistent with the theory that immigrants tend to be healthier upon arrival, but that their health deteriorates over time (Newbold, 2005; Ng et al., 2005). It is argued that as immigrants and their offspring integrate into the host society, they adopt the norms, attitudes and behaviors of the new country, and experience the accompanying health consequences (Hyman, 2001). Research on cardiovascular disease points to acculturation as a contributor to the increasing risk among immigrants and the second generation (Morales et al., 2011). For instance, people of Mexican origin who were born in the United States had higher levels of hypertension, smoking, cholesterol, diabetes and obesity than their Mexican immigrant counterparts (Sundquist and Winkleby, 2000; Singh and Siapush, 2001) and consumed less ‘heart healthy diets’ (Dixon, Sundquist and Winkleby, 2000). In Canada, cardiovascular disease risks among South Asians and Chinese immigrants tend to increase with duration of residence (Chiu et al., 2012).

The consistently higher odds of circulatory disease-related hospitalization among first- and second-generation South Asians, compared with the Chinese, meant that the South Asian immigrants’ health advantage in circulatory disease is lost by the second generation; similar to those from the UK. Among the Chinese, all-cause and circulatory disease-related hospitalization risk generally increased across generations but remained significantly lower than overall G3+ Canadians. Similar findings have been reported in the United States, the UK, South Africa, the Caribbean, and Singapore (Bhopal, 2002; Kuppuswami and Gupta, 2005; Harding et al., 2008; Yusuf et al., 2001). For example, in the UK, an excess risk of coronary artery problems among first- and second-generation South Asians was reported (Shaukat and DeBono, 1994). A study of Indian immigrants in London, England found that they had higher body mass index, systolic blood pressure and fasting blood glucose than their siblings in India (Bhatnager et al., 1995). South Asians in Canada have a high prevalence of risk factors such as diabetes, which may explain some of the findings in this study (Lau, 2010; Chiu et al., 2012; Ayesha et al., 2014). By contrast, the Chinese have the most favorable circulatory disease risk factor profile of the major ethnic groups in Canada, although it worsens with duration of residence. Contrary to these findings, an Australian study reported that the risk of circulatory- and diabetes-related mortality among older South Asians decreased with duration of residence, while immigrants from the UK and Ireland experienced increasing mortality over time (Gray et al., 2007).

Regardless of where they live, people of South Asian descent tend to have one of the highest rates of circulatory disease in the world (Celermajer et al., 2012; Gopal and Yusuf, 2006). Nonetheless, results of this study revealed a lower risk of hospitalization among recent immigrants from South Asia, compared with third-plus generation Canadians. This lower hospitalization risk may reflect the selection process that involves medical screening of potential immigrants (Gukshulak and Williams, 2004). However, additional analyses (data not shown) found relatively high circulatory disease-related hospitalization rates among younger South Asians, especially G1, which is consistent with an early onset of heart problems (McKeigue et al., 1993; Prasad et al., 2011). As well, long-term male immigrants from South Asia did not differ from G3+ in the likelihood of experiencing a circulatory disease-related hospitalization. Case-control research has found that South Asians tend to be hospitalized later in the course of acute myocardial infarction (Gupta et al., 2002), which may indicate differences in care-seeking behavior and/or cultural or language problems.

This study found that people of Chinese descent, both G1 and G2, had significantly lower odds of circulatory disease-related hospitalization than G3+, even with adjustment for education and income. Consistent with these results, an analysis of linked census and mortality data (Ng and LHAD Research Team, 2011) revealed lower circulatory disease mortality rates among recent and long-term immigrants (G1) from East Asia (Hong Kong, Japan, Macao, Mongolia, North Korea, People's Republic of China, Taiwan, Singapore, South Korea), compared with the Canadian-born population (largely G3+). The same study showed that South Asian male immigrants who arrived after 1971 also had significantly lower circulatory disease mortality rates, but South Asian female immigrants' mortality rates were similar to those of Canadian born women. The latter was not consistent with the significantly lower hospitalization rates for G1 South Asian women found in this analysis. This indicates potential underutilization of circulatory disease-related health care by female immigrants from South Asia.

Those from the UK provide a good contrast, as they offered an alternative pattern of convergence unlike the more recent immigrants of South Asian and Chinese descent. Overall ASHR and hospitalization ratios were higher than those for South Asians and the Chinese, even among recent immigrants. This overall UK pattern corroborates results from a previous mortality study; age-standardized overall mortality rates were higher for those from Western Europe compared with those from South Asia and from East Asia, even among recent immigrants (Ng and LHAD Research Team, 2011). For circulatory disease, the hospitalization odds for those from immigrants from the UK were similar to their counterparts from South Asia, a world region that has relatively high circulatory disease risk. Age-standardized circulatory disease-specific mortality rates were also similar between the South Asians and those from Western Europe, but higher than those from East Asia (Ng and LHAD Research Team, 2011).

LIMITATIONS

The limitations of the linked census-hospitalization dataset include the absence of information about diet, smoking, exercise and social capital (connectedness and support). A lack of information about non-hospital health care received from family doctors and specialists or about alternative care, which may be more prevalent among some ethnic groups, is also important because low hospitalization rates may reflect efficient use of and access to primary or alternative health care, not better health. As well, the G2 South Asian and Chinese populations are still relatively young, and their group sizes are small. For example, the unadjusted and adjusted odds of circulatory disease-related hospitalization among G2 women of South Asian descent – 0.67 and 0.71 – would seem to be significantly low, but the confidence intervals are wide. Further research is needed to determine if this is a sample size issue or if circulatory disease-related hospitalizations are actually less prevalent in this group. Finally, linkage of the long-form census with hospital records could differ by place of birth. In particular, linkage of 2006 Census results to tax data to obtain changes in postal code information, which relied on names, may yield lower linkage rates for certain subgroups (for example, Chinese). However, this would be an issue only if the link was accomplished via the additional postal code information derived from the tax data. The majority of links for this study were established in the first iteration with an exact match of the postal code on the census record.

CONCLUSION

The results of this analysis of linked census and hospital administrative data suggest that immigrants' health advantages diminish in the second generation, particularly for circulatory disease. For those of South Asian descent, similar to those from the UK, health gains were lost in the second generation, while for those of Chinese descent, the health advantage diminished but remained positive compared with the third-plus generation. These findings have potentially important implications for public health and future needs for health-care services.

NOTE

* This chapter is an adapted version of a previously published article by Ng, E., Sanmartin, C., Tu, J. and Manuel, D., 'All-cause and circulatory disease-related hospitalization, by immigrant generation status: Evidence from linked data', *Health Reports* (2015), Vol. 26, no. 10, pp. 3–9, October 2015. Published by authority of the Minister responsible for Statistics Canada. © Minister of Industry, 2017. All rights reserved. Use of this publication is governed by the Statistics Canada Open Licence Agreement, www.statcan.gc.ca/eng/reference/licence-eng. For this version, the authors added analytical results for the UK group, as part of the contribution to this paper. The authors thank David Mowat and Julie Stratton of the Office of the Medical Officer of Health Region of Peel in Ontario for reviewing an earlier version of the paper. Jack V. Tu is supported by a Tier 1 Canada Research Chair in Health Services Research, and an Eaton Family Scholar award. This does not constitute an endorsement by Statistics Canada of this product.

REFERENCES

Almeida, J., R.M. Johnson and A. Matsumoto and D. Godette (2012), 'Substance use, generation and time in the United States: the modifying role of gender for immigrant urban adolescents', *Social Science & Medicine*, **75** (December), 2069–75.

Ayesha, R., R.J. de Souza and S. Kandasamy et al. (2014), 'Cardiovascular risk among South Asians living in Canada: a systematic review and meta-analysis', *Canadian Medical Association Journal*, **2** (3), E183–E191, doi:10.9778/cmajo.20130064.

Bhatnager, D., I.S. Anand and P.N. Durrington, D.J. Patal, G.S. Wander, M.I. Mackness et al. (1995), 'Coronary risk factors in people from the Indian subcontinent living in West London and their siblings in India', *Lancet*, **345** (8947), 405–9.

Bhopal, R. (2002), 'Epidemic of cardiovascular disease in South Asians', *British Medical Journal*, **324** (7338), 625–6.

Carrière, G., P.A. Peters and C. Sanmartin (2012), 'Area-based methods to calculate hospitalization rates for the foreign born population in Canada, 2005–2006', *Health Reports*, **23** (3), 43–51.

Carriere, K.C. and L.L. Roos (1997), 'A method of comparison for standardized rates of low incidence events', *Medical Care*, **35** (1), 57–69.

Celermajer, D.S., C.K. Chow and E. Marijon, N.M. Anstery and K.S. Woo (2012), 'Cardiovascular disease in the developing world: prevalences, patterns and the potential of early disease detection', *Journal of the American College of Cardiology*, **60** (14), 1207–16.

Chiu, M., P.C. Austin and D.G. Manuel and J.V. Tu (2010), 'Comparison of cardiovascular risk profiles among ethnic groups using population health surveys between 1996 and 2007', *Canadian Medical Association Journal*, **182** (8), E301–E310.

Chiu, M., P.C. Austin and D.G. Manuel and J.V. Tu (2012), 'Cardiovascular risk factor profiles of recent immigrants vs. long-term residents of Ontario: a multi-ethnic study', *Canadian Journal of Cardiology*, **28** (1), 20–26.

Chui T., H. Maheux and K. Tran (2007), *Immigration in Canada: A Portrait of the Foreign-born Population, 2006 Census*, Catalogue 97-557-XIE, Ottawa: Statistics Canada.

Dixon, L.B., J. Sundquist and M. Winkleby (2000), 'Differences in energy, nutrient and food intakes in a US sample of Mexican-American women and men: findings from the third national health and nutrition examination survey, 1988–1994', *American Journal of Epidemiology*, **152** (6), 548–57.

Gagnon, A.J. (2002), 'Responsiveness of the Canadian health care system towards newcomers', Commission on the Future of Health Care in Canada Discussion Paper No. 40, Catalogue CP32-79/40-2002E-IN, Royal Commission on Health Care in Canada, Ottawa.

Goyal, A.S. and Yusuf (2006), 'The burden of cardiovascular disease in the Indian subcontinent', *Indian Journal of Medical Research*, **124** (3), 235–44.

Gray, L., S. Harding and A. Reid (2007), 'Evidence of divergence with duration of residence in circulatory disease mortality in migrants to Australia', *European Journal of Public Health*, **17** (6), 550–54.

Gupta, M., A.V. Doobay and N. Singh, S.S. Anand, F. Raja, F. Mawji et al. (2002), 'Risk factors, hospital management and outcomes after acute myocardial infarction in South Asian Canadians and matched control subjects', *Canadian Medical Association Journal*, **166** (6), 717–22.

Gushulak, B.D. and L.S. Williams (2004), 'National immigrant health policy: existing policy, changing needs, and future directions', *Canadian Journal of Public Health*, **95** (3), I27–I29.

Hamilton, H.A., S. Noh and E.M. Adlaf (2009), 'Adolescent risk behaviours and psychological distress across immigrant generations', *Canadian Journal of Public Health*, **100** (3), 221–5.

Harding, S., M. Rosato and A. Teyhan (2008), 'Trends for coronary heart disease and stroke mortality among migrants in England and Wales 1979–2003: slow declines notable for some groups', *Heart*, **94** (4), 463–70.

Hosper, K., V. Nierkens and M. Nicolaou et al. (2007), 'Behavioural risk factors in two generations of non-Western migrants: do trends converge towards the host population?', *European Journal of Epidemiology*, **22** (3), 163–72.

Hyman, I. (2007), 'Immigration and health: reviewing evidence of the healthy immigrant effect in Canada', Joint Centre of Excellence for Research on Immigration and Settlement (CERIS) Working Paper No. 55, CERIS, Toronto.

Hyman, I. (2001), 'Immigration and health'. Health Policy Working Paper Series Working Paper No. 01-05, Health Canada, Ottawa.

Kuppuswamy, V.C. and S. Gupta (2005), 'Excess coronary heart disease in South Asians in the United Kingdom', *British Medical Journal*, **330** (11 June), 1223–4.

Lau, D. (2010), 'Excess prevalence and mortality rates of diabetes and cardiovascular disease among South Asians: a call to action', *Canadian Journal of Diabetes*, **34** (2), 102–4.

Leão, T.S., L.M. Johansson and K. Sundquist (2006), 'Hospitalization due to alcohol and drug abuse in first- and second-generation immigrants: a follow-up study in Sweden', *Substance Use and Misuse*, **41** (3), 283–96.
Marmot, M.G. and S.L. Syme (1976), 'Acculturation and coronary heart disease in Japanese-Americans', *American Journal of Epidemiology*, **104** (3), 225–47.
Maximova, K., J. O'Loughlin and K. Gray-Donald (2011), 'Healthy weight advantage lost in one generation among immigrant elementary schoolchildren in multi-ethnic, disadvantaged, inner-city neighborhoods in Montreal, Canada', *Annals of Epidemiology*, **21** (4), 238–44.
McKeigue, P.M., J.E. Ferrie and T. Pierpoint and M.G. Marmot (1993), 'Association of early-onset coronary heart disease in South Asian men with glucose intolerance and hyperinsulinemia', *Circulation*, **87** (1), 152–61.
Morales, L.S., M. Leng and J.J. Escarce (2011), 'Risk of cardiovascular disease in first and second generation Mexican-Americans', *Journal of Immigrant and Minority*, **13** (1), 61–8.
Muennig, P., H. Jia and K. Khan (2004), 'Hospitalization for heart disease, stroke and diabetes mellitus among Indian-born persons: a small area analysis', *BMC Cardiovascular Disorders*, **4**, 19, doi:10.1186/1471-2261-4-19.
Newbold, K.B. (2005), 'Health status and health care utilization of the foreign-born in Canada: a longitudinal analysis, 1994/1995–2000/01', *Journal of Health Services Research and Policy*, **10** (2), 77–83A.
Ng, E. and LHAD Research Team (2011), 'Insights into the healthy immigrant effect: mortality by period of immigration and birthplace', Health Analysis Division Working Paper No. 8, Catalogue 82-622, Statistics Canada, Ottawa.
Ng, E., R. Wilkins, R. Gendron and J.-M. Berthelot (2005), 'Dynamics of immigrants' health in Canada: evidence from the National Population Health Survey', *Healthy Today, Healthy Tomorrow? Findings from the National Population Health Survey*, Ottawa: Statistics Canada.
Prasad, D.S., Z. Kabir, A.K. Dash and B.C. Das (2011), 'Childhood cardiovascular risk factors in South Asians: a cause of concern for adult cardiovascular disease epidemic', *Annals of Pediatric Cardiology*, **4** (2), 166–71, doi:10.4103/0974-2069.84663.
Quon, E.C., J.J. McGrath and M.-H. Roy-Gagnon (2012), 'Generation of immigration and body mass index in Canadian youth', *Journal of Pediatric Psychology*, **37** (8), 843–53.
Rotermann, M. (2011), 'The impact of considering birthplace in analyses of immigrant health', *Health Reports*, **22** (4), 37–43.
Rotermann, M., C. Sanmartin and G. Carrière, R. Trudeau, H. St-Jean, A.Saïdi et al. (2014), 'Comparing two approaches to link Census and hospital data in Canada', *Health Reports*, **25** (10), 3–14.
SAS Institute Inc. (2009), *SAS 9.2 User's Guide*, Cary, NC: SAS Institute Inc.
Shaukat, N. and D.P. DeBono (1994), 'A comparison of risk factors in south Asian and north European coronary artery patients with their young male offspring', *British Heart Journal*, **71** (5 supplement), 27.
Sheth, T., C. Nair, N. Nargundkar, S.Anand and S. Yusuf (1999), 'Cardiovascular and cancer mortality among Canadians of European, South Asian and Chinese origin from 1979 to 1993: an analysis of 1.2 million deaths', *Canadian Medical Association Journal*, **161** (2), 132–8.
Singh, G.K. and M. Siapush (2001), 'All-cause and cause-specific mortality of immigrants and native born in the United States', *American Journal of Public Health*, **91** (3), 392–9.

Statistics Canada (2010a), *Projections of the Diversity of the Canadian Population*, Catalogue 91-551-X, Ottawa: Statistics Canada.
Statistics Canada (2010b), *2006 Census Dictionary*, Catalogue 92-566-X, Ottawa: Minister of Industry.
Statistics Canada (2011), *Directive on Record Linkage,* Ottawa: Statistics Canada, accessed 30 September 2014at http://www.statcan.gc.ca/record-enregistrement/policy4-1-politique4-1-eng.htm.
Statistics Canada (2012), *Approved Record Linkages*, Linkage of the Census of Population 2006 to the Discharge Abstract Database and the Canadian Mortality Database for Purposes of the Longitudinal Health and Administrative Data Initiative, Ottawa: Statistics Canada, accessed 30 September 2014 at http://www.statcan.gc.ca/record-enregistrement/2012-eng.htm#a15.
Statistics Canada (2013), *Immigration and Ethno-cultural Diversity in Canada, National Household Survey, 2011*, Catalogue 99-010-X2011001, Ottawa: Statistics Canada.
Sundquist, J. and M. Winkleby (2000), 'Country of birth, acculturation status and abdominal obesity in a national sample of Mexican American women and men', *International Journal of Epidemiology*, **29** (3), 470–77.
Yusuf, S., S. Reddy, S. Ounpuu and S. Anand (2001), 'Global burden of cardiovascular diseases: part II: variations in cardiovascular disease by specific ethnic groups and geographic regions and prevention strategies', *Circulation*, **104** (23), 2855–64.
Zunzunnegui, M.V., M. Forster and L. Gauvin, M.F. Raynault and D.J. Willms (2006), 'Community unemployment and immigrants' health in Montreal', *Social Science and Medicine*, **63** (2), 485–500.

4. Migrant health in Australia: existing literature and new results

Nicholas Biddle and Samuel G. Weldeegzie

INTRODUCTION

This chapter reviews the existing literature on migrant health from historical and methodological perspective and expands the current analysis using the four most recent waves (2011–13) of data from the Household, Income and Labour Dynamics in Australia (HILDA) to re-examine the association between migration and self-assessed health and whether self-assessed health of migrants deteriorates the longer they stay in Australia. Using an ordered probit model, results from both cross-sectional and panel data random effects suggest that migrants from English-speaking countries have higher self-assessed health than native-born Australians while migrants from 'other' countries tend to have no difference or worse health relative to the Australian born. Furthermore, migrants' health deteriorates the longer they stay in Australia controlling for a range of covariates such as age, gender, education, employment, and income. This is consistent with previous findings from the literature not only in Australia but also in Canada and the USA.

Human migration is a ubiquitous phenomenon. From an economic point of view, as long as people anticipate better outcomes in destination countries, there will be strong incentives for them to relocate. However, migrants have to incur certain costs to be able to migrate. There are economic costs to go along with the benefits, but there may also be health costs or benefits that need to be weighed up.

Migration also affects individuals in the source and destination country. These effects, however, can be a mix of positive and negative, depending on the specific characteristics of the migrant, and the economic or social circumstances of the countries that they are migrating from and to (Collier, 2013). Although not exclusively so, net migration across countries (or the balance of in migration and out migration) tends to be from relatively poor to relatively rich countries.

One area of research on the outcomes of migration has been the changing health profile of migrants. Two key findings have emerged from this literature – the healthy migrant effect (where migrants arrive in a country with better health outcomes than the native-born population), and health assimilation (where health outcomes converge through time). In this chapter we present further support for these two explanations in the context of Australia.

Analysing the health gap between immigrants and native-born host populations is important for several reasons. First, migrants are a significant portion of the Australian population with migrants making up a very large share of the growth of the labour market in Australia over a number of years. According to Australian Bureau of Statistics (30 June 2014), 28.1 per cent (6.6 million people) of the estimated resident population was born overseas compared to 23.8 per cent (4.8 million people) ten years earlier. Second, there is a general need to understand sources of variation in health for direct policy interventions. Third, variation in health outcomes within the migrant population can tell us something about the effectiveness of migrant selection programmes. Finally, variation in health outcomes can provide indirect information about migrant decision-making, including health behaviour, health service usage, and changes in diet.

There are, however, significant methodological complexities in understanding migrant health. Cognizant of these limitations, in this chapter we update the existing literature, and provide new empirical evidence for Australia. The rest of the chapter is organized as follows. The next section provides a brief overview of the history of migration to Australia. The section that follows reviews the related literature, including a discussion of some of the methodological challenges. This is followed by a summary of the data from Australia, a discussion of the data used in our chapter, with the penultimate section presenting and discussing the results from our analysis. The final section concludes.

A BRIEF HISTORY OF MIGRATION TO AUSTRALIA

For the most part, Australia has been populated by a process of international migration. This potentially dates back to between 68 000 to 75 000 years ago, with genetic evidence suggesting that 'present-day Aboriginal Australians descend from the earliest humans to occupy Australia, likely representing one of the oldest continuous populations outside Africa' (Rasmussen et al., 2011, p. 1). Australia's more recent migrant history, however, begins with the colonization of the land mass by the British in 1788, with the Aboriginal and Torres Strait Islander population (estimated to be between 750 000 and 1 000 000 at the time) decimated by disease, frontier violence and loss of livelihood, replaced first by an Anglo-Celtic, then broader European and more recently a genuinely multicultural and multi-ethnic set of migrant waves (Biddle et al., 2015).

According to the most recent (2011) Census, 26.1 per cent of the Australian population was born overseas. Furthermore, only 58.1 per cent of the population were born in Australia themselves and had both parents born in Australia. Migrants to Australia originate from a diverse range of source countries. While the two major source countries remain England (17.3 per cent of the overseas-born population) and Australia's Pacific neighbour, New Zealand (9.2 per cent), a large and increasing share of Australia's population was born outside these English-speaking countries. This includes China (6.0 per cent of the overseas-born population), India (5.6 per cent and one of the fastest growing), Italy (3.5 per cent), and Viet Nam (3.5 per cent). This migrant profile has produced an ethnically diverse and multicultural society.

Biddle et al. (2015) outline five distinct periods of migration to Australia since colonization. A first phase up until the middle of the nineteenth century, where most migration was of convicts or Anglo-Celtic settlers, a period of relative openness with the discovery of gold in Victoria and later other colonies from the mid-nineteenth century to a major recession in the 1890s, a relatively closed population from then until just after the Second World War, a period of increased openness to other European countries from the post-war years till the 1970s, and then a rapid increase in migration from Asia.

Not only has the country of origin (and therefore ethnicity) of Australia's migration profile changed through time, but so too has the skills mix. In particular, over recent years, Australia has placed a strong premium on skills (Cully, 2011), replacing country of origin, family, and humanitarian factors as key criteria for admission.

MIGRATION AND HEALTH: MODELS AND FINDINGS

Most of the empirical research has found strong evidence that supports the 'healthy migrant effect' hypothesis where migrants tend to be relatively more healthy than residents in the host countries. Kennedy et al. (2006) discuss three main substantive reasons underlying the applicability of this hypothesis based on the existing literature: health screening of migrants by destination country prior to migration; favourable habits and behaviours of individuals in the home country prior to migration; and immigrant self-selection on personal characteristics including not only good health but also occupational skills and education. For instance, Kennedy et al. (2006) found strong evidence for positive selection of migrants on education. However, these three reasons could differ based on different visa classifications of migrants. For instance, humanitarian migrants (refugees) tend to be initially less healthy, wealthy, and educated compared with economic migrants (Beiser, 2005), implying the possibility of both negative and positive self-selection of migrants in the cases of refugees and economic migrants, respectively. In addition, there could be differences in health behaviours of these two distinct groups of migrants, both before and after migration (that is, at origin and destination countries), that could lead to different health outcomes of migrants once in the host country. Indeed, Kandula et al. (2004) argue that 'the ability of immigrants to access health-care services varies widely, depending on their immigration status, their country of origin, and their ability to navigate linguistic and cultural barriers'. Furthermore, the health screening policy for economic migrants could be significantly different for refugees or family tied migrants based on the purpose of migration (Correa-Velez et al., 2005).

Even more, there is mixed evidence as to the selection of migrants from the distribution of home population, for instance, in regards to earnings and education. For example, in an early study, Borjas (1987) found evidence of negative selection among Mexican migrants to the USA, which is contradictory to the evidence uncovered by Chiquiar and Hanson (2002) that migrants can have intermediate selection in terms of education.Kaestner and Malamud (2014) provide further evidence that Mexican migrants in the US are indeed selected from the middle of the education distribution while male migrants are selected negatively on earnings.

Concerning health status, evidence from Australia, Canada, and the USA shows that the longer the duration of stay in host countries, the higher the deterioration of migrants' health, eventually converging to health levels of the native born (for example, Frisbie et al., 2001; McDonald and Kennedy, 2004; Newbold, 2005; Biddle et al., 2007; Chiswick et al., 2008; De Maio and Kemp, 2010). Newbold (2005) analysed longitudinal data from Canada and found that while health-care utilization increases, migrant health declines converging to natives (Newbold, 2005). Contrary to this literature, evidence from Sweden suggests that immigrants with a shorter period of stay at the destination country are more likely to suffer from poor self-rated health (Leão, et al., 2009).

Chiswick et al. (2008) found significant health differences among refugees and economic migrants, and also noted a general decline of migrant health over time. However, these authors did not examine the gap between health of immigrants and native born at times when migrants arrive. Nor did they look at changes of this gap over time. Studying this gap in health between natives and different visa type migrants over time can uncover important implications concerning immigrant health and its change with increasing duration of time in the host country. For instance, we could hypothesize that if the health of economic migrants compared with natives seems better or not worse initially but then deteriorates over time, then this could imply a variety of possible processes, including shift in post-migration behaviour of migrants, the extent of assimilation to the host culture, or possibly how the health system may inadvertently by its very structure pose barriers for immigrants in terms of access to health care.

Separating out these different possible effects requires careful theoretical and empirical approaches. An important theoretical framework in the literature is a modified version of frameworks provided by Chiswick in combination with Jasso and co-authors (Chiswick, 1999; Jasso et al., 2004) in which the decision to migrate is based on the evaluation of gains over costs of migration. Using this framework, we can look at the selectivity of international migrants and the impact of migration on subsequent health trajectory of migrants.

Following Chiswick (1999), let the rate of return from migration r be:

$$r = \frac{w_b - w_a}{C_f + C_d} \tag{4.1}$$

where w_b and w_a are earnings at destination and origin country respectively. C_f is forgone earnings while C_d refers to direct cost of migration. Then, suppose earnings for a relatively healthier person ($w_{b,h}$ and $w_{a,h}$) are higher than earnings for a less healthy person ($w_{b,l}$ and $w_{b,l}$) in both destination and origin countries respectively by k fraction. This is analogous to including 'ability' as in the Chiswick (1999) in conjunction with Jasso et al. (2004):

$$w_{b,h} = (1+k)\, w_{b,l} \tag{4.2}$$

$$w_{a,h} = (1+k)\, w_{a,l} \tag{4.3}$$

At this stage, assume direct costs do not vary with health and that better health has no effect on efficiency of migration but does raise the value of forgone earnings, as healthier migrants would be assumed to earn more. Thus,

$$C_d = C_{d,h} = C_{dl} \tag{4.4}$$

$$C_{f,h} - (1+k)\, C_{f,l} \tag{4.5}$$

Then, after substituting equation (4.2) and (4.3) in (4.1), the rate of return to a healthier person (r_h) can be written as:

$$r_h = \frac{(1+k)w_{b,l} - (1+k)w_{a,l}}{(1+k)\,C_{f,l} + C_d} \tag{4.6}$$

Similarly, the rate of return for a less healthy person (r_l) is given by:

$$r_h = \frac{w_{b,l} - w_{a,l}}{C_{f,l} + C_{d,l}} \tag{4.7}$$

Remembering that, $C_d = C_{d,h} = C_{dl}$ holds.

After dividing both the numerator and denominator by (1+k), equation (4.6) could be re-written as:

$$r_h = \frac{w_{b,l} - w_{a,l}}{C_{f,l} + \dfrac{C_d}{1+k}} \tag{4.8}$$

From this, we can see that the rate of return to a healthier person is greater than the rate of return to a less healthy person as long as earnings increase with health ($k > 0$) and there are positive out-of-pocket costs of migration ($Cd > 0$).

As argued by Jasso et al. (2004) health can enter this model, as health increases earning capacity thereby reflecting healthier people are more productive or have higher inherent ability. Furthermore, healthier people can better find work and, if found, can work longer and thus earn more (Grossman, 1972; Cai and Kalb, 2006; Halla and Zweimüller, 2013). Thus, because health increases both productivity and labour supply, healthier individuals will gain more from migration and hence migrants will be positively selected. In addition, the higher the cost of migration, the more migrants will self-select on better health as higher-level health is required to achieve a threshold of income that should sufficiently cover (support) migration cost.

Apart from labour market effects, health could also be attracted through pull factors such as a better health care system in the destination country. According to Jasso et al. (2004), this could enter into the increasing utility of migration, implying a reduction in the direct cost of migration, inducing a negative self-selection of migrant health. That is, letting $C_{d,h} = u + C_{dl}$, the return to a healthier migrant (r_h) would then be lower than the return to less healthy migrants (r_l) suggesting negative self-selection of migrants on health:

$$r_h = \frac{w_{b,l} - w_{a,l}}{C_{f,l} + \dfrac{u + C_d}{1+k}} \tag{4.9}$$

MIGRATION AND HEALTH: AUSTRALIAN FINDINGS

Australian researchers have made a strong contribution to our understanding of the interaction between migration decision-making and health outcomes. Furthermore, its rather distinct migration history (summarized above) means that Australia represents an interesting counterfactual in cross-country comparisons. Australia is a relatively wealthy country, with migrants from a changing distribution of source countries, and increasingly selective migration policies. Australia also has a relatively generous public health system, with highly targeted social security arrangements.

Biddle et al. (2007) is the first major study of the healthy migrant effect and health assimilation based on self-reported health status nationally representative surveys. The authors used synthetic cohorts across three national health surveys conducted by the Australian Bureau of Statistics (ABS) in 1989/90, 1995 and 2001. They found that 'the health of Australian immigrants is better than the Australian-born population, but the longer immigrants spend in Australia, the closer their health approximates that of the Australian-born population' (Biddle et al., 2007, p. 16). The authors also found that 'there are variations for different immigrant groups and for particular chronic diseases' (Biddle, 2007, p. 16).

Anikeeva and colleagues (2010) undertook a review of the public health (generally, non-social science) literature on studies conducted in Australia between 1980 and 2008 that focused on the health status of migrants in one or more of Australia's National Health Priority Areas (NHPAs). They found that 'that the majority of migrants enjoy better health than the Australian-born population in the conditions that are part of the NHPAs, with the exception of diabetes' (Anikeeva et al., 2010, p. 159).

Kennedy et al. (2015) undertook a cross-country comparison of migrants from and to Australia, Canada, the USA and the UK. The authors found a healthy immigrant effect (HIE) across all immigrant groups in each of the destination countries in terms of both physical health and healthy behaviours. There is also evidence that the HIE is stronger for immigrants from developing countries than for those from developed countries. Across the destination countries examined, the gap between all foreign born and the native born in terms of the presence of a chronic disease was highest in the USA and lowest in the UK, with Australia and Canada being in between. In terms of self-assessed health, the difference was highest in the USA and the UK, with no difference in Canada. Australia had a small, but statistically significant difference (with migrants having better health outcomes).

There has been less attention in the recent literature on differences in mortality rates between migrant groups in Australia, as well as between migrants and the native born. In general, the research in this area tends to suggest that age-adjusted mortality rates are lower for the foreign born. Anikeeva et al. (2012) looked at cancer mortality and found that migrants generally had more favourable cancer mortality outcomes, particularly for colorectal cancer and melanoma. Migrants from Southern Europe, South Eastern Europe, Chinese Asia and Southern Asia had the greatest advantage. Anikeeva et al. (2012) also looked at a broader range of diseases and found that migrants generally displayed more favourable mortality outcomes than their Australian-born counterparts. Migrants from Southern Europe appeared to have the greatest advantage. However, some migrants appeared to be over-represented in the areas of diabetes, suicide and mental health.

DATA AND METHODOLOGY

There have been two main limitations on the empirical analysis of migrant health in Australia. One of the limitations of the work on migrant mortality in Australia is the lack of individual level data that contains relevant control variables. As outlined in the previous section, there is considerable selectivity when it comes to migration, and in particular in the case of mortality studies, the vital-statistics data does not contain any information on the migrants' socioeconomic status or health status prior to migration. The release of the 'Death Registrations to Census Linkage'[1] by the Australian Bureau of Statistics in 2016 provides an opportunity to rectify some of these limitations, although unfortunately at the time of writing this chapter, unit-record data was not available to external researchers.

Another limitation is the lack of longitudinal data that has information on a large number of migrants and the native born population. There have been a number of immigrant-specific surveys, including the Longitudinal Survey of Immigrants to Australia (LSIA)[2] and the more recent 'Building a New Life in Australia: The Longitudinal Study of Humanitarian Migrants'.[3] Both studies provide a very rich resource, but do not include a native-born comparison group and/or focus on a non-representative subset of the foreign-born population (humanitarian migrants, as opposed to those who migrant under skilled visa categories).

The major general longitudinal surveys in Australia have tended to have reasonably small migrant cohorts. This includes the major youth cohort studies (though these are useful for studying the outcomes of children of migrants) as well as the major panel studies. Fortunately, this has changed.

The sample size has been increased in the HILDA survey, thus allowing for reasonable analyses of immigrant health.

The HILDA survey is a household-based panel study, which began in 2001.[4] It collects information about economic and subjective well-being, labour market dynamics and family dynamics; and interviews are conducted annually with all adult members of each household selected. The wave 1 panel consisted of 7682 households and 19914 individuals. In wave 11, this was topped up with an additional 2153 households and 5477 individual respondents. This top-up significantly boosted the number of migrants in the study.

For our analysis, we use data from waves 11 to 14 of the survey, focusing on those adults who were observed in all four waves. Per wave, this gives us a sample of 11276 Australian residents born in Australia, 1447 born in the main English-speaking countries, referred to as Anglo-migrants, and 1634 born in another country who we define as other-migrants. It should be noted, however, that there is no information in HILDA on ethnicity or race, so this should only be taken to refer to the predominant language of the country in which the migrant is born.

The dataset is skewed towards those who moved to Australia a significant time ago. The median years since migration for Anglo-migrants is 33 years, whereas for Other-migrants it is 22 years. However, there is a not insignificant sample of recent migrants, with 188 Anglo-migrants in the sample who had arrived in Australia within the past ten years in wave 11, and a further 359 other-migrants.

This relatively large dataset (by Australian standards) allows us to compare the health outcomes of a significant number of migrants from a range of countries with those of the native born population. The longitudinal nature of the survey also allows us to look at the change in health status through time while controlling for baseline health (though not health pre-migration) and while excluding those who returned to their country of origin. This later pattern of those with poor health being more likely to return to their country of origin has the tendency to bias upwards the health profile of migrants. We cannot control completely for this in our analysis (that would require data on emigrants), but we can control for it to a certain extent in our change through time analysis.

In our analysis we use a standard measure of self-assessed health. Specifically, respondents to the HILDA are asked through a self-completed questionnaire 'In general, would you say your health is . . .?' with the options of excellent, very good, good, fair and poor. We also look at two self-reported measures of change through time. One is retrospective, with respondents asked 'Compared to one year ago, how would you rate your health in general now?' with the following options available:

1. Much better now than a year ago.
2. Somewhat better now than a year ago.
3. About the same as one year ago.
4. Somewhat worse now than one year ago.
5. Much worse now than one year ago.

The final question is about a person's view of their health into the future. Respondents are asked 'How TRUE or FALSE is each of the following statements for you?', with the third statement being 'I expect my health to get worse'. Options available are:

1. Definitely true.
2. Mostly true.
3. Don't know.
4. Mostly false.
5. Definitely false.

The variables are coded such that higher values represent better or improving health outcomes. As the three variables are categorical, we estimate the relationship between them and the main variables of interest using the ordered probit model as described briefly in Greene (2008) and in more detail in Greene and Hensher (2010). This model assumes that there is a latent (unobserved) variable that is distributed via the normal distribution. In this chapter, the latent variables would be a measure of self-assessed health or change in health. What we observe is whether an individual's value for this latent variable falls above or below a given set of thresholds. These thresholds (or cut-points) correspond to the observed categories in the data (as described above). Coefficients from the ordered probit model then correspond to the relationship between the explanatory variable (or variables) and the underlying latent variable.

We model the relationship between migration and health controlling for a parsimonious set of observable characteristics. These are:

1. Age and age squared.
2. Sex.
3. Highest level of education attainment (post-graduate degree, bachelor degree or diploma, certificate, high school, no high school).
4. Employment status (full-time, part-time, not employed).
5. Household income (high – \$100k or more per year, medium – \$60k to less than \$100k, low – less than \$40k) with negative incomes excluded.

A separate set of models is run for the migrant population only. This model has the same variables as above, with the addition of control variables for the number of years since the person first migrated to Australia. This is included in the model as a linear and a quadratic term, to take into account the fact that the health profile of migrants is likely to change at different rates for those who have been in the country for a while, compared to those who have migrated only recently.

We use a few different specifications to take into account the longitudinal nature of the data. First, we run the model on wave 11 data only. This is a simple cross-sectional model with the three health variables as outcomes, and the explanatory variables as outlined above. The second specification uses all four waves of data, and uses a random effects, ordered probit model. This model controls for the correlation through time in the outcome variables. The final model estimated further exploits the longitudinal nature of the data by looking at changing health through time. Focusing on self-assessed health, our model uses as its dependent variable the change in categories through time (modelled once again through the ordered probit model).

In the previous section, we outlined a theoretical model that suggested that there may be either positive or negative heath selection, depending on the characteristics of migrants to Australia. While we do not explicitly test different parameters of that theoretical model, the methodology outlined in this section and discussed in the next session is designed to demonstrate which of the two effects appear to be dominating.

ANALYSIS OF FINDINGS

The results of the first specification that only uses the first wave (wave 11 of HILDA in year 2011) are presented in Tables 4.1 and 4.2. The first table shows data for the entire sample. Results from this indicate that migrants from main English-speaking countries are better off in their self-reported current health compared to natives. Similarly, these groups of migrants are likely to expect to have better future health and are likely to believe that their health has improved compared to the past in relation to the native born Australians. However, relative to native born, migrants from other countries tend to report that their current health is worse than a year ago although they think their health will improve in the future compared to natives.

Looking at the migrants only in the second table, there is strong evidence for the proposition that migrants' health tends to decline the longer they stay in Australia, and this is true across all three measures of self-reported health. The relevant coefficients are all statistically significant.

Table 4.1 *Migration status and self-assessed health: cross-sectional ordered probit model*

Variables	(1) Current health	(2) Expected health	(3) Compared to past health
Age	–0.0450***	–0.0389***	–0.0209***
Age^2	0.000330***	0.000245***	9.08e–05***
Female (ref = male)	–0.00358	0.205***	0.0272
Highest education (ref = postgraduate)			
Advanced diploma and above	–0.167***	0.0382	–0.0531
Certificate	–0.413***	0.0754	–0.0865*
Year 12	–0.256***	0.101**	–0.0889*
Year 11 and below	–0.464***	0.0252	–0.146***
Undetermined	0.157	–0.389	0.402
Employment (ref = full time)			
Part-time	0.0386	–0.00974	–0.0269
Other	–0.270***	–0.224***	–0.141***
Income (ref = < 40k)			
40k–99k	0.242***	0.0618**	0.0444
> 100k	0.451***	0.120***	0.0607**
Country of birth (ref = born in Australia)			
Mainly English-speaking country	0.116***	0.0559*	0.0571*
Other	–0.0412	0.116***	–0.0782**
Constant cut1	–3.468***	–2.941***	–3.079***
Constant cut2	–2.449***	–2.015***	–1.910***
Constant cut3	–1.300***	–0.976***	0.147*
Constant cut4	–0.0727	–0.369***	0.858***
Observations	14357	14212	14312
Sample	All	All	All

Notes:
*** $p < 0.01$, ** $p < 0.05$, * $p < 0.1$ holds for all subsequent tables unless otherwise mentioned.
In this and subsequent tables 'ref' means the reference category of given variable.

We now turn to the results of the second specification in Tables 4.3 and 4.4 that used all the four waves and takes into account the correlation of health outcomes through time using the random effects model. Results are similar to the first set of findings above suggesting that migrants from English-speaking countries tend to have better health in all the three indicators as compared to native born respondents. Similarly, compared to the Australian born, migrants from other countries are more likely to have lower self-assessed health and they are likely to report that this

Table 4.2 Years since migration and self-assessed health: cross-sectional ordered probit model

Variables	(1) Current health	(2) Expected health	(3) Compared to past health
Age	–0.0354***	–0.0322***	–0.0186**
Age^2	0.000230***	0.000198***	4.78e–05
Female (ref = male)	0.0167	0.227***	–0.0178
Highest education (ref = postgraduate)			
Advanced diploma and above	–0.156**	0.0827	–0.0713
Certificate	–0.285***	0.125	–0.0614
Year 12	–0.181**	0.0738	–0.0849
Year 11 and below	–0.400***	–0.00209	–0.112
Undetermined	5.047	–1.022	–0.491
Employment (ref = full time)			
Part time	–0.000935	0.0193	0.0552
Other	–0.335***	–0.209***	–0.121**
Income (ref = < 40k)			
40k–99k	0.284***	0.0627	0.00820
> 100k	0.426***	0.109*	0.0672
Country of birth (ref = born in Australia)			
Other	–0.193***	0.0344	–0.160***
Years since immigration	–0.0242***	–0.0132***	–0.0144***
(Years since immigration)^2	0.000336***	0.000145**	0.000189***
Constant cut1	–3.683***	–2.972***	–3.380***
Constant cut2	–2.682***	–2.044***	–2.137***
Constant cut3	–1.506***	–1.019***	–0.173
Constant cut4	–0.261	–0.448**	0.511**
Observations	3079	3044	3071
Sample	Migrants only	Migrants only	Migrants only

self-assessed health has not shown an improvement compared to a year ago. However these migrants seem to remain optimistic that their health will be improving in the future as compared to native Australians.

The earlier cross-sectional evidence that suggests migrants' health deteriorates over time the longer they have lived in the destination country (Australia) is also confirmed using the random effects model (Table 4.4). Finally, we model the change in current self-reported health that controls for the same set of covariates as in the previous regressions. The results show that the short term (year by year) difference in health changes is not statistically different for migrants and non-migrants. However, these

Table 4.3 Migration status and self-assessed health: panel random effects ordered probit model

Variables	(1) Current health	(2) Expected health	(3) Compared to past health
Age	–0.0694***	–0.0516***	–0.0208***
Age^2	0.000409***	0.000238***	5.15e–05**
Female (ref = male)	–0.0106	0.318***	0.0291**
Highest education (ref = postgraduate)			
Advanced diploma and above	–0.255***	0.0447	0.0110
Certificate	–0.786***	0.0460	–0.0223
Year 12	–0.588***	0.0639	–0.0573*
Year 11 and below	–0.806***	–0.0423	–0.0727**
Undetermined	–1.058*	–0.432	–0.121
Employment (ref = full time)			
Part time	–0.0553**	–0.0173	–0.0205
Other	–0.320***	–0.145***	–0.108***
Income (ref = < 40k)			
40k–99k	0.204***	0.0842***	0.0372**
> 100k	0.391***	0.142***	0.0269
Country of birth (ref = born in Australia)			
Mainly English-speaking country	0.214***	0.128***	0.0677***
Other	–0.0915**	0.231***	–0.0580***
Constant cut1	–6.488***	–4.784***	–3.478***
Constant cut2	–4.548***	–3.215***	–2.092***
Constant cut3	–2.421***	–1.479***	0.211***
Constant cut4	–0.177*	–0.409***	1.060***
Constant sigma	2.543***	1.871***	0.328***
Observations	57 709	57 143	57 586
Number of id	18 311	18 261	18 299
Sample	All	All	All

changes in self-assessed health suggest improvements the longer the migrants have lived in Australia.

CONCLUDING COMMENTS

According to the most recent (2011) Census, 26.1 per cent of the Australian population was born overseas. Furthermore, only 58.1 per cent of the population born in Australia had both parents born in Australia. In

Table 4.4 Years since migration and self-assessed health: panel random effects ordered probit model

Variables	(1) Current health	(2) Expected health	(3) Compared to past health
Age	–0.0624***	–0.0424***	–0.0222***
Age^2	0.000304***	0.000183**	3.37e–05
Female (ref = male)	–0.0229	0.336***	–0.0258
Highest education (ref = postgraduate)			
Adv. diploma and above	–0.302***	0.138	0.0182
Certificate	–0.733***	0.215**	0.0287
Year 12	–0.607***	0.120	–0.0543
Year 11 and below	–0.831***	0.0103	–0.0709
Undetermined	–0.781	–0.664	–0.155
Employment (ref = full time)			
Part time	–0.0516	0.0216	0.0173
Other	–0.366***	–0.135***	–0.0935**
Income (ref = < 40k)			
40k–99k	0.219***	0.0650	0.0517
> 100k	0.309***	0.123**	0.0503
Country of birth (ref = born in Australia)			
Mainly English speaking country	0.368***	–0.0727	0.135***
Years since immigration	–0.0345***	–0.0157***	–0.00516
(Years since immigration)^2	0.000482***	0.000129	8.55e–05*
Constant cut1	–6.827***	–4.870***	–3.584***
Constant cut2	–4.930***	–3.303***	–2.160***
Constant cut3	–2.732***	–1.598***	0.0978
Constant cut4	–0.484*	–0.558***	0.900***
Constant sigma	2.626***	1.779***	0.365***
Observations	12156	12015	12125
Number of id	3823	3812	3819
Sample	Migrants only	Migrants only	Migrants only

addition, migrants are a significant proportion of the Australian population taking up a large share of the growth of the labour force in Australia. Thus, analysing the health gap between immigrants and natives remains an ongoing crucial question to examine.

The main findings of this study indicate that migrants from English-speaking countries have higher self-assessed health than native born, while migrants from other countries tend to have no difference or worse health relative to natives. In addition, migrants from English-speaking and other countries are more likely to expect their health to get better in the future, or not

Table 4.5 Migration and change in self-assessed health: random effects ordered probit model

Variables	(1) Change in health	(2) Change in health
Age	0.00465***	0.00155
Age squared	–4.22e–05**	–2.37e–05
Female (ref = male)	0.0263**	0.00879
Highest education (ref = postgraduate)		
Advanced diploma and above	0.0123	–0.0459
Certificate	–0.00340	–0.0814
Year 12	0.0166	–0.0443
Year 11 and below	0.00755	–0.0556
Undetermined	–0.493*	–0.452
Employment (ref = full time)		
Part time	–0.00294	–0.0139
Other	–0.0104	–0.0261
Income (ref = < 40k)		
40k–99k	–0.0235	–0.0379
> 100k	–0.0261	–0.0580
Country of birth (ref = born in Australia)		
Mainly English-speaking country)	–0.0195	
Other	–0.0291	–0.00210
Years since immigration		0.00788***
(Years since immigration)^2		–9.03e–05**
Constant cut1	–3.503***	–3.627***
Constant cut2	–2.804***	–2.823***
Constant cut3	–1.971***	–2.016***
Constant cut4	–0.698***	–0.746***
Constant cut5	0.993***	0.954***
Constant cut6	2.303***	2.238***
Constant cut7	3.142***	3.070***
Constant cut8	4.145***	
Observations	38019	8053
Sample	All	Migrant only

get worse. However, while English-speaking country migrants are more likely to think their health is improving from the immediate past, those from other countries are less likely to think so. We also find evidence that all the three self-assessed health variables get worse with the number of years since immigration to Australia, which is consistent with the previous migrant studies literature. However, there is no evidence that changes in health over time differ for migrants and non-migrant Australians over the period analysed.

The HILDA survey provides a rich source of data to analyse migrant health in Australia. As the amount of time that the boosted sample has been in Australia increases, it will be possible to get more robust information on long-term health assimilation patterns. Furthermore, it would be beneficial to analyse a more disaggregated set of migrant cohorts to Australia. The HILDA survey can be analysed by detailed country of birth, and those involved with the design of the survey may consider including visa type as a possible set of questions to be asked of migrants to Australia. Finally, as mentioned earlier in the chapter, the linked Census to deaths data is a potentially rich source of information that, when made available to external researchers, may allow for estimates of mortality differentials after controlling for observable characteristics.

NOTES

1. http://www.abs.gov.au/ausstats/abs@.nsf/mf/1351.0.55.058 (accessed 25 June 2017).
2. https://data.gov.au/dataset/the-longitudinal-survey-of-immigrants-to-australia-lsia-labour-force-subset (accessed 25 June 2017).
3. http://www3.aifs.gov.au/bnla/ (accessed 25 June 2017).
4. https://www.melbourneinstitute.com/hilda/ (accessed 25 June 2017).

REFERENCES

Anikeeva, O., P. Bi, J.E. Hiller, P. Ryan, D. Roder and G.S. Hans (2010), 'The health status of migrants in Australia: a review,' *Asia-Pacific Journal of Public Health*, **22** (2), 159–93.

Anikeeva, O., P. Bi, J.E. Hiller, P. Ryan, D. Roder and G.S. Hans (2012), 'Trends in cancer mortality rates among migrants in Australia: 1981–2007', *Cancer Epidemiology*, **36** (2), e74–e82.

Beiser, M. (2005), 'The health of immigrants and refugees in Canada', *Canadian Journal of Public Health*, **96** (supplement 2), S30–S44.

Biddle, N., S. Kennedy and J.T. McDonald (2007), 'Health assimilation patterns amongst Australian immigrants', *Economic Record*, **83** (260), 16–30.

Biddle, N., S.E. Khoo and J. Taylor (2015), 'Indigenous Australia, white Australia, multicultural Australia: the demography of race and ethnicity in Australia', in R. Saenz, D.G. Embrick, N.P. Rodriguez (eds), *The International Handbook of the Demography of Race and Ethnicity*, Dordrecht: Springer, pp. 599–622.

Borjas, G.J. (1987), 'Self-selection and the earnings of immigrants', NBER Working Paper No. 2248, National Bureau of Economic Research.

Cai, L. and G. Kalb (2006), 'Health status and labour force participation: evidence from Australia', *Health Economics*, **15** (3), 241–61.

Chiquiar, D. and G.H. Hanson (2002), 'International migration, self-selection, and the distribution of wages: evidence from Mexico and the United States, NBER Working Paper No. 9242, National Bureau of Economic Research.

Chiswick, B.R. (1999), 'Are immigrants favorably self-selected?', *American Economic Review*, **89** (2), 181–5, doi:10.1257/aer.89.2.181.
Chiswick, B.R., Y.L. Lee and P.W. Miller (2008), 'Immigrant selection systems and immigrant health', *Contemporary Economic Policy*, **26** (4), 555–78.
Collier, P. (2013), *Exodus: How Migration Is Changing Our World*, Oxford: Oxford University Press.
Correa-Velez, I., S.M. Gifford and S.J. Bice (2005), 'Australian health policy on access to medical care for refugees and asylum seekers', *Australia and New Zealand Health Policy*, **2** (1), 23.
Cully, M. (2011), 'Skilled migration selection policies: recent Australian reforms', *Migration Policy Practice*, **1** (1), 4–7.
De Maio, F.G. and E. Kemp (2010), 'The deterioration of health status among immigrants to Canada', *Global Public Health*, **5** (5), 462–78.
Frisbie, W.P., Y. Cho and R.A. Hummer (2001), 'Immigration and the health of Asian and Pacific Islander adults in the United States', *American Journal of Epidemiology*, **153** (4), 372–80.
Greene, W.H. (2008), *Econometric Analysis*, Boston, MA: Prentice Hall.
Greene, W.H. and D.A. Hensher (2010), *Modeling Ordered Choices: A Primer*, Cambridge: Cambridge University Press.
Grossman, M. (1972), *The Demand for Health: A Theoretical and Empirical Investigation*, Cambridge, MA: NBER Books, accessed 11 June 2017 at http://www.nber.org/chapters/c3484.
Halla, M. and M. Zweimüller (2013), 'The effect of health on earnings: quasi-experimental evidence from commuting accidents', *Labour Economics*, **24** (October), 23–38.
Jasso, G., D.S. Massey, M.R. Rosenzweig and J.P. Smith (2004), 'Immigrant health: selectivity and acculturation', in Norman B. Anderson (ed.), *Critical Perspectives on Racial and Ethnic Differences in Health in Late Life*, Washington, DC: National Academies Press, pp. 227–66.
Kaestner, R. and O. Malamud (2014), 'Self-selection and international migration: new evidence from Mexico', *Review of Economics and Statistics*, **96** (1), 78–91.
Kandula, N.R., Kersey and Lurie (2004), 'Assuring the health of immigrants: what the leading health indicators tell us', *Annual Review of Public Health*, **25**, 357–76.
Kennedy, S., M.P. Kidd, J.T. McDonald and N. Biddle (2015), 'The healthy immigrant effect: patterns and evidence from four countries', *Journal of International Migration and Integration*, **16** (2), 317–32.
Kennedy, S., J.T. McDonald and N. Biddle (2006), 'The healthy immigrant effect and immigrant selection: evidence from four countries', SEDAP Research Paper No. 164, McMaster University.
Leão, T. S., J. Sundquist, S.E. Johansson and K. Sundquist (2009), 'The influence of age at migration and length of residence on self-rated health among Swedish immigrants: a cross-sectional study', *Ethnicity & Health*, **14** (1), 93–105.
McDonald, J.T. and S. Kennedy (2004), 'Insights into the "healthy immigrant effect": health status and health service use of immigrants to Canada', *Social Science & Medicine*, **59** (8), 1613–27.
Newbold, B. (2005), 'Health status and health care of immigrants in Canada: a longitudinal analysis', *Journal of Health Services Research & Policy*, **10** (2), 77–83A.
Rasmussen, M., X. Guo, Y. Wang, K.E. Lohmueller, S. Rasmussen, A. Albrechtsen et al. (2011), 'An Aboriginal Australian genome reveals separate human dispersals into Asia', *Science*, **334** (6052), 94–8.

5. Mental health among immigrant background youth in Norway

Brit Oppedal

INTRODUCTION

The psychological adjustment of immigrant background children and youth has been a concern to public health officials, researchers and mental health practitioners. Much attention in the literature on immigrant children's mental health has been devoted to the period of adolescence, as this is often the developmental stage associated with the onset of, or increase in prevalence of, many psychiatric disorders such as depression, conduct problems, and eating disorders (Moffitt et al., 1996; Hankin et al., 1998; Loeber et al., 2000). However, the question of whether immigrant background children and youths are at higher risk of mental health problems compared with their non-immigrant peers remains largely inconclusive (Berry et al., 2006). Notwithstanding mental health and immigrant health being prioritized public health objectives in Norway, regular surveys of the mental health of the immigrant population in general, and of immigrant children and youths in particular, are generally lacking. This is unfortunate, given the significant changes that have occurred in the composition of the immigrant population over the past three decades.

This chapter provides an overview of research findings on the mental health of immigrant background youngsters in Norway. We use non-immigrants, that is, children with two Norwegian-born parents, as a normative reference sample. However, our main aim is not to provide information about mental health differences between immigrant and non-immigrant youth but rather to demonstrate the significant inter-group as well as intra-group variations that exist in the immigrant youth population. We use the term 'immigrant' and 'immigrant background' youth interchangeably to refer to preadolescents, adolescents and young adults who are either foreign born (first-generation immigrants) or born in Norway to two foreign-born parents (second generation). We include studies based on general immigrant populations as well as refugee groups only, in particular a section on youth who arrived in the country as unaccompanied minor asylum-seekers, that is, without being accompanied by a legal adult caretaker.

Following an introduction to the immigrant context of Norway we discuss variation in mental health problems among immigrant background children – and youths – related to gender, immigrant generation status, as well as type of migrant group and national origin. It should be noted that we examined symptoms of mental health problems, not clinically diagnosed psychiatric disorders, which have substantially lower prevalence. The concluding section suggests some directions for future research.

THE IMMIGRANT CONTEXT OF NORWAY

Norway has a population of little more than 5.2 million inhabitants. As in many other European countries, there has been a strong increase in immigration over recent decades. As of 1 January 2016, the immigrant population had reached 16.3 percent. In Oslo, Norway's capital, 33 percent of the population has an immigrant background, and immigrant background children comprise 40 percent of all elementary school children (Statistics Norway, 2016).

The five most numerous groups of foreign born immigrant children (first generation) originate from Poland, Somalia, Iraq, Lithuania, and Afghanistan, while the largest groups of children born in Norway to two immigrant parents (second generation) have a background from Pakistan, Somalia, Iraq, Vietnam, and Poland (Dyrhaug and Skyr, 2015). A ban on labor force immigration, mainly targeting unskilled workers from low-income countries, has been enforced since 1975, resulting in considerable changes in the composition of the immigrant population. The early labor force immigrants from Turkey, Morocco, and Pakistan have been outnumbered by groups with refugee and asylum-seeking backgrounds, especially from Somalia, Afghanistan, and Iraq, and more recently from Syria. Yet, the expansion of the European Union (EU) in 2004 has led to a marked increase in labor-immigration from new EU countries, particularly from Poland and Lithuania.

While the Norwegian immigration policies are strict, integration policies have proven quite successful, resulting in increased social mobility both by length of stay after resettlement, and from first to second generation (Galloway, 2006; Støren and Helland, 2009). Free health care for every citizen and free education, even at the tertiary level, are important aspects of Norway as a welfare state that facilitates social mobility. Even groups that are slow in attaining social mobility, which is currently the case for example for Turks and Somalis, tend to increase their participation over the years, and from the first to the second generation.

The same trends are true for immigrant background children and youths. Their participation in secondary and tertiary education increases with length of stay in Norway, and a larger proportion of second-generation immigrants than ethnic Norwegians attend colleges and universities (Støren and Helland, 2009). However, first-generation immigrant students have a higher rate of dropping out of school than non-immigrant Norwegian peers, while the rate for second generation is the same as for non-immigrants (Bratsberg et al., 2012). It is worth noting that youth in the most vulnerable immigrant group, those who arrived and received residence as unaccompanied minor asylum-seekers, increase their participation in education and the labor force in a relatively short time (Wiggen, 2014; Dalgard, 2016).

PREADOLESCENTS

One study of 10–13 year olds in fifth, sixth, and seventh grade of elementary school combined data from three different population-based projects on mental health, the Bergen Child Study (Heiervang et al., 2007), the Akershus Study (Van Roy et al., 2006), and the Oslo part of the Youth, Culture and Competence study (YCC) (Oppedal et al., 2008a). The total sample comprised around 13 500 children, of which 6.4 percent had an immigrant background.

All three studies collected self-report questionnaire data, with the Strength and Difficulties Questionnaire (SDQ) as the main measure of the children's mental health (Van Roy et al., 2006; Heiervang et al., 2007; Noam et al., 2014). The SDQ is a short screening instrument for mental health problems, which includes four problem sub-dimensions (emotional, conduct, hyperactivity, and peer problems) in addition to a prosocial sub-dimension (Achenbach et al., 2008; Goodman et al., 2000).

Overall Problems

The combined data from 10–13-year-old children showed an overall prevalence of mental health problems of 11.2 percent based on the SDQ total problem score (Goodman et al., 2000). The difference in prevalence between immigrant (12.3 percent) and non-immigrant children (11.1 percent) was not significant. However, the prevalence was equal for immigrant and non-immigrant girls, whereas in the boys group the prevalence was significantly higher among immigrants (16.1 percent) than among non-immigrants (11.3 percent).

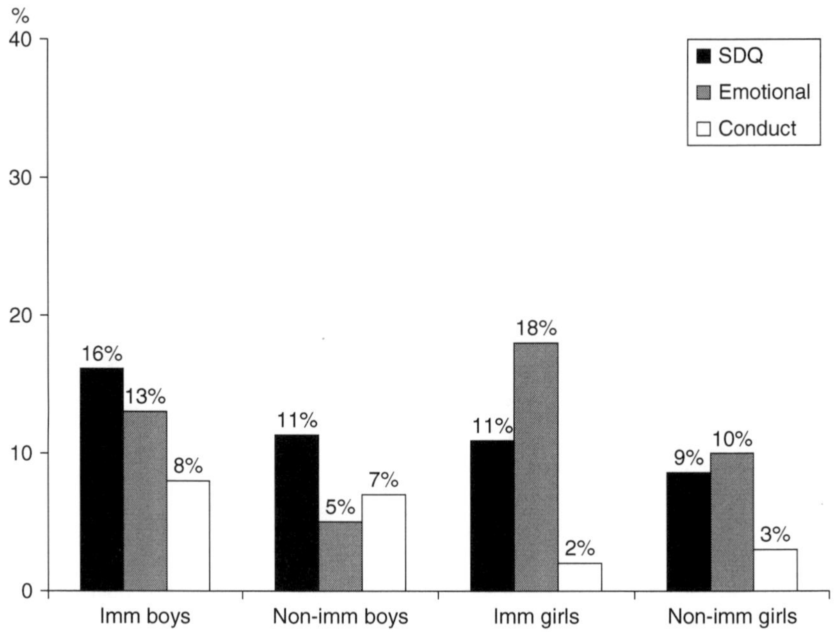

Note: Imm boys – immigrant boys; Non-imm boys – non-immigrant boys; Imm girls – immigrant girls; Non-imm girls – non-immigrant girls.

Source: Data from YCC (Oppedal et al., 2008a), the Akershus Study (Van Roy et al., 2006) and the Bergen Child Study (Heiervang et al., 2007).

Figure 5.1 Prevalence of fifth to seventh grade students with total SDQ-scores, emotional and conduct problems above the high-risk cut-off

Emotional Problems

The findings regarding overall mental health problems do, however, conceal important variations in individual dimensions of psychiatric symptoms. Both boys and girls with an immigrant background reported significantly more emotional problems than non-immigrants. Figure 5.1 shows the prevalence among boys was 13 percent and 18 percent for immigrant boys and girls respectively, compared with 5 percent and 10 percent among non-immigrants. The gender variation in emotional problems was significant in both groups. However, follow-up independent *t*-tests for each individual study sample yielded non-significant gender differences in the immigrant groups of the YCC and the Bergen Child Study, while the difference was significant for the participants of the Akershus Study. Among the non-immigrants the gender difference was significant in all three studies (table available on request from the author: brit.oppedal@fhi.no).

A female preponderance of emotional or depression problems is commonly demonstrated among adolescents, however the emergency of the gender variation typically takes place around 13–14 years (Wichstrøm, 1999; Twenge and Nolen-Hoeksema, 2002; Hankin, 2009). In this sense, the Norwegian findings among non-immigrant preadolescents, and immigrant preadolescents in the Akershus County are unexpected, and should be further examined in future studies. Moreover, there is also a need for more knowledge about the factors that cause the immigrant-status differences in emotional problems.

Externalizing Problems

The prevalence of self-reported conduct problems was generally low, and similar for immigrant and non-immigrant preadolescents. In accordance with findings from other studies (Keenan et al., 1999; Loeber et al., 2000), boys reported significantly more conduct problems than girls. Contrary to these findings, studies focusing on aggression found that immigrant boys and girls reported lower levels of reactive aggressiveness than non-immigrants. Also in accordance with other studies, boys in both groups reported more reactive aggression than girls (Vitaro et al., 1998). On the other hand, immigrants of both genders informed of higher levels of proactive affiliative aggressiveness than their non-immigrant peers (Fandrem et al., 2009). Previous studies have yielded similar results; that immigrant background children reported more proactive affiliative and less reactive aggressiveness than non-immigrants (Strohmeier et al., 2012). The authors speculated that these differences are associated with the additional challenges immigrant children and youths might experience in the formation of peer relations, however more research is needed before we can make conclusions about the immigrant-status variation in affiliative aggressiveness.

Variation by Generation Status, and National Origin

The level of mental health problems reported by first- and second-generation immigrant preadolescents was the same on all four SDQ problem subscales, and consequently also on overall mental health problems. Likewise, the level of proactive and reactive aggressiveness was also the same across generation levels in these age groups, contrary to the findings among the 14–19-year-old Austrian youths, who showed more aggressiveness among second-generation children (Strohmeier et al., 2012).

There are socio-cultural variations in what kind of and how much rule-breaking behavior society at large, educators and caretakers tolerate from children and how they sanction such behavior (Greenfield et al., 2003). A variety of other factors, such as developmental issues, construct specific characteristics, differences in immigration policies and practices, or the national group composition of the samples may also cause variation in externalizing behavior. Cross-cultural studies on the mental health of preadolescent immigrant children are therefore much needed to shed light on variation in externalizing problems between receiving countries in general, and regarding differences in externalizing symptoms according to generation status in particular.

Summary

While the overall risk for mental health problems was similar for immigrant and non-immigrant preadolescents, there was substantial variation related to gender and symptom category. Importantly, a migrant vulnerability was present in emotional, but not in externalizing problems. Non-immigrant girls reported more emotional problems than boys, however, the gender variation among immigrants was less consistent. The prevalence of all included-symptom categories was similar for foreign-born and Norwegian-born immigrant children.

ADOLESCENTS

In Norway, the shift from seventh to eighth grade at the age of 13 marks the transition from elementary to junior high school, where the students spend three years before entering senior high school which includes grades 11–13, at ages 16–18 years. Even if there are certain possibilities for individual curriculum choices during the junior high school years, differentiation of educational programs and tracking into vocational and university-bound streams does not take place until the second year of senior high school. Both transitions are associated with specific challenges that the young students have to cope with, and they take place in a developmental stage when there is an increase in mental health problems, such as depression among girls and conduct problems among boys (Wichstrøm, 1999; Lahey et al., 2000).

In junior high school, the students are for the first time evaluated with standardized grades, instead of as previously, written or oral information. The curriculum is increasingly more complex, including concepts and language that are at a higher level of abstraction. For bilingual students who may lack proficiency in the majority language, and at the same time are very ambitious (Shakya et al., 2010; Salikutluk, 2016) this may cause new mental distress. The transition to senior high school, on the other hand, is associated with educational identity developmental processes (Kalakoski and Nurmi, 1998), as at this stage the youth are faced with demands of making decisions about future vocational choices and pathways. Within this context, a mismatch between aspirations and school achievement may add to burdens of other school-related stressors associated with mental health problems (Oppedal, 2008).

The following discussion addresses variations in mental health problems among junior and senior high school students. We discuss mainly internalizing symptoms such as depression and anxiety, as they are associated with several stressors of the migration process (Keles et al., 2016a). The information reviewed is based on data from three epidemiological studies conducted around the turn of the century and together they offer a variety of perspectives on immigrant youth mental health. The School Study provided information from 451 and 472 students in eighth and ninth grades, respectively, of seven schools with a high proportion of immigrant students (Oppedal et al., 2004). The Youth Studies 2000–2004 targeted all tenth graders in six of Norway's 19 counties (N = 15931) (Norwegian Institute of Public Health, 2005). The youth part of the Akershus Study included a representative sample of all junior and senior high school students of that county (Van Roy et al., 2006).

Prevalence of Internalizing Problems during Junior High School Years

Findings from the eighth-grade students of the School Study showed that 26 percent of immigrant youth compared with 15 percent of the non-immigrants reported internalizing problems in terms of depression and anxiety symptoms, above the clinical cut-off on a 25-item version of Hopkin's Symptom Checklist (HSCL) (Derogatis et al., 1974).

Figure 5.2 illustrates the prevalence of internalizing symptoms assessed by a ten-item version of the HSCL (Strand et al., 2003) throughout the junior high school years (Oppedal, 2003). There was a steady increase in symptoms from eighth to tenth grade among both immigrant and non-immigrant girls, and a decrease among the boys. The difference in symptoms among the girls was non-significant at all grade levels. In contrast, immigrant boys had significantly higher symptom prevalence than non-immigrants, but, as can be seen, the gap was smaller in the tenth grade compared with eighth and ninth grades. The gender differences increased and were significant for non-immigrants at all grade levels. Among the immigrant youth, however, the gender difference did not reach significance until the tenth grade.

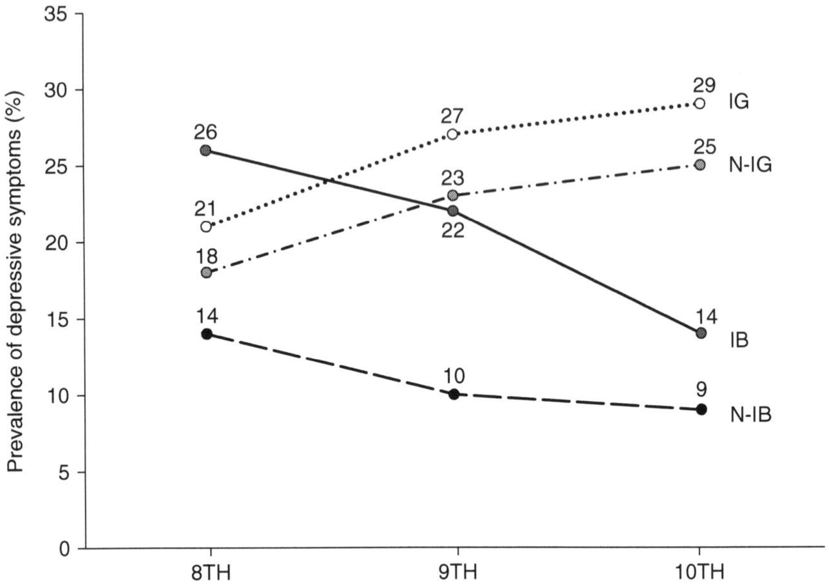

Note: N-IB – non-immigrant boys; IB – immigrant boys; N-IG – non-immigrant girls; IG – immigrant girls.

Source: School Study (Oppedal et al., 2004) and the Oslo part of the Youth Studies (Norwegian Institute of Public Health, 2005).

Figure 5.2 Prevalence of depressive symptoms during junior high school years

The increase in the prevalence of internalizing symptoms among the girls throughout junior high school, that is, from 13 to 15 years of age, is in accordance with findings from several other studies, for example, Wade et al. (2002) and Wichstrøm (1999). On the other hand, with regard to both immigrant and non-immigrant boys, there seemed to be an unexpected high level of symptoms in eighth grade with a subsequent decline over the years which was particularly strong among immigrant boys. Moreover, when compared with the proportion of preadolescent boys with clinical range symptom levels (Figure 5.2) the prevalence appeared substantially higher among these 13 year olds. These findings differ from the typical developmental trends that have been confirmed in other studies which showed a decrease in internalizing symptoms among boys aged from 12 to 13 years, with a subsequent stabilization in symptom level over the junior high school years (Hankin et al., 1998; Wichstrøm, 1999; Wade et al., 2002).

As the School Study data were collected shortly after school started in eighth grade, we may speculate that the findings imply that school-related factors associated with the transition from elementary to junior high school may be at stake, and that boys, particularly immigrant background boys, are especially susceptible to these kinds of contextual stressors. School change has been identified as an important predictor of mental health for preadolescents and young adolescents (Compas et al., 1989), in particular when transition coincides with the onset of puberty, as may be the case for many students during the transition from seventh to eighth grade. The school context involves both stressors related to school work and protective factors in terms of social support from classmates and teachers (Hankin et al., 2007; Kia-Keating and Ellis, 2007; Kuperminc et al., 2001; Oppedal, 2008; Oppedal and Roysamb, 2004). Longitudinal studies including ages and stages of school transitions and culturally diverse samples are needed to shed light on gender and immigrant-status variations in developmental trajectories of mental health.

Changes in Prevalence of Internalizing Problems from Junior to Senior High School

We used the data from 8494 junior high school students in eighth to tenth grades, and 7445 senior high school students in eleventh to twelfth grades that had participated in the Akershus Study to compare the prevalence of internalizing problems between junior and senior high school students (Figure 5.3). Unfortunately, there were too few immigrant background students, 490 (5.8 percent) and 559 (7.5 percent) respectively, to make meaningful comparisons at each grade level (Oppedal et al., 2008b). In junior high school the variation in prevalence between immigrant and non-immigrant was non-significant among both boys and girls, whereas among the high school students the difference was significant for both groups. (Chi-square statistics table available on request from the author.)

There was significantly higher symptom prevalence in senior compared with junior high school girls, and the increase was especially noticeable among the immigrant girls, from 21 percent to 33.2 percent. In the boys' group the prevalence remained the same for immigrants, while for non-immigrants there was a small but significant decrease in the prevalence of internalizing symptoms from junior to senior high school. The gender differences were significant in both groups at both school levels.

The research literature has confirmed substantial escalations in depressive symptoms in the late teenage years among girls, in contrast to a stable or decreasing prevalence among boys, resulting in increasing gender differences in this developmental stage (Hankin et al., 1998). However,

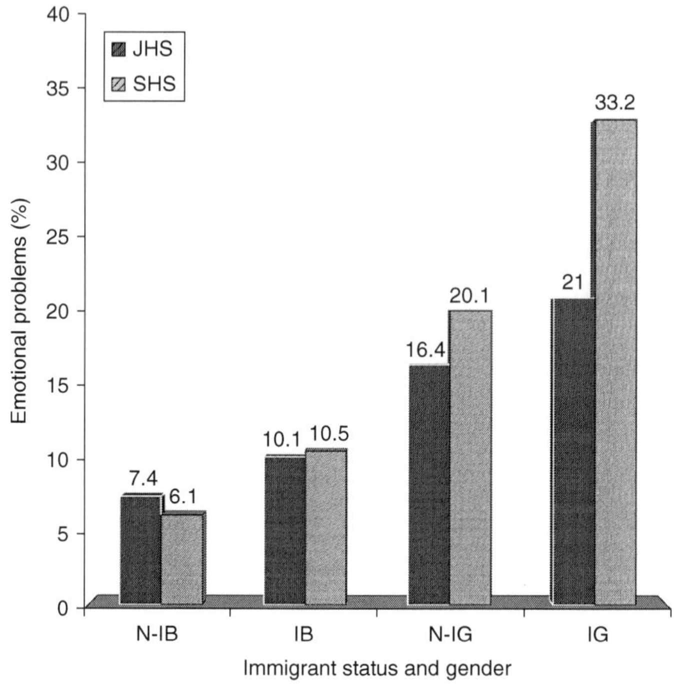

Note: N-IB – non-immigrant boys; IB – immigrant boys; N-IG – non-immigrant girls; IG – immigrant girls. JHS – junior high school; SHS – senior high school.

Source: Data from the Akershus Study (Van Roy et al., 2006).

Figure 5.3 Prevalence of emotional problems in junior and senior high school

it is worth noticing that the increase in symptoms was stronger among immigrant relative to non-immigrant girls, resulting in a highly significant difference between them in senior high school students.

Variation by Generation Status and National Origin

The combined data of the tenth graders in the Akershus Study and the Youth Studies offers a unique opportunity to investigate immigrant-status and national group variation in the immigrant youth population.

As was the case in the preadolescents group there were not significant differences in prevalence of internalizing problems between first- and second-generation immigrants participating in the Youth Studies. However, with the exception of second-generation immigrant girls, they all reported significantly more emotional problems than their non-immigrant peers. (Table of prevalence rates and Chi-square statistics available on request from the author.)

Variation in mental health problems among youth with diverse national origins has been examined from different perspectives in a series of studies based on data from the Oslo part of the Youth Studies. One study that focused on acculturation and mental health involved immigrant background youth with origins from 11 countries representing a mix of labor force and refugee sending nations. The findings demonstrated that there was significant group variation in internalizing symptoms (SDQ emotional problems) both within and across refugee background and labor force families. The groups that in general reported most problems were also found both among labor force immigrants and refugees (Turks and Pakistanis in the former, Iraqis, Iranians and Vietnamese in the latter) (Oppedal et al., 2005).

One study targeted youth from majority Muslim countries, and compared them with immigrant youth from both other non-Western and Western countries. As a group, the Muslim background youth did not differ from ethnic Norwegian youth in internalizing problems. Nevertheless there was substantial within-group heterogeneity in symptom levels, especially among the girls, as Iranian background girls had significantly more symptoms than girls with Pakistani and Somalian origins (Oppedal and Roysamb, 2007).

A third study included only participants from refugee sending nations, two of which were categorized as healthy (Somalis and Tamils) and two as vulnerable (Iranians and Vietnamese) based on the group symptom level. In the healthy groups, 6.3 percent of the boys and 18.3 percent of the girls reported symptoms in the clinical range, in contrast to 20.7 percent and 42.3 percent respectively in the vulnerable groups (Oppedal, 2008). From Figure 5.2 it can be seen that the prevalence for the tenth-grade immigrant students was 14 percent and 29 percent for boys and girls, respectively, and 9 percent and 25 percent for non-immigrants. In other words, the prevalence of the healthy refugee groups (Somalis and Tamils) was lower than among their non-immigrant, ethnic Norwegian peers. These findings clearly indicate that variation in adolescents' mental health is not consistently associated with either immigrant or refugee status.

Summary

In population-based studies, there was a higher prevalence of internalizing symptoms among immigrant than non-immigrant background youth. An increase in internalizing problems over the junior high school years resulted in significant gender variation in tenth grade that was also present in senior high school. The symptom level among the girls continued increasing in senior high school, and one of the most salient findings reported in this section was the considerable rise in emotional problems among immigrant girls from junior to senior high school. On the other hand, there was a decrease and subsequent stabilization in the symptom prevalence among the immigrant boys. The prevalence of mental health problems was the same for first- and second-generation immigrants. However, there were striking national group variations that caution against drawing general conclusions about migration as a risk factor for adolescents' mental health, and underscores the need to better understand the resources of many immigrant groups.

UNACCOMPANIED MINOR REFUGEES

The most vulnerable group of all immigrants is undoubtedly children who travel unaccompanied by a legal caretaker to seek asylum in a foreign country, called unaccompanied minor asylum-seekers. They typically originate in countries marred by war or internal conflicts, and the majority of them have been exposed to a variety of war- and catastrophe-related traumatic events (Jensen et al., 2013).

In this section we describe findings from a mixed-method longitudinal study involving a population-based representative sample of 918 youths who arrived in Norway as unaccompanied minor asylum-seekers, and were granted residence between 2000 and 2010. As the participants had been granted protection and residence, and many had reached the age of majority, we refer to them as unaccompanied refugees.

The majority were between 14 and 16 years old when they arrived in Norway, but they had spent on average 18 months traveling, implying that they were much younger when they left the countries where they used to live. Almost half the sample had not attended school before arrival in Norway, or they had only attended school for one to three years.

Around three-quarters of the youths had experienced war at first hand. On a list describing eight broad categories of traumatic events, they informed of having been exposed to on average four of them. The most frequent traumas they had experienced were that they had been hit, kicked, or shot at, or physically hurt in other ways, or that they had watched this happening to others. More than one-third of the children reported that one or both parents were dead, and another quarter did not know whether they were alive or not.

In spite of the overwhelming list of adversities described, the unaccompanied refugees express a tremendous strong will to succeed and make it in their new countries. They venture into educational career

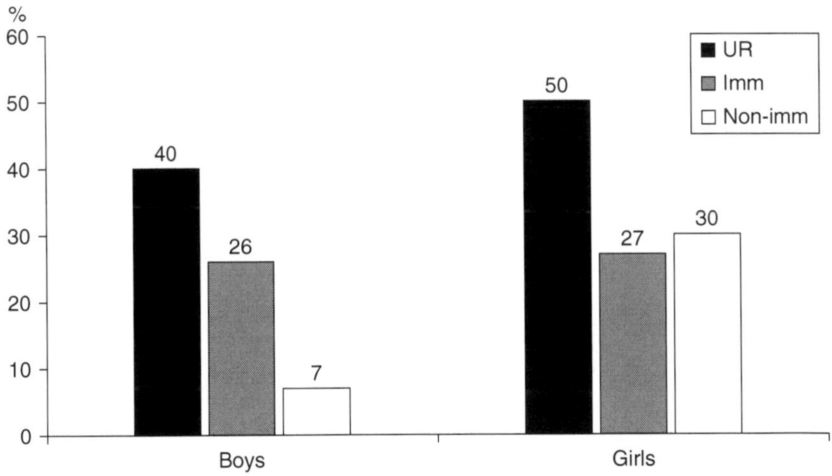

Note: UR – unaccompanied refugees; Imm – immigrant high school students with background from non-western countries; Non-imm – non-immigrant high school students.

Figure 5.4 Prevalence of clinical range internalizing symptoms in unaccompanied refugees and a reference group of immigrant and non-immigrant high school students

trajectories and participate in the work force (Oppedal et al., 2017). Importantly, the study showed that after three years of residence, unaccompanied refugees from Afghanistan were participating at the same rate as mainstream youths (Dalgard, 2016; Wiggen, 2016).

Mental Health

These positive developmental outcomes often coincide with a high level of mental health problems. In accordance with findings from other studies of unaccompanied refugees in various stages of the asylum-seeking or resettlement process (Bean et al., 2007a; Derluyn et al., 2009; Bronstein and Montgomery, 2011), the prevalence of mental health problems was high also in the present project, with an overall prevalence of clinical range depression symptoms of 41.5 percent. Girls reported significantly more symptoms than boys (Figure 5.4). Almost two-thirds of the youths had symptoms of post-traumatic stress disorder (PTSD) above the suggested clinical cut-off (Perrin et al., 2005).

While unaccompanied refugees informed of significantly higher levels of depression than immigrant and non-immigrant youth, they reported the same level of subjective well-being (Seglem et al., 2014). These findings indicate that despite more depressive symptoms than other youths and experiences of trauma and loss, unaccompanied refugees still experience a sense of contentment and well-being in their lives. One explanation of the high levels of life satisfaction reported by unaccompanied refugees may be that they compare their present situation to their situation before leaving their homeland or their fortunate situation relative to family and friends that are left behind (Seglem et al., 2014).

Stability and Change in Mental Health Problems

While on a group level, there is substantial stability in the refugees' depression symptoms, there is nevertheless significant individual variation over time (Bean et al., 2007b; Keles et al., 2016b). A study categorized the participants according to four longitudinal developmental trajectories of depression: In the healthy trajectory, participants had low scores at wave 1 that remained low over two subsequent waves one year apart; in the resilient, they reported initially high scores that decreased over time; while participants in the vulnerable trajectory had low scores initially that increased significantly over time. Participants in the clinical trajectory reported clinical level symptoms at all three waves (Keles et al., 2016b). A very high proportion of the young refugees, altogether 41.6 percent, were either in the vulnerable or clinical trajectory, implying that they were in need of supportive interventions. However, the other perspective is that as much as 58.3 percent had consistently low scores at both the second and third wave, disregarding the initial levels, which may seem amazing in such a vulnerable youth group (Keles et al., 2016b).

Summary

There is a very high prevalence of mental health problems among unaccompanied refugees compared with other immigrant and non-immigrant youth groups, after they have received residence and are resettled in Norway. Nevertheless, they report similar levels of life satisfaction as other youths, and statistics show that most of them integrate successfully into mainstream society in terms of participation in education and the work force.

DISCUSSION AND CONCLUSION

This chapter embodies the first comprehensive summary of research findings regarding the mental health of immigrant background children and youths in Norway, spanning age groups from 10 and 26 years. The main aim was to underscore research findings showing that there is more variation in mental health between and within various immigrant groups than between immigrant and non-immigrant children and youths. Ethnic Norwegians functioned as a normative group, against which we decided if immigrants had low, normal, or high problem-scores. We employed suggested clinical cut-off scores for the involved symptoms scales to indicate the prevalence of children and youths at risk for mental health problems.

Overall, the findings presented in this chapter may imply that immigrant boys are especially vulnerable with respect to internalizing problems in elementary and junior high school years, while senior high school seems to be a sensitive period for immigrant girls. Future studies should examine if differences between immigrant and non-immigrant youth in these stages are due to stronger reaction to psychosocial stressors, or to a heavier burden of such stressors among immigrants.

A 'migration morbidity association' indicating higher levels of adjustment problems among immigrant compared to non-immigrant youth was supported among boys in studies that included a variety of immigrant groups. However, the migration morbidity association was not consistent as, during the junior high school years, the differences in symptom prevalence among girls were non-significant. Moreover, we did not find the traditional gender differences in internalizing problems among immigrant junior high school students.

Boys and girls react differently to individual and contextual stressors (Hankin et al., 2007), and immigrant children and youths are presumably exposed to more stressors than non-immigrants, as they experience both general and acculturation-specific hassles (Keles et al., 2016b). Considering the importance of school achievement and school context to the mental well-being of children and youths (Kuperminc et al., 2001; Wells et al., 2003; DeSocio and Hootman, 2004; Kia-Keating and Ellis, 2007) more information about school-related predictors of mental health would contribute to our understanding of the psychosocial adjustment of immigrant children. Furthermore, information about gender variation in mental reactions to general and acculturation specific stressors among immigrant background children and youths could be very valuable in designing universal and selected preventive interventions to reduce the risk of internalizing mental health problems.

The most important findings outlined in this chapter concerned the national group differences in reported internalizing problems. Interestingly, however, the national group differences did not reach significance among preadolescent children. More research with stronger design in these age groups is needed to increase our knowledge about variation in and predictors of mental health among preadolescent immigrant children.

In the older samples national group variation was documented in several studies but there was no general support for the concept of a 'migration morbidity association' with the mental health of immigrant children and youths. Rather, the answer to the question as to whether immigrant children and youths have more mental health problems than non-immigrants depends on the national backgrounds and age groups that are in focus.

In different ways, these studies also showed that acculturation-related (for example, discrimination, ethnic identity crisis, culture competence) as well as general (for example, class support, school-related problems, intergenerational conflicts, and self-efficacy) risk and protective factors accounted for both within- and between-group variation in internalizing symptoms. The findings imply a need for a holistic, developmental approach in the study of psychosocial adjustment and mental health of immigrant background children and youths, rather than the more limited acculturation psychological perspective (Oppedal and Toppelberg, 2016).

Finally, the findings discussed in this chapter imply that concepts such as 'the immigrant paradox' and 'the migration morbidity association' are not useful in shedding light on the mental health of immigrant children and youths in Norway. Instead such generalizing concepts may contribute to stereotyping ideas and perceptions of psychosocial adjustment of immigrants. Consequently, they should be used with much caution by researchers in multicultural contexts. The findings underscore the need to better understand the dynamic interaction between macro-level policies and practices of receiving countries and the unique socio-cultural practices of different migrant groups as a context for immigrant children's well-being and mental health problems. Within this framework, there is a need for cross-cultural longitudinal and comparative research that includes different age groups and developmental transitions and that targets predictors of gender variation in the mental health of immigrant children and youths. Information from such studies can give direction to differentiated population based interventions to promote mental well-being and prevent mental health problems both at a national level and in local communities among immigrant background children and youths.

REFERENCES

Achenbach, T.M., A. Becker, M. Döpfner, E. Heiervang, V. Roessner, H.C. Steinhausen and A. Rothenberger (2008), 'Multicultural assessment of child and adolescent psychopathology with ASEBA and SDQ instruments: research findings, applications, and future directions', *Journal of Child Psychology and Psychiatry and Allied Disciplines*, **49** (3), 251–75.

Bean, T.M., I. Derluyn, E. Eurelings-Bontekoe, E. Broekaert and P. Spinhoven (2007a), 'Comparing psychological distress, traumatic stress reactions, and experiences of unaccompanied refugee minors with experiences of adolescents accompanied by parents', *Journal of Nervous and Mental Disease*, **195** (4), 288–97, doi:10.1097/01.nmd.0000243751.49499.93.

Bean, T. M., E. Eurelings-Bontekoe and P. Spinhoven (2007b), 'Course and predictors of mental health of unaccompanied refugee minors in the Netherlands: one year follow-up', *Social Science and Medicine*, **64** (6), 1204–15, doi:10.1016/j.socscimed.2006.11.010.

Berry, J.W., J.S. Phinney, D.L. Sam and P. Vedder (2006), *Immigrant Youth in Cultural Transition: Acculturation, Identity and Adaptation Across National Contexts*, Mahwah, NJ: Lawrence Erlbaum.

Bratsberg, B., O. Raaum and K. Røed (2012), 'Educating children of immigrants: closing the gap in Norwegian schools', *Nordic Economic Policy Review*, (1), 211–51.

Bronstein, I. and P. Montgomery, (2011), 'Psychological distress in refugee children: a systematic review', *Clinical Child and Family Psychology Review*, **14** (1), 44–56, doi:10.1007/s10567-010-0081-0.

Compas, B.E., V. Phares and N. Ledoux (1989), 'Stress and coping preventive interventions for children and adolescents', in L.A. Bond and B.E. Compas (eds), *Primary Prevention and Promotion in the Schools*, Newbury Park, CA: Sage, pp. 319–40.

Dalgard, A.B. (2016), 'Enslige mindreårige flyktninger i arbeid og utdanning, 2014. 90 prosent fra Afghanistan i arbeid og utdanning etter fire år' ('Unaccompanied minor refugees in the labor force and education, 2014. 90% from Afghanistan in laborforce or education after four years'), accessed 10 June 2016at http://www.ssb.no/arbeid-og-lonn/artikler-og-publikasjoner/90-prosent-fra-afghanistan-i-arbeid-og-utdanning-etter-fire-ar.

Derluyn, I., C. Mels and E. Broekaert (2009), 'Mental health problems in separated refugee adolescents', *Journal of Adolescent Health*, **44** (3), 291–7.

DeSocio, J. and J. Hootman (2004), 'Children's mental health and school success', *Journal of School Nursing*, **20** (4), 189–96, doi:10.1177/10598405040200040201.

Dyrhaug, T. and V. Skyr (2015), *Barn og unge med innvandrerbakgrunn i barnevernet 2012* (*Immigrant Background Children and Youth within the Child Welfare Services*) Statistics Norway Report 16/2015, accessed 25 JUne 2017 at https://www.ssb.no/sosiale-forhold-og-kriminalitet/artikler-og-publikasjoner/_attachment/222464?_ts=14c4ba14350.

Fandrem, H., D.L. Sam and E. Roland (2009), 'Depressive symptoms among native and immigrant adolescents in Norway: the role of gender and urbanization', *Social Indicators Research*, **92** (1), 91–109, doi:10.1007/s11205-008-9291-y.

Fazel, M., R. Reed, C. Panter-Brick and A. Stein (2012), 'Mental health of displaced and refugee children resettled in high-income countries: risk and protective factors', *Lancet*, **379** (9812), 266–82.

Galloway, T.A. (2006), 'Do immigrants integrate out of poverty in Norway?', paper presented at the Discussion, Statistics Norway, Research Department (Paper No. 482).

Goodman, R., D. Renfrew and M. Mullick (2000), 'Predicting type of psychiatric disorder from Strengths and Difficulties Questionnaire (SDQ) scores in child

mental health clinics in London and Dhaka', *European Child and Adolescent Psychiatry*, **9** (2), 129–34.
Greenfield, P.M., H. Keller, A. Fuligni and A. Maynard (2003), 'Cultural pathways through universal development', *Annual Review of Psychology*, **54**, 461–90, doi:10.1146/annurev.psych.54.101601.145221.
Hankin, B.L. (2009), 'Development of sex differences in depressive and co-occurring anxious symptoms during adolescence: descriptive trajectories and potential explanations in a multi-wave prospective study', *Journal of Cinical Child and Adolescent Psychology*, **38** (4), 460–72, doi:10.1080/15374410902976288.
Hankin, B.L., L.Y. Abramson, T.E. Moffitt, K.E. Angell, P.A. Silva and R. McGee (1998), 'Development of depression from preadolescence to young adulthood: emerging gender differences in a 10-year longitudinal study', *Journal of Abnormal Psychology*, **107** (1), 128–40, doi:10.1037/0021-843X.107.1.128.
Hankin, B.L., R. Mermelstein and I. Roesch (2007), 'Sex differences in adolescent depression: stress exposure and reactivity models', *Child Development*, **78** (1), 279–95, doi:10.1111/j.1467-8624.2007.00997.x.
Heiervang, E., K.M. Stormark, A.J. Lundervold, M. Heimann, R. Goodman, M.B. Posserud et al. (2007), 'Psychiatric disorders in Norwegian 8- to 10-year-olds: an epidemiological survey of prevalence, risk factors, and service use', *Journal of the American Academy of Child and Adolescent Psychiatry*, **46** (4),438–47, doi:10.1097/chi.0b013e31803062bf.
Jensen, T.K., K.W. Fjermestad, L. Granly and N.H. Wilhelmsen (2013), 'Stressful life experiences and mental health problems among unaccompanied asylum-seeking children', *Clinical Child Psychology and Psychiatry*, **20** (1), 106–16.
Kalakoski, V. and J.-E. Nurmi (1998), 'Identity and educational transitions: age differences in adolescent exploration and commitment related to education, occupation, and family', *Journal of Research on Adolescence*, **8** (1), 29–47, doi:10.1207/s15327795jra0801_2.
Keenan, K., R. Loeber, and S. Green (1999), 'Conduct disorder in girls: a review of the literature', *Clinical Child and Family Psychology Review*, **2** (1), 3–19, doi:10.1023/a:1021811307364.
Keles, S., O. Friborg, T. Idsøe, S. Sirin and B. Oppedal (2016a), 'Resilience and acculturation among unaccompanied refugee minors', *International Journal of Behavioral Development*, online only, doi: 0165025416658136.
Keles, S., T. Idsoe, O. Friborg, S.R. Sirin and B. Oppedal (2016b), 'The longitudinal relation between daily hassles and depressive symptoms among unaccompanied refugees in Norway', *Journal of Abnormal Child Psychology*, online only, doi:10.1007/s10802-016-0251-8.
Kia-Keating, M. and B.H. Ellis (2007), 'Belonging and connection to school in resettlement: young refugees, school belonging, and psychosocial adjustment', *Clinical Child Psychology and Psychiatry*, **12** (1), 29–43, doi:10.1177/1359104507071052.
Kuperminc, G.P., B.J. Leadbeater and S.J. and Blatt (2001), 'School social climate and individual differences in vulnerability to psychopathology among middle school students', *Journal of School Psychology*, **39** (2), 141–59, doi:http://dx.doi.org/10.1016/S0022-4405(01)00059-0.
Lahey, B.B., M. Schwab-Stone, S.H. Goodman, I.D. Waldman, G. Canino and P.J. Rathouz, et al. (2000), 'Age and gender differences in oppositional behavior and conduct problems: a cross-sectional household study of middle childhood and adolescence', *Journal of Abnormal Psychology*, **109** (3), 488–503, doi:10.1037/0021-843X.109.3.488.

Loeber, R., J.D. Burke, B.B. Lahey, A. Winters and M. Zera (2000), 'Oppositional defiant and conduct disorder: a review of the past 10 years, part I', *Journal of the American Academy of Child and Adolescent Psychiatry*, **39** (12), 1468–84, doi:http://dx.doi.org/10.1097/00004583-200012000-00007.

Moffitt, T.E., A. Caspi, N. Dickson, P. Silva and W. Stanton, W. (1996), 'Childhood-onset versus adolescent-onset antisocial conduct problems in males: natural history from ages 3 to 18 years', *Development and Psychopathology*, **8** (2), 399–424, doi:10.1017/S0954579400007161.

Noam, G., B. Oppedal, T. Idsoe and N. Panjwani (2014), 'Mental health problems and school outcomes among immigrant and non-immigrant early adolescents in Norway', *School Mental Health*, **6** (4), 279–93, doi:10.1007/s12310-014-9129-5.

Norwegian Institute of Public Health (2005), 'The youth studies', accessed 18 April 2016 at https://www.fhi.no/en/studies/regional-health-studies/ung/youth-studies-2000-2009/.

Oppedal, B. (2003), 'Adolescent mental health in multi-cultural context', doctoral thesis, University of Oslo, Oslo.

Oppedal, B. (2008), 'Psychosocial profiles as mediators of variation in internalizing problems among young immigrants with origins in countries of war and internal conflicts', *European Journal of Developmental Psychology*, **5** (2), 210–34, doi:10.1080/17405620701577850.

Oppedal, B. and E. Roysamb (2004), 'Mental health, life stress and social support among young Norwegian adolescents with immigrant and host national background', *Scandinavian Journal of Psychology*, **45** (2), 131–44, doi:10.1111/j.1467-9450.2004.00388.x.

Oppedal, B. and E. Roysamb (2007), 'Young Muslim immigrants in Norway: an epidemiological study of their psychosocial adaptation and internalizing problems', *Applied Developmental Science*, **11** (3), 112–25, doi:10.1080/10888690701454583.

Oppedal, B. and C.O. Toppelberg (2016), 'Acculturation development and the acquisition of culture competence', in D.L. Sam and J.W. Berry (eds), *The Cambridge Handbook of Acculturation Psychology*, 2nd edn, Cambridge: Cambridge University Press, pp. 71–4.

Oppedal, B., G.A. Azam, S.M. Hirsch, P. Kiamanesh, E.A. Moe and L. Jensen (2008a), 'Psykososial tilpasning og psykiske problemer blant barn i innvandrerfamilier' ('Psychosocial adaptation and psychiatric problems among children in immigrant families'), Rapport 2008/14, Norwegian Institute of Public Health, Oslo.

Oppedal, B., G.A. Azam, L. Jensen, S.M. Hirsch, P. Kiamanesh, E.A. Moe et al. (2008b), 'Psykisk Helse og Sosiokulturell Integrasjon blant Ungdom med Innvandrerbakgrunn' ('Mental health and socio-cultural integration among immigrant background youth'), working paper, Norwegian Institute of Public Health, Division of Mental Health, Oslo.

Oppedal, B., E. Guribye and J. Kroger (2017), 'Vocational identity development among unaccompanied refugee minors', *International Journal of Intercultural Relations*, https://doi.org/10.1016/j.ijintrel.2017.04.004.

Oppedal, B., E. Roysamb, and S. Heyerdahl (2005), 'Ethnic group, acculturation, and psychiatric problems in young immigrants', *Journal of Child Psychology and Psychiatry*, **46** (6), 646–60, doi:10.1111/j.1469-7610.2004.00381.x.

Oppedal, B., E. Roysamb and D.L. Sam (2004), 'The effect of acculturation and social support on change in mental health among young immigrants', *International Journal of Behavioral Development*, **28** (6), 481–94, doi:10.1080/01650250444000126.

Perrin, S., R. Meiser-Stedman, and P. Smith (2005), 'The Children's Revised Impact of Event Scale (CRIES): validity as a screening instrument for PTSD', *Behavioural and Cognitive Psychotherapy*, **33** (4), 487–98, doi:doi:10.1017/S1352465805002419.
Salikutluk, Z. (2016), 'Why do immigrant students aim high? Explaining the aspiration–achievement paradox of immigrants in Germany', *European Sociological Review*, **32** (5), 581–92, doi:10.1093/esr/jcw004.
Seglem, K.B., B. Oppedal and S. Raeder (2011), 'Predictors of depressive symptoms among resettled unaccompanied refugee minors', *Scandinavian Journal of Psychology*, **52** (5), 457–64.
Seglem, K.B., B. Oppedal and E. Roysamb (2014), 'Daily hassles and coping dispositions as predictors of psychological adjustment: a comparative study of young unaccompanied refugees and youth in the resettlement country', *International Journal of Behavioral Development*, **38** (3), 293–303. doi:10.1177/0165025414520807.
Shakya, Y.B., S. Guruge, M. Hynie, A. Akbari, M. Malik, S. Htoo, A. Khogali et al. (2010), 'Aspirations for higher education among newcomer refugee youth in Toronto: expectations, challenges, and strategies', *Refuge*, **27** (2), 65–78.
Statistics Norway (2016), 'Key figures for immigration and immigrants', accessed 10 October 2016 at https://www.ssb.no/en/innvandring-og-innvandrere/nokkeltall.
Støren, L.A. and H. Helland (2009), 'Ethnicity differences in the completion rates of upper secondary education: how do the effects of gender and social background variables interplay?', *European Sociological Review*, **26** (5), 585–601, doi:10.1093/esr/jcp041.
Strand, B.H., O.S. Dalgard, K. Tambs and M. Rognerud (2003), 'Measuring the mental health status of the Norwegian population: a comparison of the instruments SCL-25, SCL-10, SCL-5 and MHI-5 (SF-36)', *Nordic Journal of Psychiatry*, **57** (2), 113–18, doi:10.1080/08039480310000932.
Strohmeier, D., H. Fandrem, E. Stefanek and C. Spiel (2012), 'The goal to be accepted by friends as underlying function of overt aggressive behaviour in immigrant adolescents', *Scandinavian Journal of Psychology*, **53** (1), 80–88, doi:10.1111/j.1467-9450.2011.00910.x.
Twenge, J.M. and S. Nolen-Hoeksema (2002), 'Age, gender, race, socioeconomic status, and birth cohort differences on the children's depression inventory: a meta-analysis', *Journal of Abnormal Psychology*, **111** (4), 578–88.
Van Roy, B., B. Groholt, S. Heyerdahl and J. Clench-Aas (2006), 'Self-reported strengths and difficulties in a large Norwegian population 10–19 years: age and gender specific results of the extended SDQ-questionnaire', *European Child and Adolescent Psychiatry*, **15** (4), 189–94, doi:10.1007/s00787-005-0521-4.
Vitaro, F., P.L. Gendreau, R.E. Tremblay and P. Oligny (1998), 'Reactive and proactive aggression differentially predict later conduct problems', *Journal of Child Psychology and Psychiatry and Allied Disciplines*, **39** (3), 377–85.
Wade, T.J., J. Cairney and D.J. Pevalin (2002), 'Emergence of gender differences in depression during adolescence: national panel results from three countries', *Journal of the American Academy of Child and Adolescent Psychiatry*, **41** (2), 190–98, doi:http://dx.doi.org/10.1097/00004583-200202000-00013.
Wells, J., J. Barlow and S. Stewart-Brown (2003), 'A systematic review of universal approaches to mental health promotion in schools', *Health Education*, **103** (4), 197–220, doi:doi:10.1108/09654280310485546.
Wichstrøm, L. (1999), 'The emergence of gender difference in depressed mood

during adolescence: the role of intensified gender socialization', *Developmental Psychology*, **35** (1), 232–45, doi:10.1037/0012-1649.35.1.232.
Wiggen, K.S. (2014), 'Enslige mindreårige flyktninger, 2011. Arbeid, utdanning og inntekt', ('Unaccompanied minor refugees, 2011. Employment, education and income', Rapport (2014/9), Statistics Norway, Oslo, accessed 10 October 2016 at http://www.ssb.no/arbeid-og-lonn/artikler-og-publikasjoner/enslige-mindrearige-flyktninger-2011.
Wiggen, K.S. (2016), 'Personer bosatt som enslige mindreårige flyktninger i perioden 1996–2013. Tre av fire i arbeid eller utdanning' ('Individuals resettled as unaccompanied minor refugees from 1996–2013. Three of four participating in work or education'), accessed 10 October 2016 at https://www.ssb.no/arbeid-og-lonn/artikler-og-publikasjoner/tre-av-fire-i-arbeid-eller-utdanning.

6. Mental health of immigrants and refugees in Canada

Lori Wilkinson and David Ponka*

INTRODUCTION

The goal of this chapter is to review research on mental health among immigrants and refugees in Canada. We discuss the differences in mental health among these two groups, with a particular focus on adults and children as their experiences and outcomes will be different by the nature of the type of migration they experience and by their age at migration. We identify and reject, with evidence, the various misconceptions regarding mental health and newcomers as a way of better educating us about this issue in general and about immigrants and refugees in particular. We set the context by providing some demographic detail about the immigrants and refugees arriving in Canada. We then summarize the research on mental health of immigrant adults, refugee adults, immigrant children and youth, and refugee children and youth. We then examine the case of Omar and Ibrahim (true names concealed), two teen-aged brothers fleeing the war in Syria with their mother as their father was killed in the war, to show how health professionals might deal with a real-life case. We conclude by offering suggestions for future research and for a thoughtful examination of how trauma by proxy might affect caregivers.

A SHORT DEMOGRAPHIC CONTEXT OF IMMIGRANTS AND REFUGEES IN CANADA

Historically, immigrants and refugees have made and continue to make significant contributions to the diverse population of Canada. Today, immigrants and refugees make up nearly 22 percent of the population (Statistics Canada, 2012), making Canada one of the most metropolitan and diverse countries on the planet. Since 2005, over 2.6 million immigrants have entered Canada for permanent residence. This does not include the thousands of temporary workers and international students who enter the country each year who make up an additional 425 000 to 725 000 people per year. Many of those in the latter group apply to remain permanently.

Newcomers from all over the world now call Canada their home. The top three countries of origin for immigrants arriving over the past ten years are India, China and the Philippines. Together, they account for nearly 1 million of the new arrivals since 2005 (Citizenship and Immigration Canada, 2016). Those coming to Canada for work and business investment, called economic immigrants, have historically made up the largest proportion of newcomers. Between one-third and two-thirds of immigrants arrive primarily for these reasons. Family-class immigrants, those reuniting with close family members, traditionally make up between 25 percent and 33 percent of this group. Refugees, asylum seekers and other humanitarian categories comprise the remainder. Their numbers change from year to year depending on world political conditions and domestic decisions around immigration levels.

In November 2015, the newly elected Canadian government introduced measures that would bring 25 000 Syrians to Canada by 31 March 2016. Not only did they reach their goal, they exceeded it. At the time of writing, over 33 000 Syrians had arrived in Canada (Immigration, Refugees and Citizenship Canada, 2016). This was not the first time that Canada made extraordinary efforts to resettle a large number of involuntary migrants. Hungarians, Vietnamese, Kosovars, Iraqi and Karen refugees have been resettled in large numbers at varying points in time since the Second World War. Not to be lost in the Syrian arrivals, a large number of sub-Saharan Africans have also arrived in Canada in 2016, in recognition that the worldwide scale of refugee-producing situations is at an all-time high of over 19.5 million people (UNHCR, 2016). This is in addition to the 38.2 million internally displaced people and over 10 million stateless people (UNHCR, 2016). To put these numbers into perspective, that represents 1 out of every 113 people worldwide.

UNDERSTANDING HOW INTEGRATION, SETTLEMENT AND MENTAL HEALTH INTERSECT

There are many Canadians who incorrectly believe that immigrants and refugees are a drain on our social welfare resources. They believe that for refugees in particular, mental health problems will become lifelong maladies that will need to be treated and managed at great cost to the Canadian economy, and in rare incidences will pose a threat to our safety and national security. The reality is that most immigrants and refugees will not ever develop a major mental health problem, even among those who have witnessed violence and war (Beiser, 2005). This is not a recent observation. As early as 1910, Alexander Irvine (1910, p. 304), an ordained minister in the US, made this observation about the health of immigrants in his autobiography: 'it was a source of continual wonder to me that people so helpless and so neglected were as good as they were, or as healthy as they were'.

Many migrants come from the upper echelons of source countries and consequently carry with them certain benefits associated with higher socioeconomic position including better than average health. Also, the migration process by its very nature prevents the weakest immigrants and refugees from leaving their countries of origin, thus allowing those that arrive in the new country to form a selected healthy population. In addition, a formal aspect of the migration process involves passing a pre-arrival medical screening, which may serve to prevent individuals with long-term illnesses from entering a country of destination. Once in Canada, for about a decade after arrival, newcomers tend to also benefit from maintaining traditional diets brought from the old country and consequently enjoy reduced levels of obesity in relation to native-born Canadians (Sanmartin et al., 2015). Because of these features of the migration experience, researchers have proposed the term the 'healthy immigrant effect' to describe immigrants' relative physical and mental health advantage over the Canadian-born. This health-protecting feature, however, wanes with the passage of time as the immigrants become increasingly acculturated to Canadian habits and life-styles which contribute to higher rates of obesity later on.

This does not mean that immigrants and refugees are somehow insulated from poor mental and physical health. For mental health issues, the development and appearance of these tend not to happen pre-migration, nor is the migration process itself to blame. The majority of mental health problems among the newcomer population occur after their arrival and as a consequence of the uncertainties in the settlement process (Beiser, 2005; Bourque et al., 2011; Anderson et al., 2015). Most of these issues develop 10 to 24 months after arrival (Beiser, 2005). To add to the complexity, Bourque et al. (2011) explain that although the rate of disorders is small, if untreated, they can be passed along to the second generation.

Beiser (2005) reminds us that newcomers, especially those who live in communities where there are not many members from their ethnic group, may feel extremely isolated which may exacerbate mental health problems. Newcomers often lack extended family that can provide much needed support to those who are suffering. Finding culturally appropriate services in a language that newcomers can understand may be very difficult for many (George et al., 2015) and this too can affect access to services.

IMMIGRANT ADULTS

In general, the rates of mental health illness are significantly lower for immigrant adults than for all other Canadians (Beiser, 2005; Kirmayer et al., 2011a) and increase after arrival as a result of being exposed to new stressors in Canada. Anderson et al. (2015) find no difference in schizophrenia rates among immigrants, refugees, and those born in Canada. Kirmayer et al. (2011a) find that alcohol and drug dependence is lower among this group of adults than it is among those born in Canada.

Country of origin has an influence on the development of some mental health illnesses. For schizophrenia and schizoaffective disorders, immigrants from Northern and Southern Europe and those from East Asia are 50 percent less likely to develop this illness compared with newcomers from other places (Anderson et al., 2015). Prior research (Hickling and Rodgers-Johnson, 1995; Bhugra et al., 1996; Mahy et al., 1999; Hanoeman et al., 2002) shows that the incidences of these diseases were elevated compared to what they were in their country of origin, meaning that migration and post-migration experiences may influence their development within some migrant populations. Beiser (2005) warns, however, that there is likely little effect of country of origin on the development of mental health problems among immigrants. This is because most of the studies that find source-country differences are not longitudinal and what they are likely finding is 'time in Canada' effects. For instance, findings of cross-sectional studies that indicate Africans have higher rates of mental health problems likely are really finding that it is newly arrived immigrants suffering from mental health problems.

It is important to emphasize often it is the most poorly conducted studies that show the highest rates of mental illness, and methodologically rigorous studies that show much lower rates (Bourque et al., 2011; Close et al., 2016). Some of the studies do not use random sampling techniques and/or have small convenience-sized samples. As a result when these studies are used to report rates of mental illness, the numbers are significantly inflated which fuels the misperceptions about immigrants and mental health links. Bogic et al. (2015) have also identified serious deficiencies due to the inability of researchers to speak the language of the participants, thus over-estimating or misidentifying the nature of the mental health problems.

Researchers have written extensively about the factors influencing the development of mental health problems among newcomers. The consensus is that the integration process and not the migration process itself is the main contributing factor to mental health problems. These integration stressors include: prolonged poverty, periods of unemployment or under employment, loss of social status, foreign credential recognition problems, separation from family, difficulties learning a new language and culture, living in poor neighborhoods, and uncertainty about the migration decision itself (Kirmayer et al., 2011a; George et al., 2015).

Unemployment affects mental health in three ways (Beiser, 2005; George et al., 2015). First, it is inextricably linked to poverty, and this condition also increases propensity to develop mental health problems. Second, it is a frustrating, humbling experience, made more perplexing for newcomers because the promise of finding a better life in Canada can be more difficult than they imagined. Finally, lack of employment is linked to the development of addictions to alcohol, cigarettes, gambling, and illegal drugs, and that these three outcomes are a more lethal combination for newcomers. Beiser (2005) refers to this as the immigrant offshoot effect. The combination of poverty, frustration and development of addiction problems among unemployed immigrants is more likely to develop into a mental health problem than among Canadian-born unemployed persons.

Immigrants exhibit sex-differences when it comes to mental health problems. Kirmayer et al. (2011a) report that men who have difficulty learning a new language are likely to experience poor mental health outcomes because speaking good English or French is tied to having a good job, much like the immigrant offshoot effect described above. For women, post-partum depression can be a significant issue. Women are almost three times more likely to develop post-partum depression than are Canadian-born women, and it is likely to become a more entrenched problem for them owing to lack of information about post-partum depression among many immigrant communities and a reluctance to get help for this condition owing to the fear of having their children apprehended by social services (Kirmayer et al., 2011a). The good news is that women who maintain traditional health behaviors have lower risk factors for developing all sorts of mental health problems because they are less likely to participate in high-risk addictive behaviors such as smoking, alcohol and drug use (Beiser, 2005).

Accessing appropriate health services can be a challenge for newcomers. Transportation issues are particularly important for those who have newly arrived and for those living in smaller centers which may lack forms of affordable public transportation (Wilkinson et al., 2016). Culturally appropriate services are also very important, particularly when dealing with the stigma surrounding many mental health problems among some immigrant populations. Translation services are critically important as well. Some clinics are forced to rely on family members in the absence of professional interpreters. Researchers have discovered that in addition to the violation of privacy this entails, non-professional interpreters are significantly less adept at translating medical terminology correctly so communication between the clinician and patient is vastly reduced (Hansen and Houston, 2016). Professional translators should be used whenever possible because newcomers who are learning a new language may be more apt to report the physical symptoms that are linked to mental symptoms because they learn body-function words faster than emotional words. Another access problem involves the work that many newly arrived immigrants do. Those in Canada for less than three years are likely to be working in jobs where taking time off to attend a medical appointment might be impossible.

The experience of racial or ethnic discrimination has an adverse effect on mental health. The shame, stigma, disappointment, fear, and other feelings surrounding this experience can introduce or exacerbate existing mental health problems. Kirmayer et al. (2011a) find that men from Caribbean countries are more likely to develop mental health problems, likely due to higher rates of discrimination. This finding is not very surprising given the detrimental effect being victimized by discrimination has on other aspects of life including physical health, economic integration and sense of belonging (Wilkinson, 2017). Another recent study of Chinese and South Asian immigrants in Ontario reveals that Chinese Canadians have higher rates of involuntary hospital admissions, aggressive behaviors and exhibit more symptoms than those of South Asian or Canadian-born descent (Chiu et al., 2016).

REFUGEE ADULTS

Refugees face many of the same mental health challenges as immigrant adults (Beiser, 2005). Refugees typically make up between 9 percent and 20 percent of the newcomer arrivals to Canada. That number fluctuates annually owing to the status of various world conflicts. Because of these traumatic experiences, the general public sometimes assumes that all refugees are damaged, doomed to years of mental health woes, destined to become dependent on social welfare and its services. It turns out this is a false assumption. Even refugees arriving from the most gruesome and perilous conditions are more likely to be healthy than unhealthy. Recent evidence finds that among the over 20 000 Iraqi refugees that Canada sponsored between 2009 and 2014, only a small number had significant health concerns and this was a special group selected because they had serious mental or physical health problems and would unlikely be selected for permanent settlement in other countries (IRCC, 2015). Among the over 26 000 more recently arrived Syrian refugees, almost all arrived in good health (Hansen and Houston, 2016). Only two of the arrivals from Syria had 'signs of a notifiable disease . . . and were referred to public health for follow-up' (Hansen et al., 2016). It should be noted, however, that this medical screening process would only detect the most severe forms of mental health, so underlying problems may not be detected at the initial medical screening.

Post-traumatic stress disorder (PTSD), chronic pain and somatic symptoms are the conditions most prevalent among the refugee adult population (Beiser, 2005; Kirmayer et al., 2011a; IRCC, 2015). Incidence of these conditions increases as exposure to war and violence increases. For instance, Vietnamese people in Australia who witnessed three or more violent events during their refugee experience had a rate of PTSD five times higher than other refugees (Beiser, 2005). Anderson et al. (2015) also report that refugees from East Africa and Southeast Asia have higher rates of schizophrenia than other immigrants.

These conditions, however, tend to develop after their arrival in Canada and not during the migration process. The common belief is that the war conditions, witnessing or being victimized by violence ought to induce mental health problems almost immediately. It turns out that most people are more resilient and that the difficulties of integrating, particularly among forced migrants, are vastly under-estimated (George et al., 2015). Upon reflection, this makes sense. Forced migrants, by definition, would not leave their country under 'normal circumstances'. In abnormal circumstances, when people are forced from their homes under duress and threat, survival instincts may override other emotions. The struggles they must make to integrate into a new culture and way of life are complicated by loss of their past lives. Other immigrants who move to a new country do so voluntarily with the knowledge that short-term struggles will be eventually replaced by long-term success. For many refugees, starting over is not something they had planned for and this may induce some mental health problems. This idea is reinforced when we examine the list of protective factors preventing the development of mental health problems among refugee adults. According to Beiser (2005), having a good job and relationship are factors influencing positive mental health. Interestingly, underemployment has no positive or negative influence on the development of mental health issues among refugees, a finding reinforced by more recent research (George et al., 2015).

There are, however, unique structural issues that influence the propensity of refugees to develop mental health problems. They are significantly more likely to be impoverished and for much longer periods of time because they are more likely to need to learn English or French. Only three out of ten refugees know one of Canada's official languages prior to arrival. This means that the entrance into paid labor is prolonged for refugees, so the poverty/unemployment link to mental health among refugees is exacerbated. Having been exposed to trauma, war and violence also increases mental health problems. Living in a refugee camp means that life is usually put 'on hold' for adults. Most refugee camps and the countries who host the majority of the world's refugees do not allow them to work for pay – so many adults languish in the camps for years with nothing meaningful to do. Furthermore, refugee camps are not safe places. There is little in the way of policing in many camps, and assaults and theft are common. Living in these conditions adds to the sense of misery that some refugees experience. Separation from family members also adds to the stresses that refugees may face. Wondering about the safety of loved ones is a major source of anxiety.

Accessing services can be a problem for refugees. Refugees have the same linguistic and cultural challenges as other immigrant groups and they are more likely to experience these barriers. As a result, unmet health needs are a challenge. The years in refugee camps and the prolonged migration process mean that many refugees have significant unmet physical and mental health needs, which are often long term. Hansen and Houston (2016, p. 5) urge health-care practitioners that the best way to assist refugees is to '"bear witness" to the(ir) pain and suffering'. Acknowledging their trauma and experiences can be beneficial in creating a rapport with refugee patients. Understanding that the development of trust and confidence may take more time than with other patients is also important.

IMMIGRANT CHILDREN AND YOUTH

The prevalence of mental health problems among immigrant children and youth varies, but multiple studies suggest that the incidence is still lower than among Canadian-born children and youth. Research suggests that about one in ten immigrant youth experiences some sort of mental health problem compared with only 15 percent of the Canadian born population (Leitch, 2007; PHAC, 2009; Wilkinson et al., 2010; Kirmayer et al., 2011a; CMHA, 2016). It is important that any mental health problem that surfaces in childhood or in young adults be treated promptly because about 80 percent of all mental health problems in adulthood can be traced to issues in childhood (Leitch, 2007). Mental health patterns among immigrant children are very similar to those who were born in Canada. Immigrants who arrive in Canada prior to their twelfth birthday have the same rates of mental health problems as those born in Canada (Kirmayer et al., 2011a, George et al., 2015). Most newcomer children 'do exceptionally well and some surpass their native-born peers in aspiration and academic achievement' (Kirmayer et al., 2011a, p. 962).

The top mental health problems experienced by immigrant children and youth are anxiety (43 percent) and depression (27 percent) (Costello et al., 2004; Pacione et al., 2013). Some country of origin differences have been observed, for example, Vietnamese and Hong Kong Chinese children have higher rates of distress (Beiser et al., 2014; George et al., 2015) than those from other ethnic groups. Females are more likely to experience a mental health problem than males in this age group (World Health Organization, 2006; Cooper, 2013; Guruge and Butt, 2015).

Children and youth who have experienced discrimination have higher rates of mental health problems (George et al., 2015). The health of parents plays a large role in the development of health problems among children and youth. Beiser et al. (2003) find that parents who cannot speak English or French, and thus have difficulties integrating into the labor market, pass this stress along to their children. Families headed by lone females also are more likely to have children experiencing some sort of mental health problem (George et al., 2015). Among Mainland and Hong Kong Chinese and Filipino/a families, those practicing harsh parenting styles, who are experiencing integration difficulties, who have inter-generational conflict and have one parent with depressive symptoms are more likely to have children with emotional problems (Beiser et al., 2014). An older study by Ahearn and Athey (1991) reveals that the role-reversal effect can have negative mental health consequences for immigrant youth. In the short term, youth may find themselves in a pseudo-parental role, meaning that they act as translators and cultural brokers for their parents because they learn the new language much faster. As a result, they are doing 'adult' activities such as banking, health care, and other things normally done by parents. When their parents finally become fluent in the language, they try to re-take the parental role. This loss of power within the family causes inter-generational conflict and can create stress problems among some immigrant youth.

The good news is that there are some factors that protect immigrant youth and encourage good mental health. A study by Wilkinson et al. (2010) reveals that smoking, drinking and illegal drug use are significantly lower among immigrant youth and their peers who were born in Canada. Youth who know one of Canada's official languages prior to arrival, or learn that language quickly, have lower rates of mental health problems. Protection of heritage culture is also seen as a buffer against the development of various mental health problems (George et al., 2015). Arriving in Canada with an intact family, who have active affiliations with a religious group, and have a sense of cultural pride are also less likely to develop mental health problems (George et al., 2015). An immigrant paradox is also apparent among immigrant children and youth, according to Beiser (2005). Despite the fact that immigrant children and youth are three times more likely to be living in an impoverished family, they are less likely to experience emotional and behavioral problems than Canadian-born children in similar family situations.

REFUGEE CHILDREN AND YOUTH

Refugee children and youth tend to experience higher rates of adverse mental health outcomes than other newcomer youth. According to Kirmayer et al. (2011a, 2011b), refugee children and youth have ten times higher rates of PTSD than any other child group. They have higher rates of depression, distress, chronic pain and somatic symptoms. Adjustment disorders, sleep disturbances, nightmares, grief reactions, inattention, social withdrawal, and somatization are seen at increased rates among refugee children and youth (Pacione et al., 2013). The belief is that these mental health problems may be linked to having witnessed or possibly experienced torture and other forms of violence. According to Pacione et al. (2013), the rates of PTSD among those who have been abducted, forced to hide or among those who have hurt or killed other family members are much higher than expected. Those who have experienced rape, death of a parent or who were forced to fight have high rates of depression (Pacione et al., 2013). PTSD might actually be a normal response to violence in these cases. Refugee children and youth who do develop these problems tend to have a more difficult time recovering (Lustig et al., 2004; Carlson, 2005).

As with their parents, there are country of origin differences among children. Among the over 20000 Iraqi refugees arriving in Canada between 2009 and 2014, the most common mental health condition among children and youth was cognitive delays, autism and PTSD (IRCC, 2015). Somali youth are more likely to exhibit depression (Guruge and Butt, 2015). Oppositional, aggressive, impulsive, hyperactive, and anti-social behaviors are more prevalent in boys, and are even more predominant among those who have witnessed violence (Pacione et al., 2013). For girls, the issues tend to be self esteem and self doubt. There appears to be no sex differences in the development of PTSD.

What differentiates the refugee youth experience of mental health from other immigrant youth is pre-arrival conditions. Refugee children and youth are significantly more likely to have serious gaps in their education prior to arrival. Once in Canada, trying to make up for lost time and to 'catch-up' with their peers can cause emotional distress. Refugee children and youth are also more likely to have experienced separation from one or both parents. This causes anxiety. As victims of war and trauma, they are more likely to have been exposed to violence and this too contributes to anxiety and other mental health conditions. Living in a refugee camp and all the unsafe conditions that go with it increase the likelihood of problems developing. There are a staggering number of unaccompanied minors and the scant evidence available suggests that their unstable living conditions and time away from family and friends contribute to mental and behavioral problems.

CLINICAL CONSIDERATIONS AND RESILIENCE FACTORS

Omar and Ibrahim

Omar and Ibrahim, the two teen-aged brothers mentioned at the beginning of the chapter, and their mother come to your clinic several months after fleeing Syria and arriving in Canada. You may be a physician, a nurse, a social worker, or other community-based health worker. As we have just seen, these brothers, as refugee youth arriving in Canada, are at increased risk of developing mental health problems, including PTSD. We have also seen that they and their mother may be at increased risk of multiple somatic symptoms, chronic pain, and schizophrenia. Regardless of whether this risk is mostly due to pre-migration exposures or because of the migration and integration process itself, we can conceptualize this process as a latent risk that may express itself under stressful integration conditions, or remain dormant, under more ideal conditions once in Canada. When they arrive at your clinic, you do not have a good sense of what might be happening with them at the moment or if mental health problems will manifest later in their integration journey.

In this sense, mental health conditions share a similarity with other conditions affecting migrants, such as tuberculosis: after a primary exposure, usually pre-migration, this disease can reactivate under stressful resettlement conditions. Similarly, refugees can face traumatizing exposures pre-arrival that may only manifest when integrating into Canadian society. Our goal, therefore, is to help promote positive integration and resilience so that these conditions are more likely to remain dormant. We thus now turn to strategies to help this family maintain resilience, and we start with clinical considerations.

The most important way to help this family initially is to establish trust with the treating team. Evidence shows that screening (enquiring about a condition in every client, as opposed to responding to obvious signs of distress, which is clearly indicated) for conditions such a major depression or PTSD too early, before a migrant trusts the clinical milieu and knows who to turn to if questions trigger traumatic memories, can unnecessarily upset clients and cause more harm than good (Kirmayer et al., 2011b). Assuming the clinician has access to an effective and culturally sensitive treatment plan, screening can be considered after a period of integration of some months (Kirmayer et al., 2011b).

While screening too early comes with these caveats, responding immediately to an impression of emotional disturbance is crucial and can also save the client and the system more complex needs, such as emergency room visits and hospitalizations. Mental illness is akin to certain physical ailments in that it can present suddenly after a period of latency. Tuberculosis infection, for example, is well known for expressing itself years after an initial asymptomatic phase, often during times of accrued stress and reduced immune response. Similarly, lived traumas can 'prime' migrants to relive their effects during times of stress in a new society.

For most mental health concerns such as mild anxiety and depression, care should be given at the primary care level by a family doctor or other provider, assuming that certain cultural accommodations are in place (Table 6.1). Most important are the knowledge of basic approaches to interviewing using a translator and the availability of a translator not related to the clients, for confidentiality purposes. Even a translator from the same cultural group as the client may be a perceived confidentiality threat owing to their proximity to their ethno-cultural community, and extra assurances or alternate arrangements may have to be arranged. An interesting line of inquiry is currently looking at the use of real-time translation applications to use in such instances (Lepeska, 2016). Other times, translators in other provinces are connected to the patient and physician by telephone when translation services cannot be accessed readily. Certainly, any efforts to communicate a few words in the client's language will be an aid to establish relationship and trust.

Although family members should be used for translation purposes only in emergency situations, every opportunity should be taken to interview families together as part of the visit, for several reasons. First, general orientation to a new medical system is done efficiently in a group setting, as clarifying questions benefit everyone present. Second, getting a family member's perspective on a client's problem – with that client's permission of course – can prove invaluable both diagnostically and therapeutically. Third, after the visit, family members can more easily compare 'notes' and clarify questions with one another because they were all in the same room. Finally, the migration experience can engender intergenerational conflict

Table 6.1 Accommodations in the clinical milieu

Strategy	Comments
Orientation to the health system, appointments, procedures etc.	Clients may not be aware of primary care having a triage or gatekeeper role in certain countries (e.g. Canada), and may need education regarding the appropriate use of emergency rooms and specialists
Translators	Do not use family members except in emergencies. Place translator in a neutral position to be able to focus on the client. Ask the translator to indicate areas of ambivalence or nuance, especially when it comes to expressions of mental suffering
Special language accommodations	Consider the use of language-specific telephone lines, signage, and patient navigators
Stepped or integrated approaches	Stepped: as much as possible, referrals to allied health and specialist should occur in environments already familiar to the client Integrated: in essence, giving the right intervention to the right client at the right time*
Establishing trust, confidentiality	Consistent providers as much as possible; extra time for visits; eliciting all concerns and approaching them over several visits
Linkage with culture-specific resources and community organizations	For a list see www.ementalhealth.ca

Note: * For a useful list of integrated approached to different mental health presentations, see http://www.camh.ca/en/hospital/care_program_and_services/ICPs/Pages/default.aspx (accessed 30 June 2017).

Source: Mental Health Commission of Canada (2016).

that a family interview can elicit and clarify. However any suspicion of vulnerability, especially among women and adolescents, should lead to a private interview as well in order to screen for domestic violence or other sensitive topics.

It is important for the clinician not to assume pathology in their immigrant and refugee clients. Pathologizing normal grief reactions or traumatic memories that do not affect present function does not serve to enhance the client–clinician relationship, nor does it serve to enhance well-being. Unfortunately it is a common human reaction (CMAJ, 2016). It is more helpful, however, to explore how hardship may have increased the client's strength, and how the migration journey may have offered new meanings and opportunities in their lives. As we shall see, the basis of narrative exposure therapy (NET) is work in placing past traumas in the context of these overarching strengths.

Promoting Resilience

The Mental Health Commission of Canada has recently released a comprehensive report on strategies to address the mental health of immigrant, refugee, ethno-cultural and racialized (IRER) populations (Mental Health Commission of Canada, 2016). This important resource argues above all for more emphasis on the social determinants of health in IRER populations, including employment, housing, and other initiatives to enhance the physical environment of new Canadians.

The *Case for Diversity* report also usefully reviews considerations for the clinical milieu that are evidence based, and suggests where more evidence is needed (Mental Health Commission of Canada, 2016). For example, although some of the cultural accommodations in Table 6.2 have, according to the report, 'cachet' and are widely accepted, evidence is still sometimes lacking beyond specific IRER populations (for example, immigrant youth) or clinical scenarios (for example, substance misuse).

Evidence is strong, however, when it comes to the use of specific approaches such as Narrative Exposure Therapy (NET) (McPherson, 2012) and Eye Movement Desensitization and Reprocessing (EMDR), especially in refugee clients. NET is a particularly compelling approach that tries to unlink the physiological response to a traumatic memory from the current and evolving reality of the client. The use of visual aids such as string to represent the client's overall life journey, stones to represent traumas, and flowers to represent hopes and aspirations have become popular, but are optional and not as evidence-based.

Finally, it is important to note innovative research that is occurring in other jurisdictions receiving high numbers of refugees. In Germany, for example, researchers are using spatial techniques such as ecological momentary assessment (Abbot, 2016) to determine whether feelings of suspicion and perceived discrimination can partially be explained by the migrant's daily movements through the built environment.

Table 6.2 Formulation of risk-factor severity, resultant symptomatology and clinical approach

Risk level	Examples of risk factors	Indicative symptomatology	Clinical approach
Low	Voluntary relocation	No effect on activities, work, school etc.	Ongoing monitoring; consider screening after some months post-arrival in selected populations
Medium	Witnessed natural disasters	Symptoms of depression, anxiety or PTSD: flashbacks, hypervigilance, avoidance; Irritability or withdrawal in children and youth	Support in primary care setting with or without extra individual or group counseling; consider referral and/or pharmacotherapy if lifestyle interventions (exercise, community activities; sleep hygiene etc.) are unsuccessful
High	Witnessed or experienced human brutality; extensive family symptomatology	Severe depression, anxiety or PTSD; Suicidal or homicidal ideation; psychosis; be on the lookout for aggressive or self-harming behaviors among youth	Early intervention, close follow-up, specialist referral; consider NET and EMDR approaches. Will likely also need pharmacotherapy

Note: NET – narrative exposure therapy; EMDR – eye movement desensitization and reprocessing.

Source: Canadian Pediatric Society (2016).

Our Case, Revisited

Omar and Ibrahim may or may not have formal PTSD. It may be somewhat academic to compile their symptoms against precise criteria for the clinical disorder, as the persistent and severe effects of their traumas will need intervention. This may involve a combination of self-care, formal counseling, and medication, depending on risk assessment (Table 6.2). What is certain however is that their migration experience has left them with certain vulnerabilities that are now translating to self-medication through abusing drugs and other potentially risky behaviors, and they need to be managed in a culturally sensitive, integrated care environment.

The brothers are at high risk according to our formulation and should be followed closely and referred for more specialized counseling, potentially including EMDR. The astute clinician will also utilize NET techniques to work with the brothers' sense of hope, aspiration, and personal meaning (Frankl, 1984) to see how the obstacles that they have overcome can actually lead to increasing resilience. Efforts should also be made to link them to community organizations that will help secure better living conditions.

Gradually, as you explore the narratives of their migration journey, the brothers improve and are able to remember their father's death as a reason to honor his memory and make their mother proud for the accomplishments in their new society.

CONSIDERATIONS FOR FUTURE RESEARCH

We have seen how the literature on the mental health of immigrant and refugees coming to Canada is quite heterogeneous. In general, studies of lesser methodological quality tend to overestimate rates of mental illness as compared to larger, more rigorous studies. Survey-type studies of newcomers themselves suffer additional problems to do with recall bias, or under- or over-reporting. That is, there is much myth and misinformation about the mental health experiences of immigrants and refugees and we hope this chapter is one step in resolving some of these misconceptions.

There are multiple, limited data sources on migration health in Canada, each with their own opportunities and shortcomings. Let us first look at the Immigration Medical Exam (IME). Not only is the IME based on self-reporting, but it is also not meant to exhaustively detect disease. Rather, it is currently geared towards reliably detecting conditions of significance to public health or public safety. In certain cases (not for refugees or family class applicants), it can also detect conditions that may place an excessive demand on the Canadian publicly funded health system.

Thus, contrary to common perception, the IME only contains a few mandatory tests, mostly geared to detecting communicable diseases, such as tuberculosis. These do not preclude migration if they prove treatable. As for mental health conditions, they would have to be very severe to be identified at the IME screening stage, and flagrant or violent to be considered a risk to public safety. This explains why this source of data, along with data available from ports of entry (Hansen et al., 2016), tends to provide a very low incidence of mental health conditions.

In future studies, data from the Interim Federal Health Program (IFHP) could be examined, although this source too has limitations. This program is only available to certain classes of migrants, namely, refugees, and as its name suggests, it is a transitional program meant to bridge clients for one year, before provincial programs become available. The program has a basic package of benefits including doctor's visits, and a supplementary benefit package that includes vision, dental, pharmaceuticals and counseling up to 20 sessions a year after proper referral and justification from a clinician.

Certain provinces assume responsibility for the basic package more quickly than others, and in some instances this occurs almost immediately upon arrival. In addition, coverage for pharmaceuticals may be assumed by provinces before the one-year threshold. This makes the IFHP as a source of data complex and heterogeneous.

Thus, there is an opportunity to create large-scale national data linkages to more precisely examine the burden of mental disease in migrants of various types. For example, the Immigrant Landing File and the Canadian Institute of Health Information administered Discharge Abstract Database would make a compelling linkage to examine differential patterns of hospital admissions related to mental health. This would only report the most severe cases of mental health conditions, those requiring hospital admission, and leave other opportunities for more work at the community-practitioner level. Recent examples of such work (Vigod et al., 2016) are compelling, and are setting the stage for future work on better understanding major movements of migrants to Canada, including that of the recent Syrian refugees.

It will take a mosaic of approaches to fill in the gaps in our understanding of the mental health of immigrants to Canada. It will be imperative for future studies to examine the factors leading to resilience in this same population. Clinical experience shows that it is hard to predict which clients will do well and which will struggle to integrate because of mental disease or other reasons. It is clear, however, that those migrants who are able to place their traumas in context, and even to draw strength from them, will thrive in their new society.

Immigrants and refugees face significant barriers in accessing the mental health system. This understanding and action towards dealing with their problems can benefit all Canadians, and change within the health care system can become more systematic. Patient navigators, for example, are increasingly being utilized to increase coordination, effectiveness and efficiency of interventions for clients with other complex needs.

Finally, we want to mention the effects that clinicians and other caregivers – including sponsoring families and members of sponsoring organizations – can experience when caring for trauma-stricken immigrants and refugees. We mention this phenomenon not to compare it to the personal traumas or tragedies faced by certain migrants, nor to minimize these in any way, but to point to an important issue variously referred to in the literature as secondary stress or compassion fatigue among clinical caregivers. The reality of caregiver burnout is real, and clinicians should be on the lookout for signs of this in themselves, and in their colleagues. Common signs include fatigue, irritability, unexplained physical symptoms and questioning your calling or choice of practice (Portnoy, 2011).

Secondary stress is treatable, but only if recognized and not ignored. As with migrants themselves, signs can be delayed. As Romeo Dallaire (2004, p. 52), the UN peacekeeper who witnessed horrific tragedies in the Rwandan genocide has eloquently written, in a passage that strikes true for migrants and their caregivers alike:

> I could not divorce myself from Rwanda. I'm not even sure I could say the war was over; I was still living it. I kept two huge filing cabinets, full of my notes, cables, documents and photos, beside my bed. Locked inside, I had the whole genocide. The presence of those files was like something alive, pulsing in the corner, waiting to strike.

CONCLUSION

It is clear from this chapter that although immigrants and refugees of all ages experience various kinds of mental health problems, there is much variation. Immigrants, regardless of their age, tend to have significantly lower rates of mental health problems and these stem mainly from the process of integration, rather than the migration process itself. Refugees tend to have much higher rates of mental health illness and these too are exacerbated by the integration process but might have their origin in the experience of violence and conflict prior to arrival. Contrary to popular belief, the development of mental health issues among the refugee population occurs after resettlement, usually in the first six to 24 months. That is, refugees do not arrive in Canada with major mental health problems; these tend to develop later as a result of both integration and pre-arrival experiences and events.

The challenges to addressing the mental health needs of immigrant and refugee populations share some similarities and differences. Language proficiency, extended rates of poverty and unemployment, and integration into a new culture are common themes for both groups. Clinicians who are aware of these issues should be better able to address the mental health needs of this group. The issues for refugees are exacerbated by pre-arrival experiences, the role reversal between parent and child in some families and the experience of violence and trauma. More specialized and extended care may be needed.

NOTE

* The views expressed in this chapter are those of the authors and do not necessarily represent the views of Immigration, Refugees and Citizenship Canada.

REFERENCES

Abbot, A. (2016), 'German psychiatrist plans to scan the brains of refugees', *Nature News*, 4 August, accessed 20 October 2016 at http://www.nature.com/news/german-psychiatrist-plans-to-scan-the-brains-of-refugees-1.20340.

Ahearn, F.L. and J.L. Athey (1991), 'The mental health of refugee children: an overview', in F. Ahearn and J. Athey (eds), *Refugee Children: Theory Research and Services*, Baltimore, MD and London: Johns Hopkins University Press.

Anderson, K.K., J. Cheng, E. Susser, K.J. McKenzie and P. Kurdyak (2015), 'Incidence of psychotic disorders among first-generation immigrants and refugees in Ontario', *Canadian Medical Association Journal*, **187** (9), E279–E286, doi:10.1503/cmaj.14120.

Beiser, M. (2005), 'The health of immigrants and refugees in Canada', *Canadian Review of Public Health*, **96** (2), 30–44.

Beiser, M., A.M. Goodwill, P. Albanese, K. McShane and N. Nowakowski (2014), 'Predictors of immigrant children's mental health in Canada: selection, settlement contingencies, culture or all of the above?', *Social Psychiatry and Epidemiology*, **49** (5), 743–56, doi:10.1007zs00127-013-0794-8.

Beiser, M., L. Simich and K.A.S. Wickrama (2003), 'Sponsorship and resettlement success', *Journal of International Migration and Integration*, **4** (3), 203–16.

Bhugra, D., M. Hilwig and B. Hossein (1996), 'First-contact incidence of rates of schizophrenia in Trinidad and one-year follow-up', *British Journal of Psychiatry*, **169** (5), 587–92.

Bogic, M., A. Njoku and S. Priebe (2015), 'Long-term mental health of war-refugees: a systematic literature review', *BMC International Health and Human Rights*, **15** (29), 2–41, accessed 18 October 2016 at https://bmcinthealthhumrights.biomedcentral.com/articles/10.1186/s12914-015-0064-9.

Bourque, F., E. Van Der Ven and A. Malla (2011), 'A meta analysis of the risk for psychotic disorders among first- and second-generation immigrants', *Psychological Medicine*, **41** (5), 897–910, accessed 3 November 2016 at https://www.researchgate.net/profile/Elsje_Van_Der_Ven/publication/45388223_A_meta-analysis_of_the_risk_for_psychotic_disorders_among_first-_and_second-generation_immigrants_Psychol_Med/links/0c96053be6759a67d6000000.pdf.

Canadian Medical Association Journal (CMAJ) (2016), Editorial, 'Don't automatically label Syrian refugees as mentally ill', *Canadian Medical Association Journal*, 22 February, accessed 20 October 2016 at http://www.cmaj.ca/content/early/2016/02/22/cmaj.109-5239.full.pdf.

Canadian Mental Health Association (CMHA) (2016), 'Fast facts about mental

illness', accessed 9 November 2016 at http://www.cmha.ca/media/fast-facts-about-mental-illness/#.V64CwKKPssY.
Canadian Pediatric Society (2016), 'Caring for kids new to Canada', accessed 20 October 2016 at http://www.kidsnewtocanada.ca/mental-health/ptsd.
Carlson, J.M. (2005), 'Mental health and health related quality of life in tortured refugees', working paper, Faculty of Health Sciences University of Copenhagen, Copenhagen.
Chiu, M., M. Lebenbaum, A.M. Newman, J. Zaheer and P. Kurdak (2016), 'Ethnic differences in mental illness severity: a population-based study of Chinese and South Asian patients in Ontario, Canada', *Clinical Psychiatry*, **77** (9), 1108–16.
Citizenship and Immigration Canada (2016), *Facts and Figures 2015: Immigration Overview*, Ottawa: Citizenship and Immigration Canada, accessed 20 October 2016 at http://open.canada.ca/data/en/dataset/2fbb56bd-eae7-4582-af7d-a197d185fc93.
Close, C., A. Kouvonen, T. Bosqui, K. Patel, D. O'Reilly and M. Donnelly (2016), 'The mental health and wellbeing of first generation migrants: a systematic-narrative review of reviews', *Global Health*, **12** (47), 47–60, accessed 17 December 2016 at http://www.ncbi.nlm.nih.gov/pubmed/27558472.
Cooper, G. (2013), 'Social and emotional learning in Canada', Carthy Foundation Issue Brief, accessed at http://www.maxbell.org/sites/default/files/SELIssueBrief.pdf.
Costello, E.J., H.L. Egger and A. Angold (2004), 'Developmental epidemiology of anxiety disorders', in T.L. Morris and J.S. March (eds), *Phobic and Anxiety Disorders in Children and Adolescents: A Clinician's Guide to Effective Psychosocial and Pharmacological Interventions*, New York: Oxford University Press, pp. 61–91.
Dallaire, R. (2004), *Shake Hands with the Devil: The Failure of Humanity in Rwanda*, Toronto: Vintage Canada.
Frankl, V.E. (1984), *Man's Search for Meaning*, Toronto: Pocket Books.
George, U., M.S. Thomson, F. Chaze and S. Guruge (2015), 'Immigrant mental health, a public health issue: looking back and looking forward', *Environmental Research and Public Health*, **12** (October), 13624–48, doi:10.3390/ijerph121013624.
Guruge, S. and H. Butt (2015), 'A scoping review of mental health issues and concerns among immigrant and refugee children in Canada: looking back, moving forward', *Canadian Review of Public Health*, **106** (2), 72–8.
Hanoeman, M., J.P. Selten and R. S. Kahn (2002), 'Incidence of schizophrenia in Surinam', *Schizophrenia Research*, **54** (3), 219–21.
Hansen, L. and P. Houston (2016), 'Health considerations in the Syrian refugee resettlement process in Canada', *Canadian Communicable Disease Report Supplement*, **42** (2), S3–S7, accessed 20 October 2016 at http://www.phac-aspc.gc.ca/publicat/ccdr-rmtc/16vol42/dr-rm42-s2/ar-02-eng.php.
Hansen, L., L. Maidment and R. Ahmad (2016), 'Early observations on the health of Syrian refugees in Canada', *Canadian Communicable Disease Report Supplement*, **42** (S2), 1–3, accessed 20 October 2016 at http://www.phac-aspc.gc.ca/publicat/ccdr-rmtc/16vol42/dr-rm42-s2/ar-03-eng.php.
Hickling, F.W. and P. Rodgers-Johnson (1995), 'The incidence of first contact schizophrenia in Jamaica', *British Journal of Psychiatry*, **167** (2), 193–6.
Immigration Refugees and Citizenship Canada (IRCC) (2015), *Summary of*

Preliminary Findings: Iraqi Resettlement (2009–2014) Case Study, Ottawa: IRCC, April, acquired through access to information request.

Immigration Refugees and Citizenship Canada (IRCC) (2016), *Syrian Refugees: What We Did*, Ottawa: IRCC, accessed 3 November 2016 at http://www.cic.gc.ca/english/refugees/welcome/index.asp.

Irvine, A.F. (1910), *From the Bottom Up: The Life Story of Alexander Irvine*, New York: Doubleday, Page & Co, accessed 12 May 2016 at http://solomon.imld.alexanderstreet.com.uml.idm.oclc.org/cgi-bin/asp/philo/getobject.pl?c.3659:1.imld.3623.3630.

Kirmayer, L.J., L. Narasiah, M. Munoz, M. Rashid, A.G. Ryder, J. Guzder, et al. (2011a), 'Common mental health problems in immigrants and refugees: general approach to primary care', *Canadian Medical Association Journal*, **183** (12), 959–67.

Kirmayer, L.J., L. Narasiah, A.G. Ryder G. Burgos, P. Zelkowitz, K. Pottie and P. Kutcher. (2011b), 'Appendix 10: Depression: evidence review for newly arriving immigrants and refugees', in 'Guidelines for immigrant health – Canadian collaboration for immigrant and refugee health', *Canadian Medical Association Journal*, **198** (12), 959–67, accessed 9 February 2013 at http://www.cmaj.ca/content/suppl/2010/06/07/cmaj.090313.DC1/imm-depress-10-at.pdf.

Leitch, K.K. (2007), 'Reaching for the top: a report by the advisor on healthy children and youth, 8 mental health and chronic illness', accessed 29 September 2008 at http://www.hc-sc.gc.ca/hl-vs/pubs/child-enfant/advisor-conseillere/mental-eng.php.

Lepeska, D. (2016), 'Refugees and the technology of exile', *Wilson Quarterly*, accessed 10 August 2016 at http://wilsonquarterly.com/quarterly/looking-back-moving-forward/refugees-and-the-technology-of-exile/.

Lustig, S., M. Kia-Keating, G.W. Knight, P. Geltman, H. Ellis and D.J. Kinzie (2004), 'Review of child and adolescent refugee mental health', *Journal of the American Academy of Child and Adolescent Psychiatry*, **43** (1), 24–36.

Mahy, G.E., R. Mallet and J. Leff (1999), 'First-contact incidence rate of schizophrenia on Barbados', *British Journal of Psychiatry*, **175** (1), 28–33.

McPherson, J. (2012), 'Does narrative exposure therapy reduce PTSD in survivors of mass violence?', *Research on Social Work Practice*, **22** (1), 29–42.

Mental Health Commission of Canada (2016), *The Case for Diversity: Building the Case to Improve Mental Health Services for Immigrant, Refugee, Ethno-Cultural and Racialized Populations*, Ottawa: Mental Health Commission of Canada.

Pacione, L., T. Measham and C. Rousseau (2013), 'Refugee children: mental health and effective interventions', *Child and Adolescent Disorders*, **15**, 332–41, doi:10.1007/s11920-012-0341-4.

Portnoy, D. (2011), 'Burnout and compassion fatigue: watch for the signs', *Health Progress*, **15** (2), 47–53, accessed 10 August 2016 at http://www.compassionfatigue.org/pages/healthprogress.pdf.

Public Health Agency of Canada (PHAC) (2009), 'Report: the state of public health in Canada 2009', accessed 18 October 2016 at http://www.phac-aspc.gc.ca/cphorsphc-respcacsp/2009/fr-rc/index-eng.php.

Sanmartin, C.D., D.N. Manuel and J.V. Tu (2015), 'All-cause circulatory disease-related hospitalization, by generation status: evidence from linked data', *Health Reports*, **26** (10), Cat 82-003x. Statistics Canada, Health Analysis Division, Ottawa, accessed 8 November 2016 at http://www.statcan.gc.ca/pub/82-003-x/2015010/article/14227-eng.htm.

Statistics Canada (2012), *Population Estimates*, Ottawa: Statistics Canada.
United Nations High Commissioner for Refugees (UNHCR) (2016), *Refugee Statistics*, Geneva and New York: UNHCR, accessed 3 November 2016 at http://www.unhcr.ca/what-we-do/who-we-help/.
Vigod, S., A. Sultana, K. Fund, N. Hussain-Shamsy and C.L. Dennis (2016), 'A population-based study of postpartum mental health service use by immigrant women in Ontario, Canada', *Canadian Journal of Psychiatry*, **61** (11), 705–13, accessed 19 October 2016 at http://www.ices.on.ca/Publications/Journal-Articles/2016/January/A-population-based-study-of-postpartum-mental-health-service-use-by-immigrant-women-in-Ontario.
Wilkinson, L. (2017), 'Identity and belonging in the second generation', in S. Wilson-Forsberg (ed.), *Immigrant Youth in Canada*, Don Mills, ON: Oxford University Press (in press).
Wilkinson, L., J. Anchan, N. Arthur, E. Blum, E. Burgess Pinto, J. Fernandes et al. (2010), 'A portrait of the health and well-being of newcomer youth in the Canadian Prairies', working paper, Prairie Metropolis Centre, Edmonton.
Wilkinson, L., J. Bucklaschuk, Y.J. Shen, I.A. Chowdhury and T. Edkins (2016), 'What do we know about the settlement outcomes of immigrants to Canada?', Citizenship and Immigration Canada, Ottawa.
World Health Organization (2006), 'Health behavior in school aged children: healthy settings for young people in Canada', accessed 30 June 2017 at http://www.euro.who.int/en/health-topics/Life-stages/child-and-adolescent-health/child-and-adolescent-health2/youth-friendly-services/health-behaviour-in-school-aged-children-hbsc2.-who-collaborative-cross-national-study-of-children-aged-1115.

7. The immigrant mortality advantage in Canada*

Frank Trovato

INTRODUCTION

In Canada, the immigrant population enjoys lower death rates than do native-born Canadians (Vang et al., 2016). Canadian studies have looked at differences in general (all-cause) mortality or life expectancy (for example, Sharma et al., 1990; Chan et al., 1996; Trovato and Odynak, 2011; Omariba et al., 2014) as well as variations by cause of death (for example, Nair et al., 1990; Trovato and Odynak, 2011). Two primary questions motivate the present work: (1) is the immigrant mortality advantage a function of low death rates on few but highly influential causes, or is it a function of uniformly low mortality across all causes of death? (2) How do health selection and acculturation interact to produce the immigrant mortality advantage?

FACTORS THAT PROMOTE AND ERODE THE MIGRANT MORTALITY ADVANTAGE

The immigrant mortality advantage seems paradoxical because migrants often fall in the lower socioeconomic ranks of their host societies, and lower economic status is typically associated with higher, not lower, mortality. In the American context phrases such as 'mortality paradox' and 'epidemiological paradox' have appeared to describe the unexpected lower death rates of Hispanics and Latinos, many of whom are first generation immigrants (Markides and Coreil, 1986; Abraido-Lanza et al., 1999; Franzini et al., 2000; Singh and Siahpush, 2001; Palloni and Arias, 2004; Markides and Eschbach, 2005; Balfour et al., 2016; Singer et al., 2017). Studies based on the experience of other countries also indicate that socioeconomic differences do not explain away the migrant mortality advantage (Khlat, 1993; Khlat and Darmon, 2003; Anson, 2004; Deboosere and Gadeyne, 2005). It has been suggested that this differential may be a data artefact generated by undercounting in the vital statistics mortality data thereby artificially deflating immigrant death rates (Weitoft et al., 1999; Wallace and Kulu, 2014a). However, the consistency of this phenomenon across so many different national settings casts doubt on the artefact explanation (Brahimi, 1980; Marmot et al., 1984; Vallin, 1985; Young, 1987; Kliewer 1992; Razum et al., 1998; Abraido-Lanza et al., 1999; Palloni and Arias, 2003; Jasso et al., 2004; DesMeules, 2005; Trovato and Odynak, 2011; Wallace and Kulu, 2014b; Ikram et al., 2016).

Another hypothesis, the selection explanation, proposes that migrants represent a physically and psychologically healthy subset of people, and as such share a health and mortality advantage in relation to both their origin and destination populations (Kliewer, 1992; Khlat and Darmon, 2003; Newbold and Danforth, 2003; Jasso et al., 2004; McDonald and Kennedy, 2004; Newbold, 2005, 2009; Chiswick et al., 2008; Ng, 2011; Wallace and Kulu, 2013, 2014b; Kennedy et al., 2015; Vang et al., 2016; Wallace, 2016). The 'salmon bias' has also been mentioned as a possible contributing factor to the migrant mortality advantage. This thesis assumes that the least healthy and adaptable elements of the migrant population opt to return to the home country. To the extent that this occurs, this process would result in a filtering out of those with lower survival probabilities, and as a consequence would help raise the overall survival profile of the remaining immigrant population (Jasso et al., 2004; Palloni and Arias, 2004; Palloni and Ewbank, 2004; Markides and Eschbach, 2005; Wallace and Kulu, 2013). This type of phenomenon may prevail in settings where the geographical distance separating origin and destination countries is relatively short and where health care is less accessible by immigrants (Diaz et al., 2016). This situation would not seem applicable in Canada, as the vast majority of immigrants are from distant source countries with relatively less developed health care systems (Kliewer, 1992; Khlat, 1993; Turra and Elo, 2008; Leung, 2014).

A migrant mortality advantage may result from salutogenic features inherent in the immigrant population itself, including the maintenance of traditional norms, practices and orientations brought from the old country. It has been noted, for instance, that South European migrants enjoy low mortality from certain chronic diseases, particularly heart disease, because of their healthy Mediterranean diet (Khlat, 1993; Young, 1987; Powles, 1990). Smoking prevalence in the immigrant population may be low, thereby accounting for reduced mortality from major diseases such as lung cancer and vascular complications in particular (Geddes et al., 1993; Balzi et al., 1994; Fenelon, 2013). Immigrants may also benefit from the intensity of social supports and informal networks (Berkman and Glass, 2000; Kawachi and Berkman, 2000) present in the immigrant ethnic community. Among its many functions, the community can act as a buffer against severe distress and personal crises that may often lead to premature mortality (Trovato and Jarvis, 1986; Van Tran, 1987; Vega et al., 1987; Pescosolido and Georgianna, 1989; Egolf et al., 1992; Trovato, 1992; Wolf and Bruhn, 1998; Barranco, 2015).

On the other hand, some features of the immigrant experience may serve to erode an immigrant mortality advantage. Acculturation is thought to be one such factor (Berry, 1980).[1] With time, immigrants increasingly incorporate lifestyles and health behaviors characteristic of their adopted society. This process is thought to often result in a loss of health advantage for immigrants (McDonald and Kennedy, 2004; Abraído-Lanza et al., 2005; Newbold, 2005, 2009; Gray et al., 2007). In this connection, phrases such as 'unhealthy assimilation' and 'pathogenic process' have appeared in the literature to describe this aspect of the immigrant experience (Antecol and Bedard, 2006; De Maio, 2010; Leung, 2014; Vandenheede et al., 2015). All this suggests a close connection between increased time in the host country, level of acculturation, and increased morbidity and mortality (Antecol and Bedard, 2006; Stirbu et al., 2006; Gray et al., 2007; Delavari et al., 2013; Vandenheede et al., 2015; Balfour et al., 2016).

DYNAMIC INTERPLAY OF HEALTH SELECTION AND ACCULTURATION

As suggested in Figure 7.1, health selection and acculturation work in opposite directions in regard to health and survival. During the early phase of settlement immigrants enjoy reduced mortality risk (that is, immigrant survival advantage, ISA) as a function of their health selectivity. At this point, the effects of acculturation on health erosion would be minimal, as migrants would have limited exposure to the new environment. With increasing time they experience an increased level of acculturation and lose some of the protective effects of health selection. These counteracting dynamics of acculturation and health selection underlie a seemingly paradoxical feature of the migrant studies literature. Survey studies show varying degrees of health erosion in migrants with increased duration in the host country (Perez, 2002; McDonald and Kennedy, 2004; Newbold, 2005, 2009; De Maio, 2010). On the other hand, studies of mortality differentials generally indicate a persistence of survival advantage for immigrants (Vang et al., 2016). In actuality, both sets of studies may be capturing two complementary processes that are difficult to observe simultaneously: health studies reflect health erosion

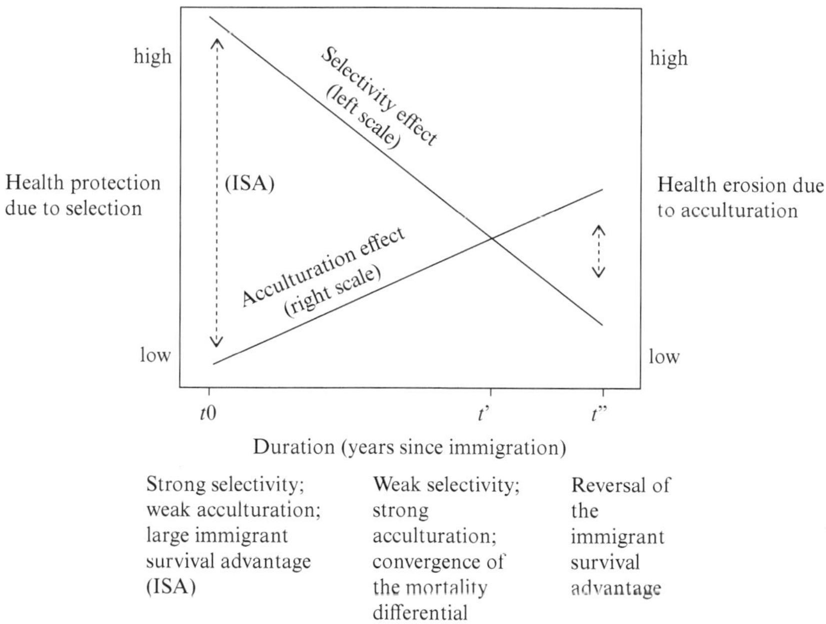

Figure 7.1 Hypothesized health selection and acculturation effects on immigrant health, showing expected change in the immigrant survival advantage (ISA)

based on retrospective accounts but cannot capture change in survival probabilities; mortality studies are able to document a migrant survival advantage but typically cannot measure erosion of health status over time.

As already noted, Figure 7.1 assumes that the protective effect of health selection on survival would be most intense early in the settlement experience and weakest at long durations post-arrival; and contrastingly, negative assimilation effects on health should be weakest early in the migration experience and strongest at long durations. It is therefore possible that these divergent dynamics could conceivably lead to mortality convergence of immigrants with their native-born hosts – that is, point *t'* in Figure 7.1. And beyond this point, there is the possibility of a reversal of the migrant mortality advantage, with the differential turning in favor of the native-born. The pace of change of the mortality differential may vary with the cause of death. For some diseases movement toward convergence may occur early in the immigrant experience and for others relatively late, or possibly not at all. Although not explicitly shown in Figure 7.1, it is also worth considering that in situations where migrants hold an initially greater risk of mortality from a given disease, acculturation may actually result in a gradual reduction in risk (Cappuccio, 2004).

DATA

The mortality data analysed in this study were taken from the Vital Statistics Mortality Data Base of Statistics Canada, accessed through its Research Data Centre at the University of Alberta. Between 2010 and 2012, there were 731 550 deaths in Canada, of which 77 percent were native born and 23 percent foreign born. Just over 4 percent of cases had missing information on the country of birth variable. These 'missing' cases were redistributed *pro rata* to the known distribution of deaths by nativity, age, sex, and cause of death. Mid-interval population counts for the computation of central death rates were initially drawn from the 2011 Canadian National Household Survey (NHS) (Statistics Canada, 2014).[2] As the NHS was conducted in early May 2011, population counts were adjusted to 1 July 2011, the midpoint of the observation period, by applying the age-sex-nativity population proportions from the NHS to the corresponding Canadian postcensal population estimates by age and sex for 1 July 2011 (Statistics Canada, 2016). On 1 July 2016, the population of Canada was 34 342 780, of which 78 percent was Canadian born and 22 percent foreign born. Consistent with the coding in the vital statistics mortality data file, the foreign-born population includes both immigrants and non-permanent residents.

DIFFERENCES IN GENERAL AND CAUSE-SPECIFIC MORTALITY

In Table 7.1 crude rates show a mortality disadvantage for immigrant males (0.60 per 1000) and a mortality advantage for females (–0.07 per 1000). These rates are distorted by group differences in age composition. The immigrant population is heavily concentrated in the prime working ages and at ages beyond 60, while the Canadian born is overrepresented at ages below 20 (figure available on request from the author). The standardized death rates, based on the total Canadian population as standard, show a mortality advantage for immigrants (–2.58 and –2.53 per 1000 for males and females, respectively).

Age patterns of cause-specific death rates by nativity and sex were examined (figure available on request from the author; see Table 7A.1

Table 7.1 Crude (CDR) and age standardized death rates (ASDRs) by sex and nativity, 2010–12

	CB males	CB females	FB males	FB females	Difference: FB–CB males	Difference: FB–CB females
CDR × 1000	7.08	7.01	7.68	6.94	0.60	–0.07
ASDRs × 1000	7.96	7.74	5.38	5.21	–2.58	–2.53

Note: In this and subsequent tables and figures, CB = Canadian born and FB = immigrants (foreign born). The standard population is the Canadian population in 2011.

in the Appendix to this chapter for the International Classification of Diseases, ICD, codes for causes of death examined). Death rates are lower in immigrants from virtually all causes analysed. Stomach cancer is a notable exception. For this disease immigrant females have relatively high death rates across virtually all age categories whereas in males, higher mortality from stomach cancer is seen only at ages 70 and above. External mortality is for the most part lower in migrants, though in the older ages immigrants tend to show higher rates of suicide in relation to their Canadian-born counterparts.

DECOMPOSITION OF DIFFERENCE IN LIFE EXPECTANCY AT AGE 20

Decomposition analysis helps to uncover the varying contribution of causes of death to group differences in life expectancy, and is therefore applied here to address the first question posed at the beginning of the chapter. The method of Preston et al. (2001, pp. 84–8) was applied to decompose difference in life expectancy at age 20 between immigrants and their Canadian-born counterparts. There were relatively few deaths below this age in the immigrant population, thus justifying the focus on this age. In Table 7.2, positive values indicate that the effect of mortality difference for a given cause serves to expand the immigrant mortality advantage, and a negative value would mean the opposite. Sex differences in expectation of life at age 20 are 4.4 and 4.8 years in favor of male and female migrants, respectively.[3] A large portion of the expectancy gap is accounted for by group differences in circulatory and cancer disease mortality. Together these categories of disease explain over 50 percent of the difference in life expectancy, with ischemic heart disease and lung

Table 7.2 Decomposition of difference in life expectancy at age 20 (e_{20}) between immigrants (FB) and Canadian born (CB); Canada 2010–2012

	Males		Females	
	(Years)	%	(Years)	%
($FBe_{20} - CBe_{20}$)	(63.5 – 59.1) = 4.4	100	(68.2 – 63.4) = 4.8	100
Contribution due to:				
Ischemic heart disease	.670	15.2	.544	11.6
Other heart disease	.233	5.3	.273	5.7
Cerebrovascular disease	.083	1.9	.177	3.7
Other circulatory diseases	.089	2.0	.080	1.7
Subtotal	*1.075*	*24.4*	*1.074*	*22.7*
Stomach cancer	–.024	–0.6	–.033	–.70
Lung cancer	.443	10.0	.641	13.4
Breast cancer	.002	0.1	.143	3.0
Prostate cancer	.105	2.4	.000	0.0
Leukemia*	.089	2.0	.057	1.2
Other malignant neoplasms	.553	12.5	.528	11.1
Subtotal	*1.168*	*26.4*	*1.336*	*28.0*
Diabetes	.136	3.1	.082	1.7
Chronic liver disease & cirrhosis	.078	1.8	.066	1.4
Subtotal	*.214*	*4.9*	*.148*	*3.1*
Motor vehicle accidents	.137	3.1	.032	0.7
Accidental falls	.041	0.9	.058	1.2
Suicide	.218	4.9	.068	1.4
Homicide	.005	0.1	.002	.04
Other accidents and violence	.204	4.6	.162	3.4
Injury undetermined	.045	1.0	.032	0.7
Subtotal	*.650*	14.6	*.354*	7.4
Other causes of death	*1.132*	*29.7*	*1.847*	*38.7*
Total	4.4	100	4.8	100

Note: * In this and subsequent tables and figures, 'Leukemia' means malignant neoplasms of lymphoid, hematopoietic and related tissues.

cancer being the dominant cause components. All other components show considerably smaller contributions. For stomach cancer there is a negative effect, indicating that its net contribution serves to reduce the migrant life expectancy advantage, though by a small degree.

ACCULTURATION AND SELECTION EFFECTS

Indirect tests of acculturation and health selection are attempted through a simulation type procedure described below. The following regression is specified:

$$r_{i(k)}^{FB} - r_{i(k)}^{CB} = \alpha + \beta t + \beta i^2 + \varepsilon_{ik}. \tag{7.1}$$

where

$(r_{i(k)}^{FB} - r_{i(k)}^{CB})$ = expected difference in death rate per person from cause k for age group i between immigrants (FB) and the Canadian-born (CB) population;

$r_{i(k)} = d_{i(k)} / P_i$, the number of deaths due to cause k for age group i divided by the corresponding population at risk (P_i);

α = regression intercept;

βt = effect of unit change in duration (t) for migrants on the mortality differential, where duration is defined as $[(t_j) - (t_0)]$, with (t_j) being an age-specific duration mean (in years) for age group x–$x+n$, and (t_0) is the mean duration for age group 0–19;[4]

βi^2 = effect of unit change in age squared on the mortality differential, where age is measured as $[i_m - i_{(0)}]^2$, with i_m being the midpoint of age group x–$x+n$, and $i_{(0)}$ the midpoint for age group 0–19;

ε_{ik}= regression residuals.

Duration is treated as an indirect measure of acculturation for the immigrant population. The input data for this variable were taken from the 2011 National Household Survey (Statistics Canada, 2014).[5] In the regressions, the Canadian born were assigned a constant value, the average duration of the immigrant population. Partial derivatives were computed to examine change in the expected mortality gap between immigrants and the native born over different values of duration spanning year 1 (that is, first year after arrival) to year 35 post-arrival. These estimates were then graphed to better visualize how the predicted mortality differential changes with increased duration for immigrants (see Figures 7.2 and 7.3). For this aspect of the analysis the regression coefficients for duration associated with each cause of death were divided by the immigrant average duration, and the quotient added to the intercept.[6] This term was then multiplied by duration:

$$(\beta_{(k)} / \mu + \alpha_{(k)}) \times t_j \tag{7.2}$$

where $\beta_{(k)}$ is the duration coefficient for cause of death k, μ is the mean duration for the immigrant population; $\alpha_{(k)}$ is the regression intercept for an equation pertaining to cause k; and t_j indexes a duration value (j = 1, 5, 10, 15, 20, 25, 30, and 35 years post-arrival).

Canadian studies suggest that after about ten or fifteen years post-arrival migrants begin approximating the health status of the native born population (Perez, 2002; Newbold and Danforth, 2003; Newbold, 2009; De Maio and Kemp, 2010; Omariba et al., 2014). Since age is statistically controlled in the regressions, the duration coefficients can be thought of as providing a test of the net effect of time in the host country, on the relative risk of death for a hypothetical cohort of migrants. The mortality advantage for immigrants should be most pronounced in the year after arrival and weakened significantly by the 35th year.

An indirect test of health selection is also conducted by comparing the magnitude and direction of estimated duration effects at two specific points in time, years 1 and 35, for three broad cause-of-death categories: 'chronic'; 'external'; 'other'; as well as 'total' (all-cause) mortality. The expectation is that at $t = 1$ health selection would be most intense in affording a mortality advantage for migrants, and at $t = 35$, this effect would be significantly diminished or non-existent. Ideally, these expectations would be tested against longitudinal cohort data. The data used in this investigation are cross-sectional; therefore results are best interpreted as suggestive, serving as possible starting points for further study.

Acculturation Effects: Males

Figure 7.2 shows predicted duration effects for the different causes of death pertaining to expected differences in cause-specific mortality risk between migrant and native-born males. These estimates allow us to assess whether the mortality advantage for migrants is uniform across causes of death and whether the time trajectories of predicted differences vary in degree of intensity and direction (see Table 7.3 for the regression equations). It can be seen, for instance, that the upward pace of change is especially intense for ischemic heart disease and the other three vascular causes, as well as for diabetes, prostate cancer, and 'other' malignancies. On the other hand, the leukemia slope is visibly less steep. These effects are consistent with the proposition that the negative effects of acculturation on migrant mortality risk vary in intensity depending on the disease. Since these estimates all increase with duration, it can be surmised that over time the mortality differentials for these causes shifts increasingly toward a point of convergence with the native born.

From these derivations it appears that the acculturation process may entail variable degrees of erosion of the immigrant mortality advantage, though it seems this process may not be as rapid as suggested by some of the migrant studies literature (Antecol and Bedard, 2006; De Maio and Kemp, 2010; De Maio, 2012). For instance, in the case of ischemic heart disease the migrant advantage in males is estimated to persist into the

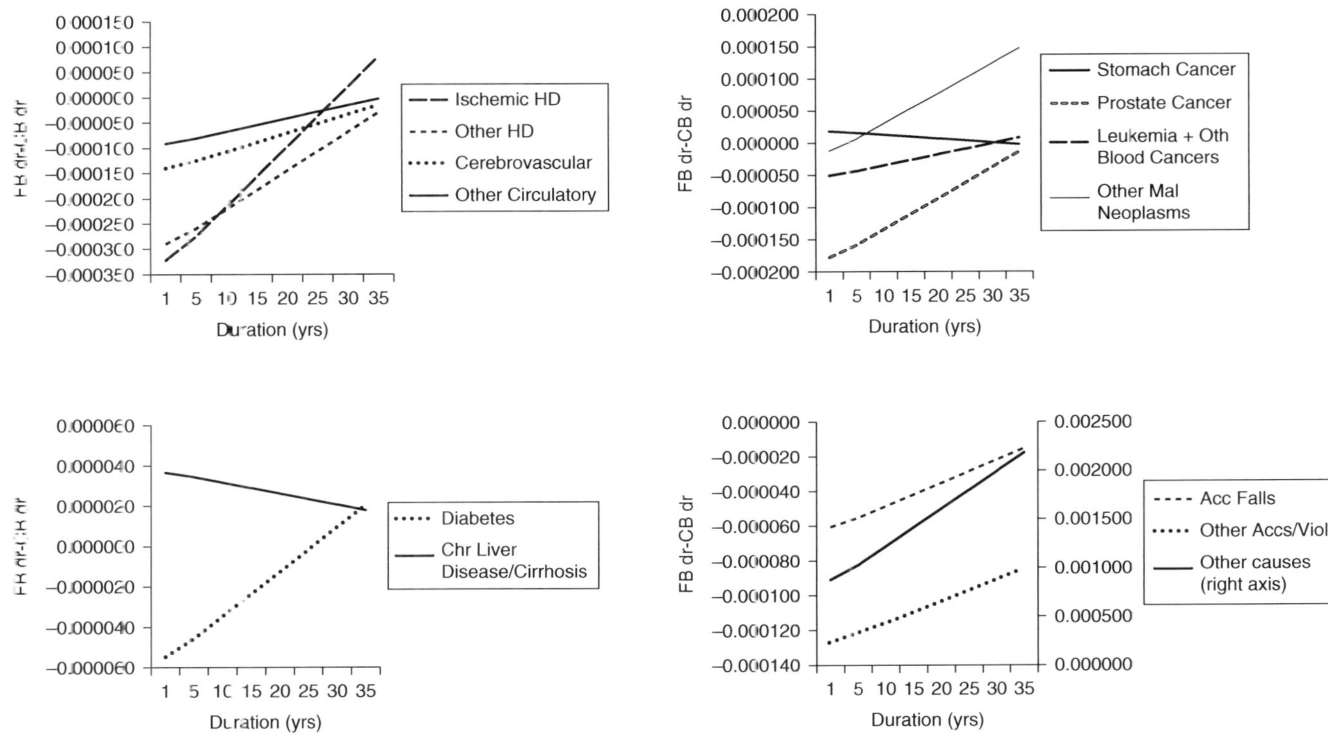

Figure 7.2 Predicted male FB–CB differences in cause-specific death rates by duration (significant effects only)

twenty-fifth year after arrival. Being a leading killer, this cause of death would certainly account for a large portion of the difference in general (all-cause) mortality between nativity groups. For the other three vascular diseases in the analysis there is some remaining advantage for the immigrants even at 35 years' duration.

The trends in Figure 7.2 suggest a gradual and possibly underlying multistage process in the progression of cardiovascular disease consistent with the perspective of Gillum (1999, 2001). Immigrants progress through various incremental stages of acculturation, initially enjoying low levels of vascular disease (for example, hypertension and atherosclerosis) and eventually reaching a peak incidence point owing to the accumulated influences of a high fat diet, salt intake, and tobacco consumption. At an advanced stage, rates of vascular disease may start to decline due to better knowledge and awareness, greater vigilance, and medical management.

For stomach cancer the estimated slope shows a declining trend of this differential. As noted previously, the difference is initially positive (higher immigrant mortality) but as seen here it reduces with time, and eventually crosses into the negative range of the *y*-axis at 30 years' duration (lower immigrant mortality). This scenario is consistent with the notion mentioned earlier that in situations in which the initial mortality difference does not favor migrants, increasing levels of acculturation may have a beneficial effect, to lower the risk towards that of the host population.

Typically, stomach cancer follows a fairly long latency period between the timing of infection and its morbid manifestations (Spallek et al., 2012; Arnold et al., 2013). For immigrants, the genesis of the disease may form early in the home country, and only later manifests itself post-settlement. Diet and tobacco consumption are two important factors contributing to cancer of the stomach, though often *Helicobacter pylori* infection is also implicated, along with the possibility of a genetic predisposition. Nonetheless, acculturation may actually help lower the risk of premature death due to this disease.

The category 'other cancers' encompasses a multitude of malignancies. In Figure 7.2 immigrant men share a favorable situation early after arrival, but by the fifth year of residence in the new country the differential turns unfavorable. Negative acculturation may play some role in this reversal, but cannot explain it completely, as the interval since immigration is too short. It is likely that many neoplasms under this category may have been formed early in the home country.

Predicted effects for diabetes and chronic liver disease/cirrhosis move in opposite directions. The latter differential remains consistently in the positive range of the *y*-axis, notwithstanding its declining trend. However, the migrant mortality advantage from diabetes, though declining, persists for over two decades before reaching convergence at 25 years' duration. The pace of change for this mortality discrepancy seems fairly rapid, and this is consistent with much of the literature concerning the problem of diabetes in migrant populations (Antecol and Bedard, 2006; Delavari et al., 2013). What makes diabetes so insidious is its close connection to other major chronic disorders (Chambers et al., 2017). The increase in mortality from diabetes likely reflects the effects of rapid weight gain as part of the acculturative process.

Montesi et al. (2016) pose an interesting thesis for the fairly rapid propensity in migrants to develop this disease. High morbidity and mortality from diabetes, they argue, underlies the fact that many migrants in rich countries grew up in deprived conditions in their homelands. Consequently, their bodies have been programmed to tackle hunger and starvation. When exposed to the rich and plentiful environment of the host society immigrants fall into a highly obesogenic set of conditions characterized by high fat diets in particular, and a predominantly sedentary way of life, all of which are closely connected to weight gain and diabetes among other chronic ailments.

Of the external causes, only two differentials were found to be statistically significant for males (see Table 7.3): accidental falls and 'other' accidents and violence. These effects remain in the negative range of the *y*-axis but reduce in magnitude with increased duration. Male migrants experience a movement toward the risk of their native born counterparts all the while maintaining a mortality advantage, even at 35 years' duration. The residual cause category (see the right axis of the bottom right graph in Figure 7.2) subsumes many causes of death and therefore does not lend to straightforward interpretation. Nonetheless, the corresponding slope for the expected mortality differential persists in the positive range of the *y*-axis. This indicates a relative disadvantage for immigrant men even though the disadvantage reduces over time. Thus, acculturation in this case would seem to afford a beneficial effect.

Acculturation Effects: Females

Predicted duration effects for females are shown in Figure 7.3 (see Table 7.4 for the regression equations). In many respects they are similar to those noted for males. Concerning the vascular diseases, relative risks start out in the negative range of the *y*-axis and tend to increase with duration. Unlike the situation for males, however, predicted differentials for ischemic heart disease and 'other' circulatory converge earlier, at 20 years' duration. Relative risks for 'other' heart disease and cerebrovascular mortality cross into the positive range at durations 25 and 30 years, respectively. (In

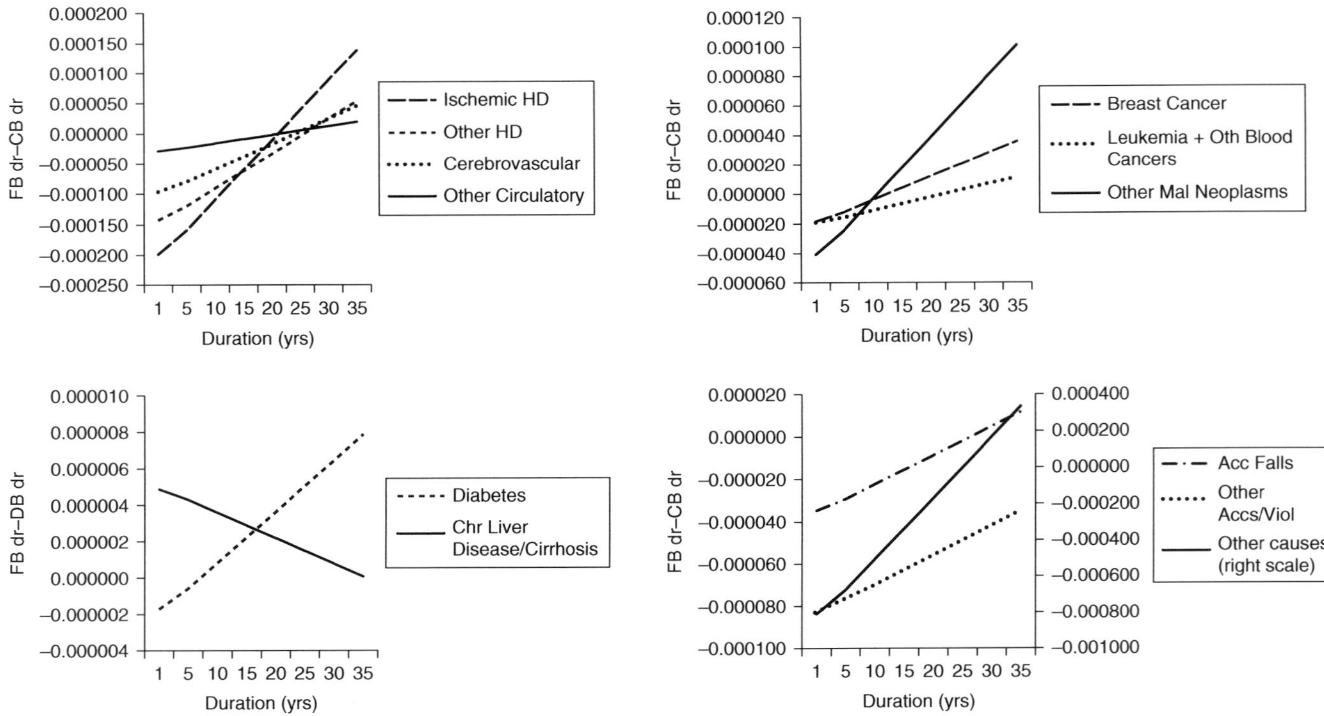

Figure 7.3 Predicted female FB–CB differences in cause-specific death rates by duration (significant effects only)

males there was absence of convergence for these two causes.) Finally, by the third decade in the host country the expected differential in vascular-related mortality changes in favor of native-born females.

Only three of the cancer differentials were statistically significant for females (see Table 7.4). The steepest change is seen for the 'other' cancer category. Differences in mortality due to breast cancer and leukemia rise less steeply. Convergence for breast cancer and 'other' cancers occurs at ten years' duration and for leukemia at 25 years. Breast cancer represents one of the most common malignancies in women, though is generally less common in immigrants especially among those from less developed countries (Arnold et al., 2013). Among the protective factors known against this disease are higher parity and longer breastfeeding. As many immigrants are from developing regions, these two features contrast sharply with women in host societies where fertility rates have been low for a long time and breastfeeding is limited. The situation concerning this differential conforms to expectations suggested in Figure 7.1, which predicts an initial lower relative risk for migrants and a movement with time toward convergence with the native born.

For diabetes and chronic liver disease, the predicted differentials are for the most part in the positive range of the *y*-axis, meaning in favor of native-born females. A crossover is seen for diabetes and chronic liver disease/cirrhosis at 15 years' duration, the former moving upward, the latter downward over time. In the case of diabetes, female immigrants tend to lose their mortality advantage relatively early, at 10 years' duration. Notwithstanding its downward trend, no convergence is seen for chronic liver disease/cirrhosis. Although the steep upward trend for the diabetes differential is similar to that observed for males, the situation with females seems more problematic because convergence occurs so early. Convergence in males was seen at 25 years' duration; unhealthy acculturation therefore seems to be more intense in females with respect to diabetes (Antecol and Bedard, 2006). As mentioned previously, the root causes of this may involve a combination of factors associated with the mismatch between the less obesogenic environment of the home country and the more obesogenic context of the adopted society, the change being more problematic for females (Bateson, et al. 2004; Gluckman and Hanson, 2004; Shapira, 2013).

Of the two significant external types of mortality, accidental falls, and 'other' accidents/violence show increases over time. Unlike the situation with males, here the differential due to accidental falls converges with the native-born fairly late, at 25 years' duration. Similar to males the mortality difference in 'other' accidents/violence remains in the negative range of the *y*-axis throughout the observation period even though the trend is clearly upward toward convergence. For 'other' causes, convergence is seen at 30 years (in men no convergence was noted).

HEALTH SELECTIVITY EFFECTS

The analysis now turns to indirect tests of health selection, relying again on the information in Tables 7.3 and 7.4 and the application of equation 7.2. Recall that consideration is given to the idea that health selectivity for immigrants should be at a maximum in year 1 after arrival, the partial coefficient for duration 1 being viewed as an indirect indicator of 'initial selectivity'. At duration 35, the terminal point of observation, a differential in favor of immigrants would signify 'remaining selectivity'. These two indexes are operationalized by summing the partial duration derivatives at these two distinct time points for causes of death falling under 'chronic', 'external', and 'other' (residual); as well as 'total' (general mortality). These estimates are shown in Figure 7.4. Negative values on the *y*-axis suggest the presence of positive health selection for immigrants (that is, the effect serves to reduce immigrant mortality relative to the native-born), while positive values would indicate the opposite – a loss of selectivity effect.

At duration 1, both male and female immigrants enjoy varying degrees of selective protection against the risk of death across these four categories of mortality. The effects are stronger in males. At duration 35 there is remaining selectivity in men with respect to 'external', 'other', and 'total' mortality, but not for the 'chronic' category. In females, with the exception of 'external' mortality, at this late stage of the migration experience the selection protective effect has all but vanished, and the relative risk for total mortality favors the Canadian born. The situation with 'chronic' mortality is interesting, as in both sexes there is a notable initial protective selection effect at duration 1 which is lost by the 35th year. The loss is visibly more pronounced in females.

CONCLUSION

A number of conclusions emerge from this analysis: (1) in relation to native-born Canadians the immigrant population shows lower mortality from virtually all causes of death examined, the exception being stomach cancer for which immigrants share a higher risk; (2) the immigrant population enjoys a substantial advantage in life expectancy – at age 20, the gap is 4.4 and 4.8 years in favour of male and female migrants, respectively; (3) this survival advantage obtains from immigrants' reduced mortality from virtually all

Table 7.3 Regressions of differences in cause-specific death rates; males (rates per person)

$Y = FB_{(males)} - CB_{(males)}$	Observed difference in death rates	Equations and fit statistics								
		Intercept	$\beta_{duration}$	P	β_{age}	P	R^2	$F_{reg.}$	df	P
Ischemic heart disease	–.001081	–.000335	.00025800	.003	–.000003000	.000	.89	46.5	2/12	.000
Other heart disease	–.000435	–.000298	.00016600	.008	–.000002000	.002	.76	18.5	2/12	.000
Cerebrovascular	–.000181	–.000144	.00008000	.018	–.000000740	.005	.62	12.6	2/12	.001
Other circulatory	–.000166	–.000094	.00005700	.002	–.000000545	.000	.83	35.2	2/12	.000
Stomach cancer	.000046	.000019	−.00001300	.001	.000000133	.000	.89	48.9	2/12	.000
Lung cancer	–.000628	.000195	.00001400	.620	–.000000479	.032	.91	60.3	2/12	.000
Breast cancer	–.000004	–.000002	.00000100	.048	–.000000011	.001	.64	13.3	2/12	.001
Prostate cancer	–.000241	–.000183	.00010500	.003	–.000000970	.001	.76	23.2	2/12	.000
Leukemia	–.000148	–.000053	.00003800	.001	–.000000384	.000	.87	49.8	2/12	.000
Other malignant neoplasms	–.000799	–.000017	.00010200	.001	–.000001000	.000	.96	182.2	2/12	.000
Diabetes	–.000214	–.000057	.00004800	.006	–.000000498	.000	.87	40.6	2/12	.000
Chronic liver dis. & cirrhosis	–.000066	.000037	−.00001200	.004	.000000068	.020	.76	19.2	2/12	.001
Motor vehicle accidents	–.000061	–.000078	.00000400	.376	–.000000025	.405	.07	0.5	2/12	.646
Accidental falls	–.000065	–.000062	.00002900	.044	.000000267	.017	.48	7.6	2/12	.008
Suicide	–.000080	–.000105	−.00000900	.212	.000000093	.093	.47	5.4	2/12	.022
Homicide	–.000003	–.000003	.00000044	.739	–.000000004	.664	.04	0.3	2/12	.779
Other accidents/violence	–.000149	–.000128	.00002700	.046	–.000000251	.015	.60	9.1	2/12	.004
Injury undetermined	–.000016	–.000024	−.00000085	.562	.000000011	.314	.38	3.6	2/12	.058
Other causes of death	–.002401	–.001500	.00083500	.003	–.000008000	.000	.83	28.2	2/12	.000

Note: *P* indicates level of significance.

Table 7.4 Regressions of differences in cause-specific death rates; females (rates per person)

$Y = FB_{(females)} - CB_{(females)}$	Observed difference in death rates	Equations and fit statistics								
		Intercept	$\beta_{duration}$	*P*	β_{age}	*P*	R^2	$F_{reg.}$	df	*P*
Ischemic heart disease	–.000665	–.000209	.00021100	.038	–.000002000	.009	.70	11.9	2/12	.001
Other heart disease	–.000333	–.000149	.00012300	.034	–.000001000	.009	.64	10.6	2/12	.002
Cerebrovascular	–.000230	–.000101	.00008900	.042	–.000000833	.012	.61	9.5	2/12	.003
Other circulatory	–.000098	–.000030	.00003000	.001	–.000000291	.002	.77	20. 4	2/12	.000
Stomach cancer	.000027	–.000004	.00000034	.735	.000000010	.166	.85	41.9	2/12	.000
Lung cancer	–.000609	.000239	–.00002800	.413	–.000000123	.611	.80	23.7	2/12	.000
Breast cancer	–.000161	–.000020	.00003400	.006	–.000000355	.000	.87	40.4	2/12	.000
Leukemia	–.000071	–.000020	.00001900	.001	–.000000192	.000	.88	45.0	2/12	.000
Other malignant neoplasms	–.000549	–.000045	.00008900	.001	–.000000989	.000	.94	95.4	2/12	.000
Diabetes	–.000075	–.000002	.00000600	.022	–.000000086	.000	.93	82.6	2/12	.000
Chronic liver dis. & cirrhosis	–.000046	.000005	–.00000300	.002	.000000003	.592	.96	149.2	2/12	.000
Motor vehicle accidents	–.000011	–.000020	.00000100	.186	–.000000009	.259	.19	1.4	2/12	.275
Accidental falls	–.000073	–.000036	.00002900	.060	–.000000272	.020	.56	7.5	2/12	.008
Suicide	–.000019	–.000032	–.00000300	.126	.000000035	.036	.58	8.4	2/12	.005
Homicide	–.000001	–.000001	.00000014	.835	–.000000001	.844	.01	.02	2/12	.977
Other accidents/violence	–.000117	–.000084	.00003000	.056	–.000000277	.019	.55	7.4	2/12	.008
Injury undetermined	–.000011	–.000014	–.00000099	.458	.000000010	.310	.20	1.5	2/12	.261
Other causes of death	–.002232	–.000844	.00071700	.015	–.000007000	.003	.74	16.8	2/12	.000

Note: *P* indicates level of significance.

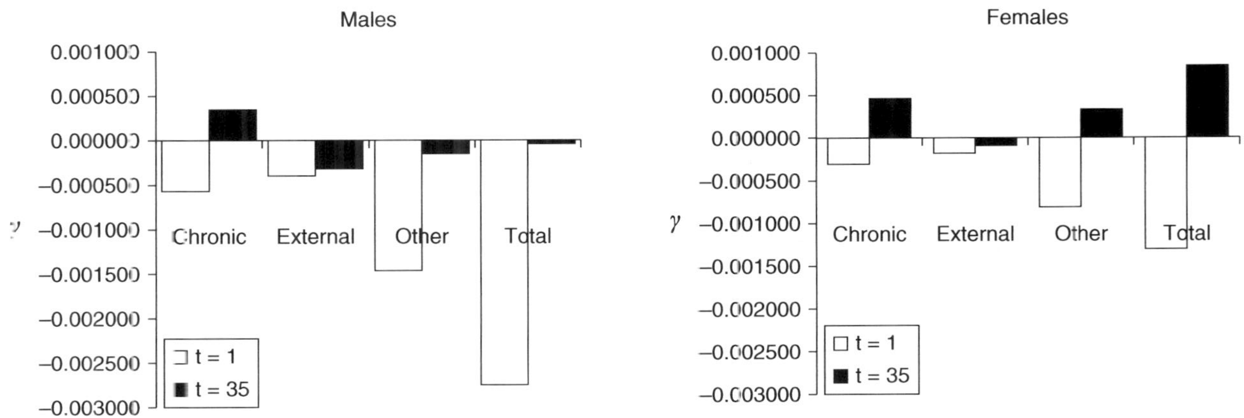

Note: γ = selectivity, measured as the sum of estimated duration effects within each type of mortality: 'Chronic' (ischemic heart disease, other heart disease, cerebrovascular, other circulatory; stomach cancer, lung cancer, prostate cancer, leukemia, other cancers, diabetes, chronic liver disease/cirrhosis); 'External' (motor vehicle accidents, accidental falls, suicide, homicide, other accidents/violence, injury undetermined); 'Other' (all other causes of death); and 'Total' (sum of all estimated duration coefficients across all causes of death). Negative values of γ indicate a protective selection effect for immigrants; positive values indicate the opposite.

Figure 7.4 Estimated health selection effects at durations 1 and 35 years

causes of death examined, the largest contribution being due to ischemic heart disease, other vascular ailments, and cancer; (4) acculturation, as indexed by duration of time in Canada, was found to have an eroding effect on immigrants' mortality advantage, though the intensity of effect varies with the cause of death; (5) convergence with the native-born population, if it occurs at all for a specific cause of death, tends to occur later in males as compared to females; (6) the risk of death due to most external causes does not vary significantly by nativity, though in some cases, such as accidental falls and 'other', with time the migrant mortality risk moves increasingly toward that of the native born; (7) indirect test of health selection suggested that this is an important source of protection for immigrants, its effect lasting for some types of mortality up to 25 years post-arrival (for example, ischemic heart disease for males), though lasting much shorter in some other cases, notably diabetes, and breast cancer in females; and (8) by 35 years' duration post-arrival the protective effect of health selection on total mortality is lost in females, whereas there persists a small protective effect in males.

Taken together these findings are consistent with the proposed framework concerning the interplay of duration and health selectivity in regard to change in mortality risk in migrant populations. Although the framework was specified in linear form, in the real world the implied dynamics likely follow nonlinear patterns. Nonlinear specifications should therefore be attempted in future research based on longitudinal data. Concerning acculturation, the literature has tended to emphasize its negative features; however, acculturation may also have beneficial effects on immigrant health. More attention should be devoted to this possibility (Landrine and Klonoff, 2004; Gray et al., 2007). Finally, the health selection phenomenon also requires further exploration. This property of immigrant populations does not appear to be static. Depending on the disease, migrants may lose their survival advantage relatively early, while in other cases the protective effects of selection can persist for many years post-arrival. This is another important hypothesis worth pursuing.

NOTES

* This research was supported by funds to the Canadian Research Data Centre Network (CRDCN) from the Social Science and Humanities Research Council (SSHRC), the Canadian Institute for Health Research (CIHR), the Canadian Foundation for Innovation (CFI) and Statistics Canada. Although the research and analysis are based on data from Statistics Canada, the opinions expressed do not represent the views of Statistics Canada or the Canadian Research Data Centre Network (CRDCN).

1. Acculturation has four components: (1) integration – maintaining attitudes and behaviors from the original culture but also adopting values and behaviors of the dominant culture; (2) assimilation – entirely adopting the values and behaviors of the dominant

culture; (3) separation – rejecting the ways of the dominant culture and keeping the cultural practices and behaviors of the original culture; and (4) marginalization – not identifying with the original culture or the dominant/mainstream culture (Berry, 1980).
2. The NHS is a large sample of Canadians that responded voluntarily to the 2011 long form census.
3. Life tables for the decomposition were constructed using the method of Chiang (1984).
4. The starting age group is 0–19, as death counts for migrants across most causes of death below age 20 are sparse.
5. Inclusion of duration as an external variable assumes that the unknown distribution of duration for foreign-born decedents matches perfectly the duration distribution of migrants that had participated in the NHS.
6. This operationalization assumes that the average duration captures the total duration experience for immigrants and, by dividing the duration regression slope by this average, one obtains an approximate annual rate of change of the expected mortality differential. The means for males and females are 21.70547 and 21.28693 respectively.

REFERENCES

Abraido-Lanza, A.F., B.P. Dohrenwend, D.S. Ng-Mak and J.B. Turner (1999), 'The Latino mortality paradox: a test of the salmon bias and healthy migrant hypothesis', *American Journal of Public Health*, **89** (10), 1543–8.

Abraido-Lanza, A.F., M.T. Chao and K.R. Florez (2005), 'Do healthy behaviors decline with greater acculturation? Implications for the Latino mortality paradox', *Social Science & Medicine*, **61** (6), 1243–55.

Anson, J. (2004), 'The migrant mortality advantage: a 70 month follow-up of the Brussels population', *European Journal of Population*, **20** (3), 191–218.

Antecol, H. and K. Bedard (2006), 'Unhealthy assimilation: why do immigrants converge to American health status levels?', *Demography*, **43** (2), 337–60.

Arnold, M., M.J. Aarts, S. Siesling, M. van der Aa, O. Visser and J.W. Coebergh (2013), 'Diverging breast and stomach cancer incidence and survival in migrants in The Netherlands, 1996–2009', *Acta Oncologica*, **52** (6), 1195–201, doi:10.3109/0284186X.2012.742962.

Balfour, P.C., J.M. Ruiz, G.A. Talavera, M.A. Allison and C.J. Rodriguez (2016), 'Cardiovascular disease in Hispanics/Latinos in the United States', *Journal of Latina/o Psychology*, **4** (2), 98–113.

Balzi, D., M. Geddes, A. Brancker and D.M. Parkin (1994), 'Cancer mortality in Italian migrants to Canada', *Tumori*, **80** (1), 19–23.

Barranco, R.E. (2015), 'Suicide, religion, and Latinos: a macrolevel study of U.S. Latino suicide rates', *Sociological Quarterly*, **57** (2), 256–81.

Bateson, P., D. Barker, T. Clutton-Brock, D. Deb, B. D'Udine, R.A. Foley et al (2004), 'Developmental plasticity and human health', *Nature*, **430** (22 July), 419–21.

Berkman, L.F. and T. Glass (2000), 'Social integration, social networks, social support, and health', in L.F. Berkman and I. Kawachi (eds), *Social Epidemiology*, Oxford: Oxford University Press, pp. 137–73.

Berry, J.W. (1980), 'Acculturation as varieties of adaptation', in A.M. Padilla (ed.), *Acculturation: Theory, Models and Some New Findings*, Boulder, CO: Westview Press, pp. 9–25.

Brahimi, M. (1980), 'La mortalite des estrangers en France', *Population*, **35** (3), 603–22.
Breton, R. (1964), 'Institutional completeness of ethnic communities and the personal relations of immigrants', *American Journal of Sociology*, **70** (2), 193–205.
Cappuccio, F.P. (2004), 'Commentary: epidemiological transition, migration, and cardiovascular disease', *International Journal of Epidemiology*, **33** (2), 387–8.
Chambers, J.C., H. Grallert, J.S. Kooner, C. Geiger, G. Matullo, J.T. Bell et al. (2017), 'Epigenome-wide association study of body mass index, and the adverse outcomes of adiposity', *Nature*, **541** (5 January), 81–100, accessed 8 January 2017 at http://www.nature.com/doifinder/10.1038/nature20784.
Chan, J., R. Wilkins and E. Ng (1996), 'Health expectancy by immigrant status', *Health Reports*, **8** (3), 29–37.
Chiang, C.L. (1984), *The Life Table and its Applications*, Malabar, FL: Robert E. Krieger.
Chiswick, B.R., Y. L. Lee and P. W. Miller (2008), 'Immigrant selection systems and immigrant health', *Contemporary Economic Policy*, **26** (4), 555–78.
De Maio, F. (2010), 'Immigration as pathogenic: a systematic review of the health of immigrants to Canada', *International Journal for Equity in Health*, **9** (1), 27.
De Maio, F.G. (2012), 'Understanding the health transitions of immigrants to Canada: research priorities', *Journal of Health Care for the Poor and Underserved*, **23** (3), 958–62.
De Maio, F.G. and E. Kemp (2010), 'The deterioration of health status among immigrants to Canada', *Global Public Health*, **5** (5), 462–78.
Deboosere, P. and S. Gadeyne (2005), 'Adult migrant mortality advantage in Belgium: evidence using census and register data', *Population*, **60** (5–6), 655–98.
Delavari, M., A.L. Sonderlund, B. Swinburn, D. Mellor and A. Renzaho (2013), 'Acculturation and obesity among migrant populations in high income countries: a systematic review', *BMC Public Health*, **13** (458).
DesMeules, M., J. Gold, S. McDermott, Z. Cao, J. Payne and B. Lafrance et al. (2005), 'Disparities in mortality patterns among Canadian immigrants and refugees, 1980–1998: results of a national cohort study', *Journal of Immigrant Health*, **7** (4), 221–32.
Diaz, C.J., S.M. Koning and A.P. Martinez-Donate (2016), 'Moving beyond salmon bias: Mexican return migration and health selection', *Demography*, **53** (6), 2005–30.
Egolf, B., J. Lasker, S. Wolf and L. Potvin (1992), 'The Roseto effect: a 50-year comparison of mortality rates', *American Journal of Public Health*, **82** (8), 1089–92.
Fenelon, A. (2013), 'Revisiting the Hispanic mortality advantage in the United States: the role of smoking', *Social Science & Medicine*, **82** (C), 1–9.
Franzini L., J.C. Ribble and A.M. Keddie (2000), 'Understanding the Hispanic paradox,' *Ethnicity and Disease*, **11** (3), 496–518.
Geddes, M., D. Balzi, E. Buiatti, M. Khlat and D. Parkin (1993), *Cancer in Italian Migrant Populations*, IARC Scientific Publications No. 123, Lyon: International Agency for Research on Cancer.
Gillum, R.F. (1999), 'Stroke mortality in blacks: disturbing trends', *Stroke*, **30** (August), 1711–15.
Gillum, R.F. (2001), 'The epidemiology of cardiovascular disease in black Americans', *New England Journal of Medicine*, **335** (1), 1597–9.
Gluckman, P.D, and M. Hanson (2004), 'Living with the past: evolution, development, and patterns of disease', *Science*, **305** (5691), 1733–6.

Gray, L., S. Harding and A. Reid (2007), 'Evidence of divergence with duration of residence in circulatory disease mortality in migrants to Australia', *European Journal of Public Health*, **17** (6), 550–54.
Ikram, U.Z., K. Malmusi, K. Juel and A. Kunst (2015), 'Association between integration policies and immigrants' mortality: an explorative study across three European countries', *Plos One*, **10** (6), e0129916, doi:10.1371/journal.pone.0129916.
Jasso, G., S.D. Massey, M.R. Rosenzweig and J.P. Smith (2004), 'Immigrant health: selectivity and acculturation', in N.B. Anderson (ed.), *Critical Perspectives on Racial and Ethnic Differences in Health in Late Life*, Washington, DC: National Academies Press, pp. 227–66.
Kawachi, I. and L. Berkman (2000), 'Social cohesion, social capital, and health', in L.F. Berkman and I. Kawachi (eds), *Social Epidemiology*, Oxford: Oxford University Press, pp.174–90.
Kennedy, S., M.P. Kidd, J.T. McDonald and N. Biddle (2015), 'The healthy immigrant effect: patterns and evidence from four countries', *Journal of International Migration & Integration*, **16** (2), 317–32.
Khlat, M. (1993), 'Mortalité des Levantins en Australie', *Population*, **48** (4), 1072–81.
Khlat, M. and N. Darmon (2003), 'Is there a Mediterranean migrants mortality paradox in Europe?', *International Journal of Epidemiology*, **32** (6), 1115–18.
Kliewer, E. (1992), 'Epidemiology of diseases among migrants', *International Migration*, **30** (supplement), 141–65.
Landrine, H. and E.A. Klonoff (2004), 'Culture change and ethnic-minority health behavior: an operant theory of acculturation', *Journal of Behavioral Medicine*, **27** (6), 527–55.
Leung, L.A. (2014), 'Health and unhealthy assimilation: country of origin and smoking behavior among immigrants', *Health Economics*, **23** (12), 1411–29.
McDonald, J.T. and S. Kennedy (2004), 'Insights into the "healthy immigrant effect": health status and health service use of immigrants to Canada', *Social Science & Medicine*, **59** (8), 1613–27.
Markides, K.S. and J. Coreil (1986), 'The health of Hispanics in the southwestern United States: an epidemiological paradox', *Public Health Reports*, **101** (3), 253–65.
Markides, K.S. and K. Eschbach (2005), 'Aging, migration, and mortality: current status of research on the Hispanic paradox', *Journal of Gerontology B. Psychology and Social Sciences*, **60** (2), 68–75.
Marmot, M.G., A.M. Adelstein and L. Bulusu (1984), *Immigrant Mortality in England and Wales, 1970–78. Cause of Death by Country of Birth*, Studies on Medical and Population Subjects no. 47, London: Her Majesty's Stationery Office.
Montesi, L., M.T. Caletti and G. Marchesini (2016), 'Diabetes in migrants and ethnic minorities in a changing world', *World Journal of Diabetes*, **7** (3), 34–44.
Nair, C., M. Nargundkar, H. Johansen and J. Strachan (1990), 'Canadian cardiovascular disease mortality: first generation immigrants versus Canadian born', *Health Reports*, **2** (3), 203–28.
Newbold, B. (2005), 'Health status and health care of immigrants in Canada: a longitudinal analysis', *Journal of Health Services Research & Policy*, **10** (2), 77–83.
Newbold, B. (2009), 'The short-term health of Canada's new immigrant arrivals: evidence from LSIC', *Ethnicity & Health*, **14** (3), 315–36.

Newbold, K.B. and J. Danforth (2003), 'Health status and Canada's immigrant population', *Social Science & Medicine*, **57** (November), 1981–95.
Ng, E. (2011), 'The healthy immigrant effect and mortality rates', *Health Reports*, **22** (4), 25–9.
Omariba, W.R., E. Ng and B. Vissandjée (2014), 'Differences between immigrants at various durations of residence and host population in all-cause mortality, Canada 1991–2006', *Population Studies*, **68** (3), 339–58.
Palloni, A. and E. Arias (2004), 'Paradox lost: explaining the Hispanic adult mortality advantage', *Demography,* 41, 385–415.
Palloni, A. and D.C. Ewbank (2004), 'Selection processes in the study of racial and ethnic differentials in adult health and mortality', in N.B. Anderson, R.A. Bulatao and B. Cohen (eds), *Critical Perspectives on Racial and Ethnic Differences in Health in Later Life*, New York: National Academies Press, pp. 171–226.
Perez, C.E. (2002), 'Health status and health behaviour among immigrants', *Health Reports*, (13), supplement, Statistics Canada, Ottawa.
Pescosolido, B.A. and S. Georgianna (1989), 'Durkheim, suicide, and religion: toward a network theory of suicide', *American Sociological Review*, **54** (1), 33–48.
Powles, J.W. (1990), 'The best of both worlds: attempting to explain the persisting low mortality of Greek migrants to Australia', in J. Caldwell, S. Findlay, P. Caldwell and G. Santow (eds), *What We Know about Health Transition*, Canberra: Australian National University, pp. 584–94.
Preston, S.H., P. Heuveline and M. Guillot (2001), *Demography: Measuring and Modeling Population Processes,* Oxford: Blackwell.
Razum, O., H. Zeeb, H.S. Akgun and S. Yilmaz (1998), 'Low overall mortality of Turkish residents in Germany persists and extends into a second generation: merely a healthy migrant effect?', *Tropical Medicine and International Health*, **3** (4), 297–303.
Shapira, N. (2013), Women's higher health risks in the obesogenic environment: a gender nutrition approach to metabolic dimorphism with predictive, preventive, and personalised medicine', *EPMA Journal*, **4** (1), accessed 26 June 2017 at https://link.springer.com/article/10.1186/1878-5085-4-1.
Sharma, R.D., M. Mikalowski and R.B.P. Verma (1990), 'Mortality differentials among immigrant populations in Canada', *International Migration*, **28** (4), 443–50.
Singer, E., R. McElroy, and P. Muennig (2017), 'Social capital and the paradox of poor but healthy groups in the United States', *Journal of Immigrant Minority Health*, **19**, 716–22. DOI 10.1007/s10903-016-0396-0 (published online 23 March 2016).
Singh, G.K. and M. Siahpush (2001), 'All-cause and cause-specific mortality of immigrants and native born in the United States', *American Journal of Public Health*, **91** (3), 392–99.
Spallek J., M. Arnold, O. Razum, K. Juel, G. Rey, P. Deoboosere et al. (2012), 'Cancer mortality patterns among Turkish immigrants in four European countries and in Turkey', *European Journal of Epidemiology*, **27** (12), 915–21.
Statistics Canada (2014), 'National Household Survey (NHS) – Main Survey – 2014 National Household Survey Test (Field Procedures Test)', accessed 12 May 2016 at http://www.statcan.gc.ca/eng/survey/household/5178.
Statistics Canada (2016), CANSIM database, 'Table 051-0001, Estimates

of population, by age group and sex for July 1, Canada, provinces and territories, annual', accessed 9 May 2016 at http://www5.statcan.gc.ca/cansim/a26?lang=eng&id=510001.

Stirbu, I., A. Kunst, F.A. Vlems, O. Visser, V. Bos, W. Deville et al. (2006), 'Cancer mortality rates among first and second generation migrants in the Netherlands: convergence toward the rates of the native Dutch population', *International Journal of Cancer*, **119** (11), 2665–72.

Trovato, F. (1992), 'Violent and accidental mortality among four immigrant groups in Canada, 1970–72', *Biodemography and Social Biology*, **39** (1–2), 82–101.

Trovato, F. and G.K. Jarvis (1986), 'Immigrant suicide in Canada: 1971 and 1981', *Social Forces*, **65** (2), 433–57.

Trovato, F. and Odynak, D. (2011), 'Sex differences in life expectancy in Canada: immigrant and native-born populations', *Journal of Biosocial Science*, **43** (3), 353–67.

Turra, C.M. and I.T. Elo (2008), 'The impact of salmon bias on the Hispanic mortality advantage: new evidence from Social Security Data', *Population Research and Policy Review*, **27** (October), 515–30.

Van Tran, T. (1987), 'Ethnic community supports and psychological well-being of Vietnamese refugees', *International Migration Review*, **21** (3), 833–44.

Vallin, J. (1985), 'La mortalite des immigres en Engleterre et Galles' ('The mortality of immigrants in England and Wales'), *Population*, **40** (1), 156–61.

Vandenheede, H., D. Willaert, H. De Grande, S. Simoens and C. Vanroelen (2015), 'Mortality in adult immigrants in the 2000s in Belgium: a test of the "healthy-migrant" and the "migration-as-rapid-health-transition" hypotheses', *Tropical Medicine and International Health*, **20** (12), 1832–45.

Vang, Z.M., S. Jennifer, F. Astrid and A. Gagnon (2016), 'Are immigrants healthier than native-born Canadians? A systematic review of the healthy immigrant effect in Canada', *Ethnicity & Health*, **22** (3), 1–33.

Vega, W.A., B. Kolody and J.R. Valle (1987), 'Migration and mental health: an empirical test of depression risk factors among immigrant Mexican women', *International Migration Review*, **21** (3), 512–30.

Wallace, M. (2016), 'Adult mortality among the descendants of immigrants in England and wales: does a migrant mortality advantage persist beyond the first generation?', *Journal of Ethic & Migration Studies*, **42** (9), 1558–77, doi:org/10.1080/1369183x.2015.1131973.

Wallace, M. and H. Kulu (2013), 'Migration and health in England and Scotland: a study of migrant selectivity and Salmon bias', *Population, Space & Place*, **20** (8), 694–708, http://dx.doi.org/10.1002/psp.1804.

Wallace, M. and H. Kulu (2014a), 'Low immigrant mortality in England and Wales: a data artefact?' *Social Science & Medicine*, **120** (November), 100–109.

Wallace, M. and H. Kulu (2014b), 'Mortality among immigrants in England and Wales by major causes of death, 1971: a longitudinal analysis of register-based data', *Social Science & Medicine*, **147**, 209–21.

Weitoft, G.R., A. Gullberg, A. Hjern and M. Rosen (1999), 'Mortality statistics in immigrant research: method for adjusting underestimation of mortality', *International Journal of Epidemiology*, **28** (4), 756–63.

Wolf, S. and J.G. Bruhn (1998), *The Power of Clan: A 25-Year Prospective Study of Roseto, Pennsylvania*, New Brunswick, NJ: Transaction.

Young, C.M. (1987), 'Migration and mortality: the experience of birthplace groups in Australia', *International Migration Review*, **21** (3), 531–54.

APPENDIX

Table 7A.1 Causes of death categories used in this study and corresponding ICD-10 codes

No.	Cause of death (ICD-10 titles)	ICD-10 codes
1	Ischemic heart diseases	I20–I25
2	Other heart disease	I00–I09, I10, I11, I12, I13, I26–I51
3	Cerebrovascular diseases	I60–I69
4	Other circulatory diseases	I70–I99
5	Malignant neoplasm of stomach	C16
6	Malignant neoplasm of trachea, bronchus and lung	C33–C34
7	Malignant neoplasm of breast	C50
8	Malignant neoplasm of prostate	C61
9	Malignant neoplasms of lymphoid, haematopoietic and related tissues	C81–C96
10	Other malignant neoplasms	Remainder C00–C97
11	Diabetes mellitus	E10–E14
12	Chronic liver disease and cirrhosis	K70, K73–K74
13	Motor vehicle accidents	V02–V04, V090, V092, V12–V14, V190–V192, V194–V196, V20–V79, V803–V805, V810–V811, V820–V821, V83–V86, V870–V878, V880–V888, V890, V892
14	Falls	W00–W19
15	Intentional self-harm (suicide)	X60–X84, Y870
16	Assault (homicide)	X85–Y09, Y871
17	Other accidents and violence	All other external cause not in 13, 14, 15 and 16
18	Injury/events of undetermined intent	Y10–Y34, Y87.2, Y899
19	All other causes of death including unknown	Remainder of A00–Y89

8. Mortality trends, patterns, and differentials among immigrants in the United States*

Gopal K. Singh and Lihua Liu

INTRODUCTION

The United States (US) has seen a substantial increase in its immigrant population over the past several decades in both absolute numbers and as a percentage of the total population. The immigrant population increased more than four-fold, from 9.6 million in 1970 to 43.3 million in 2015 (Singh et al., 2013a; US Census Bureau, 2016). The proportionate share of the immigrant population has also risen sharply, from 4.7 percent in 1970 to 13.5 percent in 2015 (Larsen, 2003; Singh and Miller, 2004; US Census Bureau, 2016). The rapid increase in the immigrant population in recent decades reflects large-scale immigration from Latin America and Asia (Singh et al., 2013a). Consequently, the immigrant population in the United States has become more heterogeneous over time in its ethnic and country-of-origin composition. Currently, 51 percent of US immigrants are from Latin America, 13 percent from Asia, and 5 percent from Africa. Europeans who accounted for 75 percent of all US immigrants in 1960 represented only 11 percent of the immigrant population in 2015 (US Census Bureau, 2016). Since 2008, immigrants from Asia have outnumbered those from Latin America (Waters and Pineau, 2015; US Census Bureau, 2016).

With the increasing availability of health, disease, and mortality statistics for the foreign-born population in both the administrative records and sample surveys, many US studies have examined health and mortality patterns among immigrant (foreign-born) and US-born (native-born) populations, including some analyses showing differentials over time (Kestenbaum, 1986; Singh and Yu, 1996; Hummer et al., 1999a, 1999b; Singh and Siahpush, 2001, 2002; Singh and Miller, 2004; Singh and Hiatt, 2006; Singh et al., 2011; Singh et al., 2013a, 2013b; Singh and Lin, 2013a, 2013b; Mehta et al., 2016). In this chapter, we examine mortality and life expectancy trends and differentials among immigrant and US-born populations by age, sex, race/ethnicity, and cause of death. The mortality trends and differentials presented are based on death certificate and population data from the National Vital Statistics System (NVSS) and decennial censuses, whereas nativity differentials in all-cause and cause-specific mortality risks are based on prospective data from the National Longitudinal Mortality Study (NLMS). The chapter begins by describing trends and differentials in life expectancy, followed by presentation and discussion of infant, child, and adult mortality differentials. Nativity patterns and differentials in mortality are discussed next in terms of what we know about immigrant and native-born differences in health status, chronic disease morbidity, hypertension, disability, injuries, mental health, health-risk behaviors such as obesity, physical inactivity, diet, smoking, alcohol use, health care access and use, and socioeconomic and demographic characteristics. Next, we discuss the theoretical perspectives that have been advanced for interpreting persistent and/or widening nativity differentials in health and mortality. The chapter ends with some observations on the health and mortality conditions of refugees and undocumented immigrants in the United States.

TRENDS AND DIFFERENTIALS IN LIFE EXPECTANCY, 1979–2013

The US national mortality database, a component of the NVSS, has been the primary source of mortality analyses and surveillance by age, sex, race/ethnicity, cause of death, immigrant status, marital status, socioeconomic status, and place of residence for over a century (Singh et al., 2013a; Xu et al., 2016). Nativity/immigrant status in the mortality file is determined by decedent's state/country of birth (Singh and Hiatt, 2006; Singh et al., 2013a; NCHS, 2016). For mortality analysis, individuals born outside the 50 states, DC, and US territories are considered foreign-born and referred to as immigrants (Singh and Hiatt, 2006; Singh et al., 2013a).

Table 8.1 includes data on overall nativity differentials in life expectancy from 1979 to 2013. Life expectancy estimates were calculated by the standard life table methodology by converting age-specific mortality rates (for 19 age groups: fewer than 1, 1–4, 5–9, . . ., 75–79, 80–84, and 85 years and older) into life table probabilities of dying. Infant mortality rates stratified by maternal nativity status were used to approximate the probability of dying in the first year of life (Singh and Hiatt, 2006).

During 2011–13, immigrants had an overall life expectancy of 84.0

Table 8.1 *Life expectancy (in years) by sex and immigrant status, United States, 1979–2013*

	1979–81		1989–91		1999–2001		2011–13		Absolute difference[a]			
	US-born	Foreign-born	US-born	Foreign-born	US-born	Foreign-born	US-born	Foreign-born	1979–81	1989–91	1999–2001	2011–13
Both sexes												
At birth	73.9	76.2	75.3	78.1	76.6	80.0	78.4	84.0	2.3	2.8	3.4	5.6
At age 25	50.8	53.0	51.9	54.7	52.9	56.1	54.5	59.9	2.2	2.8	3.2	5.4
At age 45	32.3	34.1	33.4	35.9	34.2	37.0	35.8	40.6	1.8	2.5	2.8	4.8
At age 65	16.8	17.1	17.4	18.6	17.8	19.3	19.3	22.7	0.3	1.2	1.5	3.4
Males												
At birth	70.1	72.8	71.7	74.9	73.8	77.8	76.0	81.8	2.7	3.2	4.0	5.8
At age 25	47.3	50.1	48.6	51.8	50.2	54.1	52.2	57.8	2.8	3.2	3.9	5.6
At age 45	29.1	31.6	30.6	33.5	31.9	35.2	33.9	38.7	2.5	2.9	3.3	4.8
At age 65	14.3	15.1	15.2	16.7	16.0	17.9	18.0	21.2	0.8	1.5	1.9	3.2
Females												
At birth	77.8	79.4	78.8	81.1	79.4	82.0	80.8	85.9	1.6	2.3	2.6	5.1
At age 25	54.3	55.7	55.0	57.2	55.3	57.8	56.7	61.7	1.4	2.2	2.5	5.0
At age 45	35.3	36.4	36.0	37.9	36.3	38.4	37.7	42.1	1.1	1.9	2.1	4.4
At age 65	18.8	18.8	19.2	20.1	19.3	20.3	20.5	23.8	0.0	0.9	1.0	3.3

Notes:
[a] Difference in life expectancy in years between foreign- and US-born individuals.
US-born or native-born are individuals born in the 50 states, District of Columbia, Puerto Rico, and other US territories. Immigrants refer to those born elsewhere.
The total number of deaths used to calculate life expectancies for US- and foreign-born individuals were as follows: 5 223 160 and 625 396 in 1979–81; 5 850 910 and 553 013 in 1989–91; 6 581 830 and 583 335 in 1999–2001; and 6 987 024 and 668 293 in 2011–13.

Source. Based on data from the US National Vital Statistics System, 1979–2013 (NCHS, 2016).

years, compared with 78.4 years for the US-born population. Nativity differentials in life expectancy at birth increased between 1979 and 2013. On average, immigrants lived longer than the US-born by 2.3 years in 1979–81, 2.8 years in 1989–91, 3.4 years in 1999–2001, and 5.6 years in 2011–13. The immigrant/US-born gap in life expectancy at age 65 increased from 0.3 years in 1979–81 to 3.4 years in 2011–13. Nativity differentials in life expectancy were larger for men than for women at each age and in each time period. The life expectancy estimates for immigrant and US-born populations at age 65 in Table 8.1 are consistent with those derived from the linked Social Security and Medicare records for the 2000–2009 time period (Mehta et al., 2016).

In the United States, immigrants in most major racial/ethnic groups have higher life expectancy than their US-born counterparts (Singh and Miller, 2004; Singh and Hiatt, 2006; Singh et al., 2013a). However, nativity differentials in life expectancy vary substantially by race/ethnicity. For example, during 1999–2001, the nativity differential was greatest for black immigrants (both sexes combined) who had 7.4 years longer life expectancy than US-born blacks (78.6 versus 71.2 years). Among the foreign-born population (both sexes combined), Asian/Pacific Islander (API) immigrants had the highest life expectancy (83.0 years), followed by Hispanic immigrants (81.6 years), black immigrants (78.6 years), and white/European immigrants (78.1 years) (Singh and Hiatt, 2006; Singh et al., 2013a). Life expectancy disparities, when stratified by ethnicity and sex, were quite wide, ranging from a low of about 67 years for US-born black men to a high of 86 years for US-born API women (Singh and Hiatt, 2006).

Differences in age-specific survivor functions for immigrant groups indicate that, regardless of gender, the US-born population not only had worse survival experiences than the immigrant population in 2011–13 but they experienced similar survival probabilities as those enjoyed by the immigrant population three decades earlier (figure available from authors on request). Although a formal decomposition analysis is needed to identify which major causes of death have contributed most to the widening nativity differentials in life expectancy, the available evidence from previous analyses of cause-specific mortality differentials seems to indicate cancer, cardiovascular disease (CVD), diabetes, respiratory diseases, unintentional injuries, and suicide as the most prominent causes accounting for the life expectancy gap (Singh and Hiatt, 2006).

TRENDS AND DIFFERENTIALS IN INFANT MORTALITY BY AGE AND CAUSE OF DEATH, 1985–2013

National linked birth and infant death files, another component of the NVSS, are generally used to compute infant mortality rates and risks in the US according to immigrant status and other socio-demographic and medical risk factors (Mathews et al., 2015). As shown in Table 8.2, during 2011–13, the infant mortality rate for US-born mothers was 6.32 per 1000 live births, 38 percent higher than the rate of 4.59 for immigrant mothers. The infant mortality rate declined faster for immigrant mothers compared with US-born mothers, which contributed to the widening nativity differentials in infant mortality between 1985 and 2013. Nativity differentials in infant mortality were greatest for black infants, and infant mortality rates varied greatly among various ethnic-immigrant groups in the United States. During 2011–13, the infant mortality rate ranged from a low of 2.38 per 1000 live births for Chinese immigrants to a high of 11.86 for US-born blacks.

Even after controlling for infant- and maternal-risk factors such as maternal age, race/ethnicity, marital status, birth order, maternal education, prenatal care, and smoking during pregnancy, infants born to immigrant mothers continue to have significantly lower risks of infant mortality than those born to US-born mothers (Singh et al., 2013a). Similar nativity patterns have been observed for other birth outcomes such as low birthweight and preterm birth (Singh and Yu, 1996; Singh and Miller, 2004).

Neonatal mortality refers to infant deaths in the first 27 days of life, whereas post-neonatal mortality refers to infant deaths between 28 days and 1 year of age. Nativity differentials in post-neonatal mortality are larger than those in the neonatal period. Socioeconomic, behavioral, and environmental influences on infant mortality are greater in the post-neonatal period than in the neonatal period. During 2011–2013, the neonatal mortality rate for US-born mothers was 4.14 per 1000 live births, 23 percent higher than the rate of 3.37 for immigrant mothers. The post-neonatal mortality rate for US-born mothers was 2.18 per 1000 live births, 80 percent higher than the rate of 1.21 for immigrant mothers (data not shown).

The leading causes of infant death in the United States are congenital anomalies (birth defects), short gestation and low birthweight (LBW), and sudden infant death syndrome (SIDS). During 2011–13, infants born to immigrant mothers had 25 percent lower risk of mortality from LBW/prematurity and 74 percent lower risk of SIDS mortality than those born to US-born mothers. No significant nativity differentials existed in rates of infant mortality from birth defects (data not shown).

Table 8.2 *Infant mortality rates (IMRs) per 1000 live births for major ethnic-immigrant groups and nativity differentials in infant mortality, United States, 1985–2013*

	1985–88 (N = 15 207 754)			1999–2002 (N = 16 023 367)			2011–13 (N = 11 797 322)			
Ethnic-immigrant group	Infant deaths	IMR	Rate ratio[a]	Infant deaths	IMR	Rate ratio[a]	Infant deaths	IMR	Rate ratio[a]	% Decline IMR 1985–2013
Total population			1.24*			1.39*			1.38*	
US-born[b]	133 903	10.08		90 253	7.21		57 658	6.32		37.3
FB[c]	15 626	8.12		18 119	5.17		12 260	4.59		43.5
Non-Hispanic White			1.11*			1.25*			1.33*	
US-born	84 099	8.32		51 083	5.74		30 551	5.12		38.5
FB	3 543	7.52		2 414	4.59		1 522	3.86		48.7
Non-Hispanic Black			1.31*			1.43*			1.60*	
US-born	40 443	18.07		29 073	13.84		17 232	11.86		34.4
FB	2 356	13.75		2 528	9.71		1 793	7.41		46.1
American Indian/AN	1 834	13.10		1 398	9.04		902	8.51		35.0
Asian or Pacific Islander			1.24*			1.45*			1.29*	
US-born	629	8.77		842	6.39		842	4.94		43.7
FB	2 715	7.08		2 892	4.40		2 892	3.83		45.9
Chinese			1.30*			0.96			0.96	
US-born	61	7.26		36	2.96		50	2.69		62.9
FB	353	5.58		353	3.08		303	2.38		57.3
Japanese			1.18			1.47*			1.60	
US-born	126	7.19		75	5.37		23	3.93		45.3
FB	91	6.08		77	3.65		39	2.46		59.5
Filipino			1.34*			1.04			0.94	

US-born	110	9.09		135	5.84		110	4.39		51.7
FB	502	6.78		559	5.62		343	4.67		31.1
Hawaiian	220	10.79		189	8.84		19	6.82		36.8
Other Asian/Pacific Islander			1.12*			1.51*			1.31*	
US-born	116	8.55		360	6.83		202	5.52		35.4
FB	1765	7.65		1888	4.51		1609	4.22		44.8
Asian Indian						1.81*			1.25	
US-born				27	7.28		82	4.85		
FB				394	4.02		631	3.88		
Korean						0.83			1.18	
US-born				8	3.26		33	4.18		
FB				146	3.92		138	3.54		
Vietnamese						1.22			1.03	
US-born				8	4.80		33	3.72		
FB				239	3.95		194	3.61		
Samoan						1.56			1.03	
US-born				32	10.12		35	10.60		
FB				22	6.49		27	10.25		
Hispanic			1.18*			1.28*			1.20*	
US-born	6548	9.17		7965	6.41		7200	5.55		39.5
FB	7046	7.78		10276	4.99		6589	4.63		40.5
Mexican			1.17*			1.25*			1.12*	
US-born	3889	8.77		5364	6.14		4050	5.26		40.0
FB	4244	7.47		7282	4.90		4207	4.69		37.2
Puerto Rican			1.12*			1.05			1.06	
US-born	961	11.61		1243	8.33		1017	6.96		40.1
Foreign-born	763	10.38		639	7.95		356	6.54		37.0

Table 8.2 (continued)

Ethnic-immigrant group	1985–88 (N = 15 207 754)			1999–2002 (N = 16 023 367)			2011–13 (N = 11 797 322)			% Decline IMR 1985–2013
	Infant deaths	IMR	Rate ratio[a]	Infant deaths	IMR	Rate ratio[a]	Infant deaths	IMR	Rate ratio[a]	
Cuban			1.45*			1.15*			1.13*	
US-born	59	10.36		110	4.62		113	4.34		58.1
FB	246	7.13		124	4.01		104	3.83		46.3
Central and South American			0.91			1.15*			1.07*	
US-born	40	7.02		283	5.52		295	4.48		36.2
FB	1 459	7.68		1 987	4.82		1 396	4.20		45.3
Other Hispanic			1.07			1.40*			1.26*	
US-born	1 599	9.06		965	6.65		1 724	5.93		34.5
FB	334	8.48		243	4.76		527	4.70		44.6

Notes:
* $p < 0.05$.
FB = foreign-born. IMR = infant mortality rate.
[a] Rate ratio = ration of rate for the US-born in each ethnic group to that for the corresponding immigrant group.
[b] US-born are those born in the 50 states and the District of Columbia.
[c] Foreign-born are those born elsewhere.

Source: Data derived from the 1985–2013 US National Linked Birth and Infant Death data files (Mathews et al., 2015).

Decomposition analysis indicated that 22 percent of the nativity differential in infant mortality can be attributed to the excess SIDS mortality among the US-born. More than 40 percent of the nativity gap in infant mortality can be attributed to the higher mortality among infants of US-born mothers from perinatal conditions, a broad cause-of-death category that includes prematurity and LBW, infections, maternal complications of pregnancy, and respiratory distress syndrome (data not shown).

TRENDS AND DIFFERENTIALS IN CHILD AND YOUTH MORTALITY, 1979–2013

During 2011–13, immigrant children aged 1–14 years had 6 percent lower all-cause mortality than US-born children (15.6 versus 16.6 deaths per 100 000 population). During 1979–81, child mortality rates were similar for immigrant and US-born children (27.6 versus 27.3 per 100 000). During 2011–13, immigrant men aged 15–24 had 22 percent lower all-cause mortality and immigrant women 34 percent lower all-cause mortality than their US-born counterparts. Nativity differentials in youth mortality widened over time as mortality declined faster among immigrant youth than US-born youth during 1979–2013 (Singh and Hiatt, 2006).

TRENDS AND DIFFERENTIALS IN ALL-CAUSE AND CAUSE-SPECIFIC MORTALITY, 1979–2013

During 2011–13, both male and female immigrants experienced 34 percent lower all-cause age-adjusted mortality than their US-born counterparts (Table 8.3). This pattern held for non-Hispanic whites, blacks, APIs, and Hispanics, although the nativity differential was greatest for black immigrants who had approximately 50 percent lower all-cause mortality than US-born blacks. Similar ethnic-nativity patterns in all-cause were observed previously for the 1989–91 and 1999–2001 time periods (Singh and Hiatt, 2006). Nativity differentials in all-cause mortality in the United States have increased consistently over time as mortality rates for immigrants have declined faster than those for the US-born.

Ethnic-nativity patterns in CVD and all-cancer mortality in the United States are generally similar to those in all-cause mortality with a few exceptions. Overall, male and female immigrants had, respectively, 29 percent and 26 percent lower CVD mortality than their US-born counterparts during 2011–13 (Table 8.3). Immigrants also had lower

Table 8.3 Average annual age-adjusted death rates for selected major causes of death by nativity/immigrant status, USA, 2011–13

	Male					Female				
	US-born		Foreign-born		Rate	US-born		Foreign-born		Rate
Cause of death	Rate	SE	Rate	SE	Ratio	Rate	SE	Rate	SE	Ratio
All-cause mortality	911.99	0.48	602.99	1.07	0.66*	655.18	0.35	434.24	0.8	0.66*
Non-Hispanic White	851.98	0.28	695.21	1.14	0.82*	657.10	0.22	537.61	0.87	0.82*
Black	1081.24	0.99	536.02	2.26	0.50*	729.05	0.64	377.61	1.5	0.52*
Asian/Pacific Islander	602.70	2.40	429.65	1.02	0.71*	409.48	1.81	306.21	0.7	0.75*
Hispanic	748.81	1.24	577.39	1.09	0.77*	510.36	0.89	404.14	0.8	0.79*
Cardiovascular diseases (CVD)	281.80	0.27	199.26	0.63	0.71*	192.60	0.19	142.14	0.4	0.74*
Heart disease	225.99	0.24	153.27	0.55	0.68*	141.07	0.16	101.50	0.4	0.72*
Stroke	38.02	0.10	32.69	0.26	0.86*	36.91	0.08	29.60	0.20	0.80*
All cancers combined	208.36	0.23	148.99	0.53	0.72*	147.12	0.17	107.50	0.38	0.73*
Lung cancer	59.37	0.12	33.43	0.25	0.56*	39.26	0.09	18.11	0.15	0.46*
Colorectal cancer	18.30	0.07	14.53	0.16	0.79*	13.00	0.05	10.22	0.11	0.79*
Prostate cancer	20.43	0.08	16.15	0.18	0.79*					
Breast cancer						22.02	0.07	16.16	0.14	0.73*
Stomach cancer	3.93	0.03	7.22	0.11	1.84*	2.00	0.02	4.21	0.07	2.10*
Liver and IBD cancer	9.11	0.05	10.87	0.14	1.19*	3.56	0.03	5.04	0.08	1.42*
Diabetes	26.51	0.08	21.62	0.20	0.82*	15.07	0.14	18.33	0.06	0.82*
Pneumonia and influenza	18.67	0.07	16.22	0.19	0.87*	13.75	0.05	11.02	0.12	0.80*
COPD	51.64	0.12	22.74	0.22	0.44*	41.79	0.09	15.55	0.14	0.37*
Liver cirrhosis	14.09	0.06	9.65	0.12	0.69*	7.17	0.04	4.28	0.07	0.60*

Nephritis/kidney diseases	16.91	0.07	11.74	0.16	0.69*	11.83	0.05	7.46	0.10	0.63*
Alzheimer's disease	20.72	0.08	13.72	0.18	0.66*	27.24	0.07	18.29	0.15	0.67*
HIV/AIDS	3.47	0.03	2.18	0.05	0.63*	1.37	0.02	0.61	0.03	0.44*
Other infectious diseases	20.83	0.07	14.51	0.17	0.70*	16.62	0.06	11.32	0.13	0.68*
Unintentional injuries	57.94	0.12	31.79	0.25	0.55*	29.72	0.08	13.83	0.16	0.47*
Motor vehicle accidents	17.01	0.07	11.66	0.14	0.69*	6.68	0.04	4.58	0.10	0.69*
Non-motor-vehicle injuries	40.93	0.10	20.13	0.20	0.49*	23.04	0.07	9.25	0.13	0.40*
Suicide	22.15	0.08	10.68	0.13	0.48*	5.86	0.04	3.10	0.07	0.53*
Homicide	8.88	0.05	5.38	0.10	0.61*	2.33	0.02	1.46	0.10	0.63*

Notes:
Death rates are per 100 000 population, and age-adjusted by the direct method to the 2000 US standard population.
SE = standard error.
Rate ratio = ratio of mortality rate for immigrants to that for the US-born.
US- or native-born are individuals born in the 50 states, DC, Puerto Rico, and other US territories.
Immigrants refer to those born elsewhere.
* $p < 0.05$.

Source: Derived from the US National Vital Statistics System (NCHS, 2016).

CVD mortality than the US-born in earlier time periods; however, the gap in CVD mortality has widened over time in favor of immigrants (Singh and Hiatt, 2006). Previous studies have shown lower CVD mortality among black and Hispanic immigrants compared to their US-born counterparts; however, non-Hispanic white and API immigrant women appear to have higher CVD mortality rates than their US-born counterparts (Singh and Hiatt, 2006; Singh et al., 2013a). The increased CVD mortality risk is found among Japanese and Filipino immigrant men and women but not among Chinese immigrants (Singh and Miller, 2004).

In 2011–13, male and female immigrants had at least 27 percent lower overall cancer mortality than their US-born counterparts did (Table 8.3). In earlier studies, API and Hispanic immigrants had the lowest all-cancer mortality rates of all groups, and immigrants in each broad racial/ethnic group generally had lower cancer mortality rates then their US-born counterparts (Singh and Hiatt, 2006; Singh et al., 2013a).

Nativity differentials are particularly pronounced in tobacco-related cancers such as lung and esophageal cancers (Singh and Miller, 2004; Singh and Hiatt, 2006; Singh et al., 2013a). In 2011–13, lung cancer mortality was 44 percent lower among male immigrants and 54 percent lower among female immigrants compared to the US-born (Table 8.3). This pattern is generally found for most ethnic groups in the United States, although immigrants in certain Asian subgroups such as Chinese and Japanese women, based on 1986–94 data, appeared to have higher lung and esophageal cancer mortality rates than their US-born counterparts (Singh and Miller, 2004). This needs to be confirmed with more recent data.

Compared with the US-born, immigrants experience substantially lower risk of mortality from other major cancers such as colorectal, prostate, breast, kidney, non-Hodgkin's lymphoma, and brain cancers (Singh and Hiatt, 2006). Table 8.3 shows 21–27 percent lower mortality risks in 2011–13 from colorectal, prostate and breast cancers among immigrants compared to the US-born. Comparison of recent estimates with data from the earlier time periods shows widening disparities in colorectal and breast cancer mortality between immigrants and the US-born (Singh and Hiatt, 2006).

Previous studies have shown increased risks of cervical cancer mortality in immigrant women, particularly among API immigrants (Singh and Miller, 2004; Singh and Hiatt, 2006). Higher cervical cancer mortality in immigrant women is consistent with their lower use of Pap smear and higher incidence of cervical cancer in Asian Americans, particularly Vietnamese Americans. These ethnic-immigrant differences may also reflect disparities in human papillomavirus infection (Singh and Hiatt, 2006).

Time trend data have shown consistently higher rates of stomach and liver cancer mortality among immigrants than the US-born, with the absolute risk of stomach and liver cancer mortality being particularly high among immigrant and US-born Asians, Hispanics, and blacks (Singh and Miller, 2004; Singh and Hiatt, 2006; Singh et al., 2013a). In 2011–13, immigrant men and women had an approximately two times higher rate of mortality from stomach cancer than their US-born counterparts did (Table 8.3). During the same time period, immigrant men and women had, respectively, 19 percent and 42 percent higher liver cancer mortality than US-born men and women. Higher liver and stomach cancer mortality rates in the above ethnic-immigrant groups have been partly attributed to their higher incidence of hepatitis-B virus and *Helicobacter pylori* infection (Singh and Hiatt, 2006; Singh et al., 2013a).

As for disparities in other chronic diseases, mortality from diabetes, chronic obstructive pulmonary disease (COPD), liver cirrhosis, kidney diseases, and Alzheimer's disease in 2011–13 was significantly lower among immigrants, compared to the US-born (Table 8.3). Nativity differentials in COPD mortality, for which smoking is a major risk factor, have increased consistently over time, with immigrant men experiencing a 34 percent lower mortality risk in 1979–81 and 56 percent lower risk in 2011–13; for women, the differential increased from 38 percent lower mortality risk among immigrants in 1979–81 to 63 percent lower risk in 2011–13 (Singh and Hiatt, 2006; Table 8.3).

Risks of mortality from HIV/AIDS and other infectious diseases are markedly lower in immigrants than the US-born. Immigrants have half the rate of mortality from unintentional (motor vehicle and non-motor-vehicle) injuries compared to the US-born, with the nativity differentials in mortality widening over time. Differentials in suicide mortality also widened over time, with immigrants overall experiencing about 50 percent lower suicide risk than their US-born counterparts. However, nativity patterns in suicide mortality have been shown to vary by ethnicity and sex. Data from 1989–91 and 1999–2001 indicate lower rates of suicide among Asian, black, and Hispanic immigrant men, and higher rates of suicide among non-Hispanic white and Asian immigrant women, compared to their US-born counterparts (Singh and Hiatt, 2006). Data from 1986–94 indicate a two-fold higher suicide risk among Chinese and Japanese immigrant women and an approximately 50 percent higher suicide risk among Chinese and Japanese immigrant men, compared to their US-born counterparts (Singh and Miller, 2004). In 2011–13, homicide rates for immigrant men and women were about 40 percent lower than those for the US-born (Table 8.3). However, ethnic-specific data for 1999–2001 indicated 89 percent and 36 percent higher homicide rates for non-Hispanic white immigrant men and women, respectively, compared to the US-born. Although the absolute risk of homicide among APIs is the lowest among all the major racial/ethnic groups in the United States, API immigrant men, but not women, have a significantly higher homicide rate than US-born API men (Singh and Hiatt, 2006). During 1986–94, API immigrant men overall and Chinese and Filipino immigrant men, in particular, had a two-fold higher risk of homicide victimization than their US-born counterparts (Singh and Miller, 2004).

Immigrant Mortality Patterns Based on the National Longitudinal Mortality Study

The 1979–2011 NLMS is a longitudinal dataset for examining socioeconomic, occupational, and demographic factors associated with all-cause and cause-specific mortality in the United States (Sorlie et al., 1995; US Census Bureau, 2012). Nativity patterns in mortality based on the NLMS are generally consistent with those derived from the NVSS, although the ability to control for the baseline socioeconomic and demographic characteristics using a cohort approach is clearly an advantage. Additionally, the analysis based on the NLMS is not subject to the numerator-denominator inconsistency problem that can influence results based on the NVSS (Singh and Hiatt, 2006; Singh et al., 2013a). Moreover, in the NLMS, the racial/ethnic detail is based on self-reports as obtained in the CPS and decennial census.

The analysis of the 1979–2011 public-use NLMS file using various population cohorts and a mortality follow-up of 11 years is presented in Table 8.4. Nativity differentials in all-cause mortality appears to narrow by age. After controlling for socio-demographic covariates, immigrants aged 20–44 years had 52 percent lower risk of mortality than the US-born. Immigrants aged 45–64 and 65 years and over had 47 percent and 35 percent lower adjusted risk of mortality than their US-born counterparts, respectively. Adjusted nativity differentials in mortality were larger for men than women, and for blacks and Hispanics than for APIs and non-Hispanic whites (Table 8.4).

Previous analyses of NLMS have indicated large ethnic-immigrant disparities in all-cause mortality and cause-specific mortality, with mortality risks being lowest among black, API, and Hispanic immigrants (Singh and Siahpush, 2002). Analysis of the most recent follow-up data from the 1979–2011 NLMS indicates a similar ethnic-nativity

Table 8.4 *Age- and covariate-adjusted mortality risks (derived from Cox regression models) for immigrants relative to US-born men and women, by age, sex, and race/ethnicity: the US National Longitudinal Mortality Study, 1979–2011, 11-year mortality follow-up*

	Age adjusted[a]			Covariate adjusted[b]		
Age group (years), sex, or race/ethnicity	Hazard ratio	95% CI		Hazard ratio	95% CI	
Population aged 20+	0.62	0.61	0.64	0.68	0.66	0.70
Population aged 20-44	0.59	0.55	0.63	0.48	0.45	0.52
Population aged 45-64	0.58	0.55	0.60	0.53	0.51	0.55
Population aged 65+	0.66	0.64	0.68	0.65	0.63	0.67
Men aged 20+	0.59	0.57	0.61	0.63	0.61	0.66
Women aged 20+	0.67	0.65	0.69	0.73	0.70	0.76
Non-Hispanic Whites aged 20+	0.73	0.71	0.75	0.74	0.72	0.77
Non-Hispanic Blacks aged 20+	0.42	0.37	0.47	0.47	0.41	0.53
Asian/Pacific Islanders aged 20+	0.68	0.61	0.75	0.70	0.62	0.78
Hispanics aged 20+	0.61	0.58	0.64	0.59	0.56	0.62

Notes:
[a] Adjusted for age only.
[b] Adjusted for age, sex, race/ethnicity, marital status, rural/urban residence, geographic region, education, occupation, and family income.

Source: Based on US Census Bureau (2012).

pattern. Black, API, Mexican, and non-Hispanic white immigrants aged 20 years and over had, respectively, 47 percent, 50 percent, 58 percent, and 26 percent lower risks of all-cause mortality than US-born non-Hispanic whites of equivalent socioeconomic and demographic background (Figure 8.1).

Overall, adult immigrants have lower adjusted risks of mortality than the US-born from CVD, heart disease, stroke, all cancers combined and lung, colorectal, prostate, and breast cancers, diabetes, pneumonia and influenza, COPD, cirrhosis, nephritis, and Alzheimer's disease, HIV/AIDS and other infectious diseases, unintentional injuries, suicide, and firearm injuries (Table 8.5). For many of the chronic diseases, controlling for sociodemographic factors reduced nativity differentials in mortality, however, marked differences persisted. The excess risk of stomach cancer mortality in immigrants is mostly accounted for after controlling for race/ethnicity, socioeconomic status, and other demographic covariates. However, immigrants maintained 27 percent higher risk of liver cancer mortality than

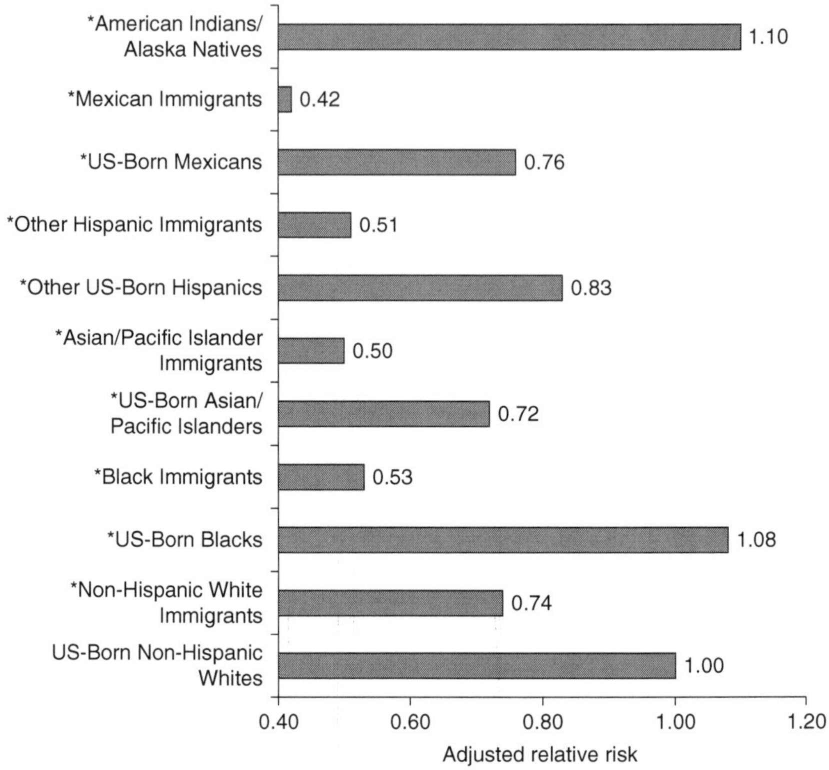

Notes:
Adjusted by Cox regression for age, sex, marital status, education, occupation, family income, rural/ urban residence, and geographic region.
* $p < 0.01$, US-born non-Hispanic whites as the reference group.
Number of deaths during the 11-year follow-up = 154 087.

Source: Based on US Census Bureau (2012).

Figure 8.1 Ethnic-immigrant differentials in US all-cause mortality (hazard ratio or relative risk) among those aged 20+ years: the US National Longitudinal Mortality Study, 1979–2011 (N = 1 283 880)

the US-born even after controlling for socio-demographic covariates. No significant differences in homicide risk were found between immigrants and the US-born after controlling for socio-demographic differences. These patterns are largely consistent with those observed in the previous follow-up of the NLMS cohorts (Singh and Siahpush, 2001).

Table 8.5 *Age- and covariate-adjusted mortality risks (derived from Cox regression models) for immigrants relative to US-born men and women aged 20+ years, by major causes of death: the US National Longitudinal Mortality Study, 1979–2011, 11-year mortality follow-up*

Cause of death	Age-adjusted[a]			Covariate-adjusted[b]		
	Hazard ratio	95% confidence interval		Hazard ratio	95% confidence interval	
Cardiovascular diseases (CVD)	0.60	0.58	0.63	0.69	0.58	0.63
Heart disease	0.60	0.58	0.63	0.68	0.65	0.72
Stroke	0.61	0.56	0.67	0.70	0.63	0.77
All cancers combined	0.62	0.59	0.65	0.71	0.68	0.75
Lung cancer	0.43	0.39	0.47	0.57	0.51	0.63
Colorectal cancer	0.65	0.57	0.74	0.77	0.66	0.89
Prostate cancer	0.62	0.51	0.75	0.71	0.58	0.88
Breast cancer	0.68	0.59	0.79	0.82	0.69	0.97
Stomach cancer	1.32	1.08	1.62	1.05	0.83	1.34
Liver and IBD cancer	1.87	1.52	2.31	1.27	0.97	1.66
Diabetes	0.80	0.70	0.91	0.63	0.54	0.73
Pneumonia and influenza	0.65	0.57	0.74	0.62	0.53	0.72
COPD	0.35	0.30	0.40	0.44	0.38	0.51
Liver cirrhosis	0.81	0.68	0.97	0.63	0.51	0.77
Nephritis/kidney diseases	0.66	0.54	0.81	0.62	0.49	0.78
Alzheimer's disease	0.79	0.64	0.98	0.92	0.73	1.16
HIV/AIDS	1.00	0.82	1.22	0.72	0.57	0.92
Other infectious diseases	0.74	0.61	0.90	0.75	0.60	0.93
Unintentional injuries	0.61	0.54	0.69	0.68	0.59	0.79
Motor vehicle accidents	0.62	0.51	0.74	0.68	0.55	0.85
Non-motor-vehicle injuries	0.60	0.51	0.71	0.69	0.57	0.83
Suicide	0.49	0.40	0.61	0.61	0.48	0.79
Homicide	1.33	1.01	1.61	0.92	0.68	1.24
Firearm injuries	0.54	0.43	0.67	0.62	0.48	0.80

Notes:
[a] Adjusted for age only.
[b] Adjusted for age, sex, race/ethnicity, marital status, rural/urban residence, geographic region, education, occupation, and family income.

Source: Based on US Census Bureau (2012).

DISCUSSION

Life expectancy and mortality patterns for immigrants and the native-born vary considerably in the United States. Overall, immigrants have higher life expectancy and lower infant, child, youth, and adult mortality rates than the US-born. The foreign-born population in the United States is a very heterogeneous group, and the nativity/immigrant patterns in life expectancy and age- and cause-specific mortality vary greatly across different racial/ethnic groups. Immigrants currently live 5.6 years longer than the US-born, with the immigrant advantage in life expectancy at birth increasing from 2.3 years in 1979–81 to 5.6 years in 2011–13. The nativity gap (or the immigrant advantage) in life expectancy at birth has increased by 2.2 years for the total population and by 2.5 years for women in just a decade.

Ethnic-nativity patterns in life expectancy revealed a disparity of 19 years in 1999–2001 – ranging from a low of 67 years for US-born black men to a high of 86 years for US-born API women. A 20-year gap in life expectancy has previously been noted between the most and least advantaged populations in the United States and between Australians and Aboriginal and Torres Strait Islander peoples (Marmot, 2005). Some studies have found even greater disparities in life expectancy at birth and at older ages when considering detailed Asian subgroups and country/region of birth categories for the US foreign-born population (Singh and Miller, 2004; Mehta et al., 2016). Estimates for a more recent time period need to be developed to examine whether ethnic-nativity disparities in life expectancy have continued to widen.

A number of explanations have been suggested for higher life expectancy, better health, and lower mortality rates among immigrants. First, people immigrating to the United States may be healthier than those who remain in their countries of origin. This is referred to as the 'healthy immigrant effect' or positive immigrant selectivity (Singh and Siahpush, 2001, 2002; Singh and Miller, 2004; Singh and Hiatt, 2006). Second, immigrants have lower prevalence of many health-risk behaviors than the native-born, including lower rates of smoking, drinking, obesity, and better diet (Singh and Siahpush, 2001, 2002; Singh and Hiatt, 2006; Singh et al., 2011; Singh and Lin, 2013a; Singh et al., 2013a). Third, immigrants appear to have higher levels of social and familial support and social integration compared with the native-born (Singh and Yu, 1996; Singh and Miller, 2004; Singh and Hiatt, 2006; Singh et al., 2013a). This is particularly evident when suicide rates for certain ethnic-immigrant groups are compared with those for the native-born. Trovato and Jarvis (1986), for example, found lower rates of suicide among Italian, Portuguese, and Irish immigrants (the groups with presumably higher levels of social integration given their Catholic religious background) and higher suicide rates among English-Welsh, Scottish, German, and American immigrants (groups known to have lower levels of community integration) compared with the Canadian-born population. The 'Roseto effect' involving a study of an Italian American community in Pennsylvania has also been cited as evidence for the protective effects of social integration and social support on mortality and survival (Egolf et al., 1992). Fourth, socioeconomic characteristics might partly account for nativity differentials and trends in health and mortality outcomes. Although immigrants are generally better educated, they have higher unemployment and poverty rates and lower rates of health insurance coverage than the US-born (Singh and Hiatt, 2006; Singh and Lin, 2013b; Singh et al., 2013a; US Census Bureau, 2016). However, previous studies and analyses presented in this chapter indicate only a modest contribution of socioeconomic factors in explaining nativity differentials in infant mortality, all-cause mortality, and mortality from chronic diseases and injuries (Singh and Yu, 1996; Singh and Siahpush, 2001, 2002; Singh and Hiatt, 2006; Singh et al., 2013a).

Errors in the reporting of immigrant or foreign-born status in vital records, census, and sample surveys such as the Current Population Survey, American Community Survey, and National Health Interview Survey may also contribute to the reported life expectancy, mortality, and health differentials between immigrants and the native-born (Singh and Siahpush, 2001; Singh and Hiatt, 2006; Singh et al., 2013a). However, the consistency of findings of lower immigrant mortality and longer life expectancy based on both vital statistics and longitudinal data across various settings and over time appears to rule out potential data biases as a major explanation for reported nativity differentials in mortality.

Growing ethnic heterogeneity of the immigrant population as well as its migration selectivity and continuing advantages in social and behavioral characteristics have been suggested as factors explaining the widening health and mortality gaps between immigrants and the US-born (Singh and Hiatt, 2006). Socioeconomic and behavioral-risk profiles of the immigrant population relative to the US-born population have become more favorable over time (Singh and Hiatt, 2006; Singh et al., 2011; US Census Bureau, 2016). Trend data on obesity, smoking, hypertension, and chronic disease prevalence show a widening gap, with immigrants showing increasingly lower rates of behavioral and health risks over time compared with the US-born population (Singh and Hiatt, 2006; Singh et al., 2011; NCHS, 2016). The racial/ethnic composition of the immigrant population in the United States has undergone substantial change, largely due to a tremendous increase in the skilled migration from such Asian countries as China, India, South Korea, Taiwan, the Philippines, and Vietnam following the Immigration Act of 1965 (Singh and Miller, 2004; Singh and Hiatt, 2006; Singh et al., 2013a).

As the US immigrant population has become more diverse in its ethnic and country-of-birth composition, both acculturation and cultural pluralism have been suggested as complementary theoretical perspectives for explaining changing behavioral and health inequalities between immigrants and the native-born (Alba and Nee, 1997; Gans, 1997; Singh and Miller, 2004; Singh and Hiatt, 2006). Acculturation, the process by which immigrants adopt behavioral and lifestyle practices of the native-born (often measured by duration of residence in the host country since the time of immigration), plays a major role in modifying the social, behavioral, and health characteristics of immigrants, particularly of Asian and Hispanic immigrant groups, which generally leads to a decline in their health and mortality advantage over time (Chen et al., 1996; Singh and Siahpush, 2002; Singh and Hiatt, 2006; Singh and Miller, 2004; Singh et al., 2013a; Mehta et al., 2016). However, acculturation effects may vary by ethnicity, and health and mortality advantage of certain immigrant groups in the United States, particularly those of Asian and Hispanic origins, may persist into the second generation or beyond (Hummer et al., 1999a, 1999b; Singh and Siahpush, 2002; Singh and Miller, 2004; Singh and Hiatt, 2006; Singh and Lin, 2013b; Singh et al., 2013b). For many Asian and Hispanic immigrants, acculturation may not necessarily accompany other forms of assimilation, such as social and structural assimilation (Alba and Nee, 1997; Singh and Hiatt, 2006). In this regard, cultural pluralism, whereby groups retain significant ties to their ethnic and cultural heritage, may provide a more adequate explanation of why immigrants continue to maintain better health status or lower mortality than do their US-born counterparts (Gans, 1997; Singh and Siahpush, 2002; Singh and Hiatt, 2006).

Refugees, Asylum Seekers (Asylees), and Undocumented/Unauthorized Immigrants

Few studies have examined refugee and asylee health; and to our knowledge, no studies have looked at mortality patterns among undocumented immigrants in the United States.[1] Clearly, this remains an important area for further research. Here, we offer a few observations on these immigrant categories in the hope of stimulating further interest. Refugees and asylees, similar to the general immigrant population, are younger than the US native-born population. They come from diverse regions of the world and bring with them specific health risks and disease. Limited findings suggest that refugees and asylees have similar infectious disease burden and prevention needs, both had higher prevalence of latent tuberculosis infection, hepatitis B and HIV seropositivity than the US population (Chai et al., 2013). Some studies have found higher rates of chronic disease and poorer overall health status among refugees when compared with other immigrant populations and age-matched US peers (Wong et al., 2011; Yun et al., 2012). Country of origin was found to be highly associated with the long-term morbidity associated with obesity, hypertension, type-2 diabetes, and tobacco use among refugees and asylees (Dookeran et al., 2010; Nguyen and Rehkopf, 2016). However, mortality data specific to refugees and asylees in the United States are not available.

CONCLUSION

Life expectancy and mortality patterns vary greatly among ethnic-nativity groups in the United States, with consistently better outcomes for immigrants than for the US-born. The life expectancy and survival advantage for immigrants relative to the US-born has increased over time. All-cause mortality is 34 percent lower and life expectancy at birth 5.6 years longer for immigrants compared with the US-born. Except for a few causes of death such as stomach and liver cancers, mortality from most causes of death, including chronic and infectious diseases, injuries, suicide, and violence, are substantially lower in immigrants than in the US-born population. Ethnic-nativity patterns show wide disparities in mortality and survival – a 19-year lower life expectancy at birth for US-born black men compared with immigrant and US-born API women and a 3.5 times higher all-cause mortality rate for US-born black men compared with immigrant API women. The most important factors indicated in the literature for the immigrant survival advantage in relation to the US-born include the healthy migrant effect, increased skilled and highly selective immigration from Asia, lower prevalence of health risk factors in migrants, especially smoking, obesity, heavy drinking, and poor nutrition/diet; higher levels of familial and social supports available to immigrants, as well as lower disability and disease prevalence. Consideration of these factors together with the broader social determinants such as social and material conditions, physical and built environments, and healthcare access and use of quality health services is needed to understand fully the marked ethnic-immigrant differentials in health and mortality reported here. Unfortunately, existing federal administrative databases and sample surveys such as the NVSS, NLMS, and linked census and mortality databases, do not include legal and refugee status of immigrants. Therefore, it is currently not possible to derive mortality and life expectancy estimates for this important segment of the immigrant population and to examine whether refugees, asylees, and undocumented immigrants experience similar health, mortality, and survival advantages as the general immigrant population in the United States.

NOTES

* The views expressed are the authors' and not necessarily those of the Health Resources and Services Administration or the US Department of Health and Human Services.

1. The numbers of refugees and asylees admitted to the United States vary by year. In 2014, about 70000 new refugees were authorized to come into the United States and 24000 individuals granted asylum status (Mossaad, 2016). In 2016, more than 70000 refugees were admitted. Regarding undocumented migrants, there were an estimated 11.1 million such cases in the United States in 2014, accounting for about one-quarter of the total foreign-born population (Waters and Pineau, 2015; Passel and Cohn, 2016).

REFERENCES

Alba, R., and V. Nee (1997), 'Rethinking assimilation theory for a new era of immigration', *International Migration Review*, **31** (4), 826–74.

Chai, S.J., J. Davies-Cole and S.T. Cookson (2013), 'Infectious disease burden and vaccination needs among asylees versus refugees, District of Columbia', *Clinical Infectious Diseases*, **56** (5), 652–8.

Chen, J., R. Wilkins and E. Ng (1996), 'Health expectancy by immigrant status, 1986 and 1991', *Health Reports*, **8** (3), 29–38.

Dookeran, N.M., T. Battaglia, J. Cochran and P.L. Geltman (2010), 'Chronic disease and its risk factors among refugees and asylees in Massachusetts, 2001–2005', *Preventing Chronic Disease*, **7** (3), A51.

Egolf, B., J. Lasker, S. Wolf and L. Potvin (1992), 'The Roseto effect: a 50-year comparison of mortality rates', *American Journal of Public Health*, **82** (8), 1089–92.

Gans, H.J. (1997), 'Toward a reconciliation of "assimilation" and "pluralism": the interplay of acculturation and ethnic retention', *International Migration Review*, **31** (4), 875–92.

Hummer, R.A., M. Biegler, P.B. De Turk, D. Forbes, W.P. Frisbie, Y. Hong Y. and S.G. Pullam (1999a), 'Race/ethnicity, nativity and infant mortality in the United States', *Social Forces*, **77** (3), 1083–118.

Hummer, R.A., R. G. Rogers, C.B. Nam and F.B. LeClere (1999b), 'Race/ethnicity, nativity and US adult mortality', *Social Science Quarterly*, **80** (1), 136–53.

Kestenbaum, B. (1986), 'Mortality by nativity', *Demography*, **23** (1), 87–90.

Larsen, L.J. (2003), 'The foreign-born population in the United States: 2003', Current Population Reports, Washington, DC: US Census Bureau, pp. 20–551.

Marmot, M. (2005), 'Social determinants of health inequalities', *Lancet*, **365** (9464), 1099–104.

Mathews, T.J., M.F. MacDorman and M.E. Thoma (2015), 'Infant mortality statistics from the 2013 period linked birth/infant death data set', *National Vital Statistics Reports*, **64** (9), 1–30.

Mehta, N.K., I.T. Elo, M. Engelman, D.S. Lauderdale and B.M. Kestenbaum (2016), 'Life expectancy among US-born and foreign-born older adults in the United States: estimates from linked Social Security and Medicare data', *Demography*, **53** (4), 1109–34.

Mossaad, N. (2016), 'Refugees and asylees: 2014. Annual flow report', Policy Directorate, DHS Office of Immigration Statistics, accessed 30 September 2016 at https://www.dhs.gov/sites/default/files/publications/Refugees%20%26%20Asylees%20Flow%20Report%202014_508.pdf.

National Center for Health Statistics (NCHS) (2016), National Vital Statistics System, Mortality Multiple Cause-of-Death Public Use Data File Documentation, US Department of Health and Human Services, Hyattsville, MD, accessed 12 May 2016 at http://www.cdc.gov/nchs/nvss/mortality_public_use_data.htm.

Nguyen, M.T. and D.H. Rehkopf (2016), 'Prevalence of chronic disease and their risk factors among Iranian, Ukrainian, and Vietnamese refugees in California, 2002–2011', *Journal of Immigrant and Minority Health*, **18** (6), 1274–83, doi:10.1007/s10903-015-0327-5.

Passel, J.S. and D. Cohn (2016), 'Unauthorized immigrant population stable for half a decade', Pew Research Center, accessed 30 September 2016 at http://www.pewresearch.org/fact-tank/2016/09/21/unauthorized-immigrant-population-stable-for-half-a-decade/.

Pew Research Center (2016), 'Key facts about the world's refugees', accessed 30 September 2016 at http://www.pewresearch.org/fact-tank/2016/09/15/key-facts-about-the-worlds-refugees.

Singh, G.K. and R.A. Hiatt (2006), 'Trends and disparities in socioeconomic and behavioral characteristics, life expectancy, and cause-specific mortality of native-born and foreign-born populations in the United States, 1979–2003', *International Journal of Epidemiology*, **35** (4), 903–19.

Singh, G.K. and S.C. Lin (2013a), 'Dramatic increases in obesity and overweight prevalence among Asian subgroups in the United States, 1992–2011', *ISRN Preventive Medicine*, 29 October, 1–12, doi:10.5402/2013/898691.

Singh, G.K. and S.C. Lin (2013b), 'Marked ethnic, nativity, and socioeconomic disparities in disability and health insurance among US children and adults', *BioMed Research International*, 22 October, 1–17, doi:10.1155/2013/627412.

Singh, G.K. and B.A. Miller (2004), 'Health, life expectancy, and mortality patterns among immigrant populations in the United States', *Canadian Journal of Public Health*, **95** (3), I14–I21.

Singh, G.K. and M. Siahpush (2001), 'All-cause and cause-specific mortality of immigrants and native born in the United States', *American Journal of Public Health*, **91** (3), 392–9.

Singh, G.K., and M. Siahpush (2002), 'Ethnic-immigrant differentials in health behaviors, morbidity, and cause-specific mortality in the United States: an analysis of two national data bases', *Human Biology*, **74** (1), 83–109.

Singh, G.K. and S.M. Yu (1996), 'Adverse pregnancy outcomes: differences between US- and foreign-born women in major US racial and ethnic groups', *American Journal of Public Health*, **86** (6), 837–43.

Singh, G.K., A. Rodriguez-Lainz and M.D. Kogan (2013a), 'Immigrant health inequalities in the United States: use of eight major National Data Systems', *Scientific World Journal*, 27 October, 1–21, doi:10.1155/2013/512313.

Singh, G.K., M. Siahpush, R.A. Hiatt and L.R. Timsina (2011), 'Dramatic increases in obesity and overweight prevalence and body mass index among ethnic-immigrant and social class groups in the United States, 1976–2008', *Journal of Community Health*, **36** (1), 94–110.

Singh, G.K., S.M. Yu and M.D. Kogan (2013b), 'Health, chronic conditions, and behavioral risk disparities among U.S. immigrant children and adolescents', *Public Health Reports*, **128** (6), 463–79.

Sorlie, P.D., E. Backlund and J.B. Keller (1995), 'US mortality by economic, demographic, and social characteristics: the National Longitudinal Mortality Study', *American Journal of Public Health*, **85** (7), 949–56.

Trovato, F. and G.K. Jarvis (1986), 'Immigrant suicide in Canada: 1971 and 1981', *Social Forces*, **65** (2), 433–57.

US Census Bureau (2012), *National Longitudinal Mortality Study, Reference Manual*, Washington, DC: US Census Bureau, accessed 30 September 2016 at http://www.census.gov/did/www/nlms/publications/reference.html.

US Census Bureau (2016), *The 2015 American Community Survey*, Washington, DC: US Census Bureau, accessed 30 September 2016 at http://www.census.gov/programs-surveys/acs/.

Waters, M.C. and M.G. Pineau (eds.) (2015), *The Integration of Immigrants into American Society*, Washington, DC: National Academies Press.

Wong, E.C., G.N. Marshall, T.L. Schell, M.N. Elliott, S.H. Babey and K. Hambarsoomians (2011), 'The unusually poor physical health status of Cambodian refugees two decades after resettlement', *Journal of Immigrant and Minority Health*, **13** (5), 876–82.

World Health Organization (WHO) (2016), *World Health Statistics 2016: Monitoring Health for the SDGs, Sustainable Development Goals*, Geneva: WHO.

Xu, J.Q., S.L. Murphy, K.D. Kochanek and B.A. Bastian (2016), 'Deaths: final data for 2013', *National Vital Statistics Reports*, **64** (2), 1–118.

Yun, K., E. Fuentes-Afflick and M.M. Desai (2012), 'Prevalence of chronic disease and insurance coverage among refugees in the United States', *Journal of Immigrant and Minority Health*, **14** (6), 933–40.

9. Cancer mortality among immigrants in Australia

Olga Anikeeva and Peng Bi

INTRODUCTION

This chapter presents migrant mortality patterns for the most common cancers in Australia and discusses the impact of diet, lifestyle factors and acculturation on the observed trends. Generally, Australian migrants are in better health than the Australian-born population, and have lower cancer mortality rates (Mathers, 1996; Young, 1987; Strong et al., 1998). Greek and Italian migrants in Australia have the greatest cancer mortality advantage, which can in part be explained by a considerable body of evidence that suggests that the diets of these migrant groups have a strong protective effect (Young, 1987; Kouris-Blazos et al., 1996, 1999). Greek and Italian migrants tend to cluster together in the larger Australian cities, which creates a supportive environment for traditional food preparation and consumption.

However, there are a number of specific cancers where mortality rates are higher for some migrant groups compared with the Australian-born population. The higher mortality rates tend to reflect the migrants' dietary and lifestyle habits, which many retain for some years after arrival in Australia. For example, East and Southeast Asian migrants have an approximately thirty-fold higher age-adjusted risk of dying from nasopharyngeal cancer compared with their Australian-born counterparts upon arrival, which reduces to nine-fold after 30 years of living in Australia (McCredie et al., 1999a). Migrants from the United Kingdom, the former Yugoslavia, Greece and Italy have higher age-adjusted mortality rates from cancer of the stomach and pancreas, which decreases with increasing duration of residence in Australia (McMichael et al., 1980).

COLORECTAL CANCER

Figure 9.1 shows that colorectal cancer mortality rates generally decreased over time, with the trend particularly pronounced among the

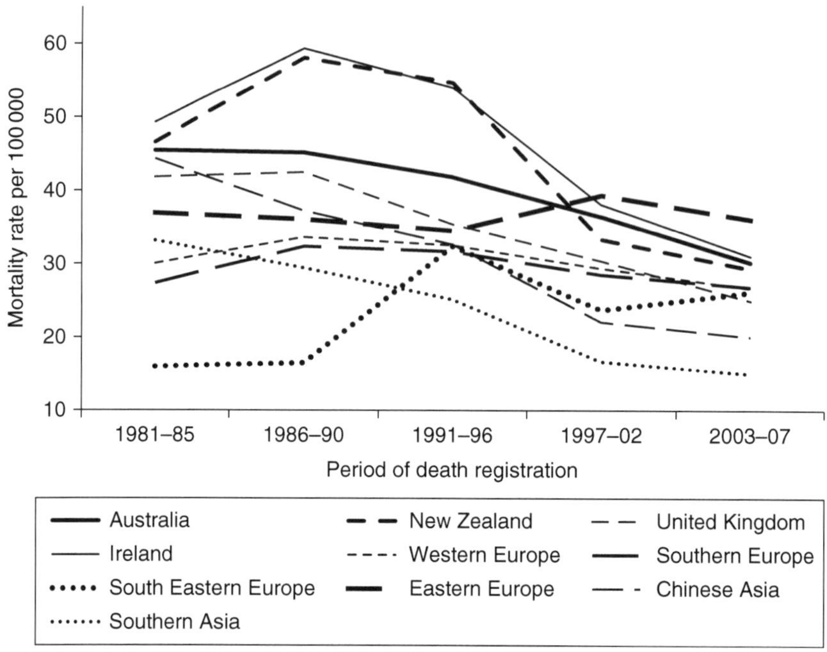

Figure 9.1 *Average annual directly age- and sex-standardized mortality rates (per 100 000) for colorectal cancer by region of birth and period of death registration; Australia, 1981–85 to 2003–07*

Australian-born and migrants from New Zealand, the United Kingdom, Chinese Asia and Southern Asia. Southern European, Chinese Asian and Southern Asian migrants had lower colorectal cancer mortality rates compared with their Australian-born counterparts (Khlat, 1995). The most likely explanation for the observed trends is the influence of a diet high in cereals, fruits, non-root vegetables, and low in fats, particularly those of animal origin (McMichael et al., 1980; McMichael and Bonett, 1981; Khlat, 1995). It is generally accepted that lack of physical activity and obesity are associated with increased colorectal cancer risk (Hanley et al., 1995; Flood et al., 2000). While it is unclear whether these migrant groups in Australia engage in more physical activity compared with the Australian-born population, earlier investigations have shown that Southern European migrants tend to engage in more manual labour occupations (Colic-Peisker, 2009), which may carry a protective effect.

Furthermore, studies have shown that well-established migrant groups in Australia, such as those born in Southern Europe, China and Southern

Asia, tend to settle in distinct areas within Australian cities (Gray et al., 2007). This creates migrant communities, which provide a supportive environment for the retention of traditional diets and lifestyle habits (Khlat, 1995), meaning that the process of acculturation and the adoption of Australian eating and exercise habits is slowed, thus enabling migrants to maintain their health advantage (Gray et al., 2007). Well-established ethnic communities provide a nurturing environment for newly arrived migrants, enabling access to traditional produce stores and community and religious centres that facilitate adherence to traditional norms and behaviours (Gray et al., 2007). This is likely to lead to an acculturation style where emphasis is placed on retaining and nurturing cultural norms and values, while at the same time developing English language proficiency and other skills that allow migrants to participate actively in the wider Australian community while maintaining their cultural identity.

However, although the process of acculturation is slowed in these groups, previous research has indicated that Southern European migrants experience an increase in colorectal cancer mortality with increasing time spent in Australia (McCredie et al., 1999b). This has been explained by the tendency for migrants to gradually adopt some Australian dietary patterns, which includes replacing certain traditional foods such as olive oil with less healthy options, including butter and margarine (McCredie et al., 1999b; Kouris-Blazos et al., 1996; Kouris-Blazos, 2002). Similar results have been noted for other migrant groups, such as those originating from East and Southeast Asia, who retain their lower risk of mortality from colorectal cancer for the first ten years spent in Australia, but after this period their mortality rates begin to converge towards Australian-born rates over the next 20 years of residence (McCredie et al., 1999a).

STOMACH CANCER

Figure 9.2 demonstrates reductions in stomach cancer mortality over time among all groups with the exception of South Eastern European and Eastern European migrants. In comparison with Australian-born individuals, European and Asian migrants had substantially higher stomach cancer mortality rates. Mortality rates were particularly high for migrants born in Southern Europe, South Eastern Europe, Eastern Europe and Chinese Asia. Previous studies have suggested that diets that are high in abrasive or irritant foods, such as complex carbohydrates and salted, pickled, cured and smoked foods, and low in fat and vitamins A and C are associated with the development of stomach cancer (McMichael et al., 1980; McMichael and Bonett, 1981; McCredie et al.,

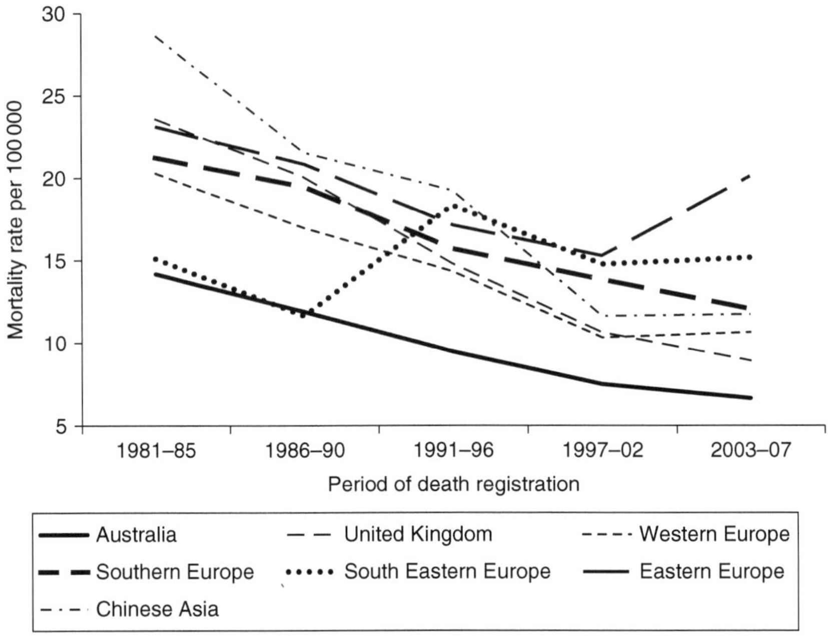

Figure 9.2 Average annual directly age- and sex-standardized mortality rates (per 100 000) for stomach cancer by region of birth and period of death registration; Australia, 1981–85 to 2003–07

1999a; Hanley et al., 1995; Tsugane, 2005). There is evidence to suggest that first-generation migrants appear to maintain their elevated risk of stomach cancer, with only modest reductions in risk over time (McCredie et al., 1999b; Kelley and Duggan, 2003). In addition to diet, infection with *Helicobacter pylori* is associated with stomach cancer, whereby infection causes the development of chronic gastritis, which can then lead to the development of stomach cancer (Hanley et al., 1995; Kelley and Duggan, 2003; Tsugane, 2005). *Helicobacter pylori* infection is particularly common in developing countries, and may in part explain the high stomach cancer mortality rates observed among migrants from Chinese Asia (Kelley and Duggan, 2003). Cigarette smoking is also an established risk factor for stomach cancer (Tsugane, 2005); however, smoking rates do not differ substantially enough between the Australian-born population and the migrant groups in explaining the migrants' excess mortality (Australia Bureau of Statistics, 2006; Lin and Ward, 2000; Hsu-Hage and Wahlqvist, 1993).

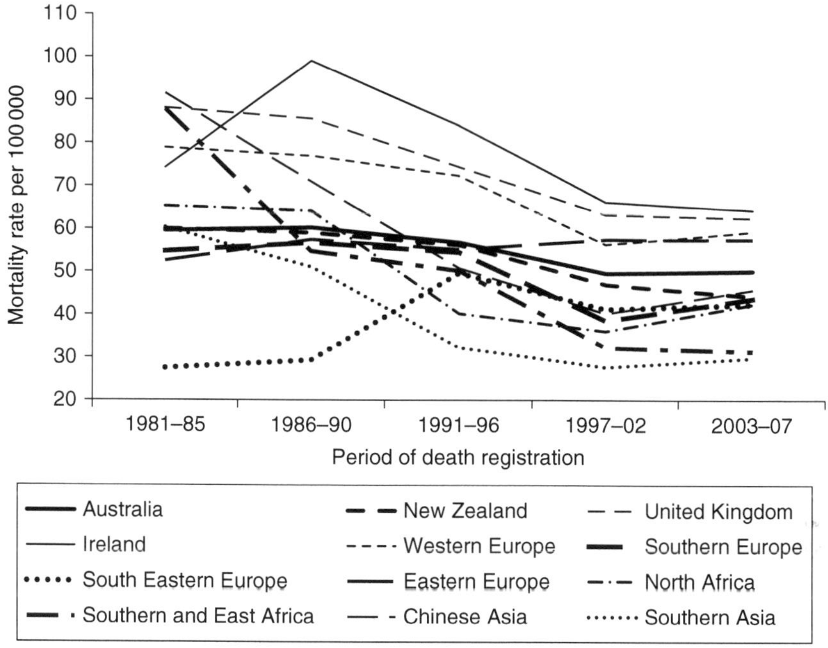

Figure 9.3 *Average annual directly age- and sex-standardized mortality rates (per 100 000) for cancer of the trachea, bronchus and lung by region of birth and period of death registration; Australia, 1981–85 to 2003–07*

TRACHEA, BRONCHUS AND LUNG CANCER

As Figure 9.3 shows, lung cancer mortality rates reduced over time; however, South Eastern European migrants experienced an increase in mortality. Migrants from the United Kingdom, Ireland, Western Europe and Eastern Europe tended to have higher rates of lung cancer mortality compared with the Australian-born population. On the other hand, migrants from Southern Europe, Southern and East Africa and Southern Asia experienced lower lung cancer mortality rates than their Australian-born counterparts (McMichael and Bonett, 1981; Khlat, 1995). The most likely explanation for differences in lung cancer mortality is lifetime smoking habits, which differ between country of birth groups (McMichael and Bonett, 1981). Lung cancer mortality rates reduce with increasing time spent in Australia for migrants originating from the United Kingdom and Ireland, Southern and Eastern Europe and Southeast Asia, which is likely due to changes in smoking habits. There are numerous anti-smoking mass-media campaigns and support services that operate in Australia, and it is likely that migrants become increasingly aware of these messages that have an impact on their smoking behaviours with time spent in the country. It is possible that differences in cigarette prices between Australia and the migrants' countries of origin also influence their tobacco use (Guindon et al., 2002; Montes and Villalbi, 2001). The high cigarette prices in Australia coupled with smoking cessation services and public health campaigns are likely to motivate migrants to quit for both health and financial reasons with increasing time spent in the country.

MELANOMA OF THE SKIN

Melanoma mortality rates (Figure 9.4) remained relatively stable over time, with only small increases observed among the Australian-born population and migrants from the United Kingdom. Australian-born individuals experienced significantly greater melanoma mortality compared with migrants from the United Kingdom, Southern Europe and South Eastern Europe. The particularly low rate of melanoma mortality among individuals born in Southern Europe can be explained by the protective effect of darker skin tone (Khlat et al., 1992). Conversely, the high mortality rates observed among Australian-born individuals highlight the importance of childhood exposure to ultraviolet radiation and the experience of sunburn early in life (Mack and Floderus, 1991; Khlat et al., 1992). It is also important to consider the impact of behavioural factors and attitudes to sun exposure. It has been shown previously that some migrant groups, particularly from cultures where a lighter complexion is seen as desirable or where concealing clothing is worn for religious reasons, continue to protect themselves by staying out of direct sunlight and shielding their skin by using sunscreens and clothing (Benson and Skull, 2007). While adult migrants typically retain these behaviours upon migration to Australia, it is possible that young children may gradually adopt attitudes towards sun exposure that are prevalent in Australia (Khlat et al., 1992). Therefore, age at migration is considered to be a more important factor in determining melanoma risk than duration of residence in Australia (Cooke and Fraser, 1985).

BREAST CANCER

As Figure 9.5 illustrates, breast cancer mortality rates declined among those born in Australia and the United Kingdom, while fluctuations

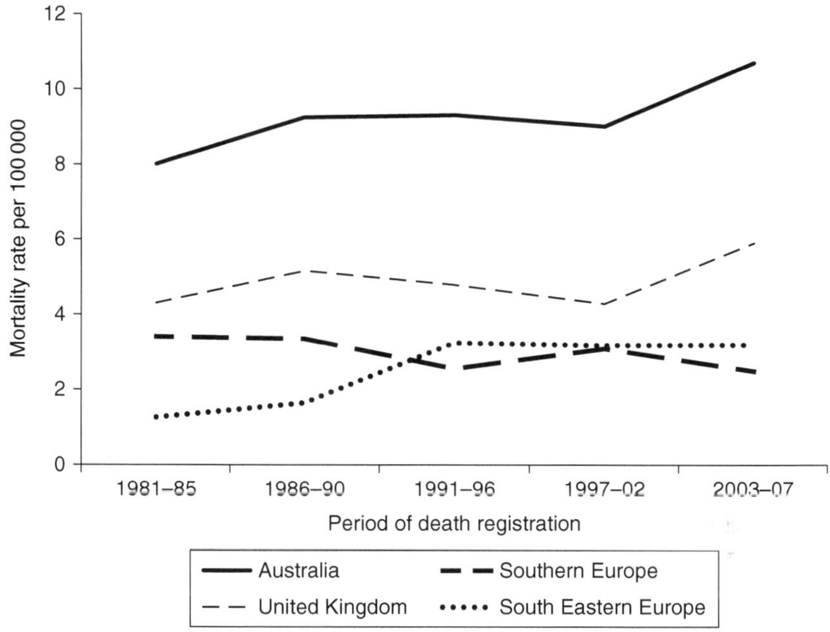

Figure 9.4 Average annual directly age- and sex-standardized mortality rates (per 100 000) for melanoma of the skin by region of birth and period of death registration; Australia, 1981–85 to 2003–07

over time were observed among other migrant groups. Mortality rates were relatively consistent across country of birth groups, with slightly lower rates observed among Southern European and South Eastern European migrants. This is consistent with earlier research studies, which found somewhat lower breast cancer mortality rates among those born in Southern Europe (McMichael and Bonett, 1981; Khlat et al., 1992; Kliewer and Smith, 1995; Bray et al., 2004). This slight difference has been attributed to Southern European migrants' lower consumption of saturated fat and total kilojoules, as well as differences in reproductive practices (McMichael and Bonett, 1981; Kliewer and Smith, 1995; Kelsey and Bernstein, 1996; Bray et al., 2004). Nulliparity, late age at first birth, late age at any birth, low parity and the use of oral contraceptives and hormone replacement therapy increase the risk of breast cancer, and tend to be more common in westernized societies such as Australia, the United States of America and the United Kingdom (Kelsey and Bernstein, 1996; Bray et al., 2004).

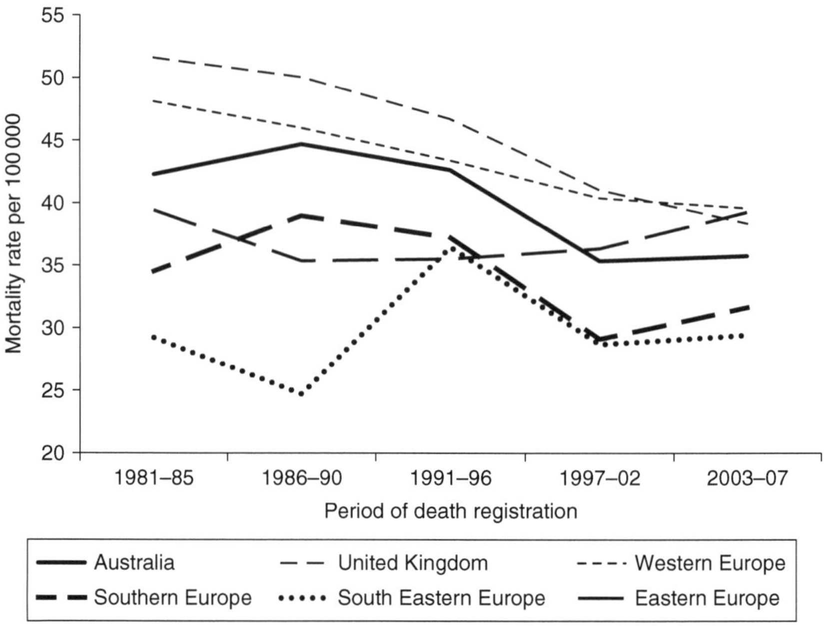

Figure 9.5 *Average annual directly age- and sex-standardized mortality rates (per 100 000) for breast cancer (female only) by region of birth and period of death registration; Australia, 1981–85 to 2003–07*

BLADDER CANCER

Figure 9.6 shows that bladder cancer mortality rates declined over time among those born in Australia and the United Kingdom. Mortality rates were significantly higher among migrants from the United Kingdom and Western Europe compared to Australian-born individuals. Southern European migrants' bladder cancer mortality rates were similar to those of the Australian-born population. The most likely explanation for these differences are variations in smoking behaviour, as high levels of smoking among migrant groups tend to parallel higher mortality owing to bladder cancer (McMichael et al., 1989; Khlat, 1995; McCredie et al., 1999b; Parkin, 2008).

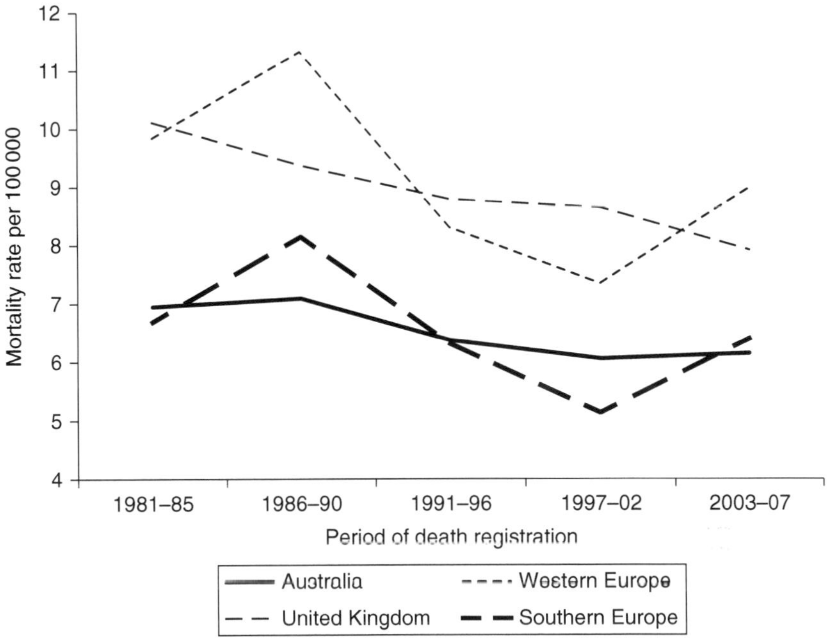

Figure 9.6 Average annual directly age- and sex-standardized mortality rates (per 100 000) for bladder cancer by region of birth and period of death registration; Australia, 1981–85 to 2003–07

CONCLUSION

Migrants generally have more favourable cancer mortality outcomes compared with their Australian-born counterparts. Southern European migrants appear to have the greatest health advantage, while Eastern European migrants have cancer mortality rates similar to or higher than the Australian-born population.

Despite their overall health advantage, migrants have higher rates of mortality from stomach and bladder cancers compared with the Australian-born population, which can in part be explained by dietary patterns and smoking behaviour (McMichael et al., 1980; McMichael and Bonett, 1981; McCredie et al., 1999b; Tsugane, 2005). There is some evidence to suggest that chronic infection with *Helicobacter pylori* increases the risk of developing stomach cancer (Hanley et al., 1995; Kelley and Duggan, 2003), with exposure early in life being particularly significant (McCredie, 1998). This has important implications for public health policy and practice in Australia, as these at-risk migrant groups may benefit from specifically designed education and prevention programmes, which could focus on risk factors specific to these groups. Providing targeted interventions, delivered through migrant resource centres or community establishments, may increase uptake of services that have the potential to prevent or delay the development of these cancers.

Duration of residence has an important impact on migrant cancer mortality trends. Dietary and lifestyle changes, as well as increased familiarity with Australian public health campaigns, influence migrant mortality outcomes. This is well illustrated by the convergence of Southern European migrants' colorectal cancer mortality rates towards those of the Australian-born population with increasing duration of residence, owing to the gradual adoption of a diet higher in saturated fat and lower in fibre (Khlat, 1995). This observation has important implications for policy and practice, in that newly arrived migrants could be targeted through migrant resource centres and cultural organizations and informed about the potentially negative health effects of replacing certain traditional foods with processed, energy-dense alternatives and adopting a more sedentary lifestyle. Migrants should be encouraged to retain their traditional diets and lifestyle habits, through health promotion programmes targeted at specific migrant groups that focus on preventing the decline in health status that occurs with increasing duration of residence (Mathers, 1996). It is particularly important that these messages are delivered as early as possible after the migrants' arrival in Australia, before acculturation and the adoption of unhealthy eating and physical activity patterns occurs (Ott, 2010).

However, increasing duration of residence can also have a positive impact on migrant cancer mortality trends, as illustrated by the reduction in lung cancer mortality among migrants from the United Kingdom and Ireland, Southern and Eastern Europe, and Southeast Asia. Lung cancer is strongly linked to smoking, and reductions in mortality with increasing time spent in Australia may be linked to exposure to smoking cessation mass-media campaigns and the impact of higher cigarette prices (McMichael and Bonnet, 1981). To further support migrants, smoking cessation information and telephone support services are made available in a range of languages in Australia.

In summary, migrants in Australia tend to have lower cancer mortality rates compared with the Australian-born population. However, for some cancers, this health advantage can deteriorate with increasing time spent in the country, owing to the gradual adoption of typical Australian lifestyle and dietary habits. For this reason, it is of critical importance that migrants are targeted through education and health promotion campaigns that encourage the retention of traditional eating and exercise habits, as well as alert migrant groups to the availability of screening services and community support organizations.

Further research is needed to understand the influence of duration of residence on migrant cancer mortality trends. In particular, this research could examine the manner in which migrant groups adopt Australian dietary and lifestyle patterns and the factors that influence the retention of traditional behaviours and eating habits. Future research could also compare cancer mortality rates between migrant groups in Australia, the migrants' countries of origin and the Australian-born population. However, obtaining the required data from migrant source countries may be problematic.

REFERENCES

Australia Bureau of Statistics (2006), 'Tobacco smoking in Australia: a snapshot, 2004–05', Report no. 4831.0.55.001, accessed 8 November 2010 at http://www.abs.gov.au/ausstats/abs@.nsf/mf/4831.0.55.001.

Benson, J. and S. Skull (2007), 'Hiding from the sun: vitamin D deficiency in refugees', *Australian Family Physician*, **36** (5), 355–7.

Bray, F., P. McCarron and D.M. Parkin (2004), 'The changing global patterns of female breast cancer incidence and mortality', *Breast Cancer Research*, **6** (August), 229–39.

Colic-Peisker, V. (2009), 'The rise of multicultural middle class: a new stage of Australian multiculturalism?', in S. Lockie, D. Bissell, A. Greig, M. Hynes, D. Marsh, L. Saha et al. (eds), *The Australian Sociological Association 2009 Annual Conference*, Canberra: TASA, Australian National University.

Cooke, K.R. and J. Fraser (1985), 'Migration and death from malignant melanoma', *International Journal of Cancer*, **36** (2), 175–8.

Flood, D.M., N.S. Weiss, L.S. Cook, J.C. Emerson, S.M. Schwartz and J.D. Potter (2000), 'Colorectal cancer incidence in Asian migrants to the United States and their descendants', *Cancer Causes & Control*, **11** (5), 403–11.

Gray, L., S. Harding and A. Reid (2007), 'Evidence of divergence with duration of residence in circulatory disease mortality in migrants to Australia', *European Journal of Public Health*, **17** (6), 550–54.

Guindon, G., S. Tobin and D. Yach (2002), 'Trends and affordability of cigarette prices: ample room for tax increases and related health gains', *Tobacco Control*, **11** (March), 35–43.

Hanley, A.J.G., B.C.K. Choi and E.J. Holowaty (1995), 'Cancer mortality among Chinese migrants: a review', *International Journal of Epidemiology*, **24** (2), 255–65.

Hsu-Hage, B.H. and M.L. Wahlqvist (1993), 'Cardiovascular risk in adult Melbourne Chinese', *Australian Journal of Public Health*, **17** (4), 306–13.

Kelley, J.R. and J.M. Duggan (2003), 'Gastric cancer epidemiology and risk factors', *Journal of Clinical Epidemiology*, **56** (1), 1–9.

Kelsey, J.L. and L. Bernstein (1996), 'Epidemiology and prevention of breast cancer', *Annual Reviews Public Health*, **17** (may), 47–67.

Khlat, M. (1995), 'Cancer in Mediterranean migrants – based on studies in France and Australia', *Cancer Causes & Control*, **6** (6), 525–31.
Khlat, M., A. Vail, M. Parkin and A. Green (1992), 'Mortality from melanoma in migrants to Australia: variation by age at arrival and duration of stay', *American Journal of Epidemiology*, **135** (10), 1103–13.
Kliewer, E.V. and K.R. Smith (1995), 'Breast cancer mortality among immigrants in Australia and Canada', *Journal of the National Cancer Institute*, **87** (15), 1154–61.
Kouris-Blazos, A. (2002), 'Morbidity mortality paradox of 1st generation Greek Australians', *Asia Pacific Journal of Clinical Nutrition*, **11** (3 supplement), S569–S575.
Kouris-Blazos, A., M.L. Wahlqvist, A. Trichopoulou, E. Polychronopoulos and D. Trichopoulos (1996), 'Health and nutritional status of elderly Greek migrants to Melbourne, Australia', *Age and Ageing*, **25** (3), 177–89.
Kouris-Blazos, A., C. Gnardellis, M.L. Wahlqvist, D. Trichopoulos, W. Lukito and A. Trichopoulou (1999), 'Are the advantages of the Mediterranean diet transferable to other populations? A cohort study in Melbourne, Australia', *British Journal of Nutrition*, **82** (1) 57–61.
Lin, M. and J.E. Ward (2000), 'Smoking among ethnic Chinese patients and their recall of quit advice by Chinese-speaking general practitioners in Sydney', *Australian and New Zealand Journal of Public Health*, **24** (4), 437–40.
Mack, T.M. and B. Floderus (1991), 'Malignant melanoma risk by nativity, place of residence at diagnosis, and age at migration', *Cancer Causes & Control*, **2** (6), 401–11.
Mathers, C. (1996), 'Health patterns of immigrants in Australia', *People and Place*, **4** (1), 8–18.
McCredie, M. (1998), 'What have we learned from studies of migrants?', *Cancer Causes & Control*, **9** (1), 1–2.
McCredie, M., S. Williams and M. Coates (1999a), 'Cancer mortality in East and Southeast Asian migrants to New South Wales, Australia, 1975–1995', *British Journal of Cancer*, **79** (7–8), 1277–82.
McCredie, M., S. Williams and M. Coates (1999b), 'Cancer mortality in migrants from the British Isles and continental Europe to New South Wales, Australia, 1975–1995', *International Journal of Cancer*, **83** (2), 179–85.
McMichael, A.J. and A. Bonett (1981), 'Cancer profiles of British and Southern-European migrants', *Medical Journal of Australia*, **1** (5), 229–32.
McMichael, A.J., A. Bonett and D. Roder (1989), 'Cancer incidence among migrant populations in South Australia', *Medical Journal of Australia*, **150** (8), 417–19.
McMichael, A.J., M.G. McCall, J.M. Hartshorne and T.L. Woodings (1980), 'Patterns of gastro-intestinal cancer in European migrants to Australia: the role of dietary change', *International Journal of Cancer*, **25** (4), 431–7.
Montes, A. and J. Villalbi (2001), 'The price of cigarettes in the European Union', *Tobacco Control*, **10** (2), 135–6.
Ott, J., A.M. Paltiel, V. Winkler and H. Becher (2010), 'The impact of duration of residence on cause-specific mortality: a cohort study from the former Soviet Union residing in Israel and Germany', *Health and Place*, **16** (1), 79–84.
Parkin, D.M. (2008), 'The global burden of urinary bladder cancer', *Scandinavian Journal of Urology and Nephrology*, **42** (218) (supplement), 12–20.
Strong, K., P. Trickett and K. Bhatia (1998), 'The health of overseas-born Australians, 1994–1996', *Australian Health Review*, **21** (2), 124–33.

Tsugane, S. (2005), 'Salt, salted food intake, and risk of gastric cancer: epidemiologic evidence', *Cancer Science*, **96** (1), 1–6.
Young, C.M. (1987), 'Migration and mortality: the experience of birthplace groups in Australia', *International Migration Review*, **21** (3), 531–54.

10. Mortality among migrants and their descendants living in England and Wales*

Matthew Wallace

INTRODUCTION

The migrant mortality advantage describes observed low mortality among migrants relative to non-migrants in developed host countries (Razum, 2008). Although an advantage has been consistently documented (Razum et al., 1998; Abraido-Lanza et al., 1999; Anson, 2004; Palloni and Arias, 2004; Deboosere and Gadeyne, 2005; Turra and Elo, 2008; Hajat et al., 2010), exactly what generates lower mortality among migrants remains unclear. Typical explanations include selection (atypically healthy people tend to move), cultural factors which positively influence health behaviours, a rapid health transition in migrants from developing countries, the remigration of ill migrants (a salmon bias effect), and censoring bias. It is vital to understand the role of the last two factors, because while the first three factors account for a 'real' advantage, the salmon bias effect and censoring bias reduce it to an artefact, generated by an inability to track migrants and produce reliable estimates of their mortality.

This chapter covers a series of articles from a project which aimed to (1) examine adult mortality (age 20+) patterns among migrants, descendants of migrants and the England and Wales-born population and (2) to investigate the causes of mortality differences between these groups. Through modelling the impact of censoring bias and investigating the salmon bias effect, the first section of the chapter determines whether the advantage can be fully explained away by bias. The second section then examines the evidence for the remaining explanations of the advantage by presenting a detailed analysis of migrant mortality by gender, age, and cause of death. The third section investigates whether a migrant mortality advantage persists among the descendants of migrants. The chapter finishes with an overall summary of the findings and identifies the research's main contribution to the literature.

DATA

The analyses use the Office for National Statistics Longitudinal Study (LS), data which contains linked census and life event data for a 1 per cent sample of England and Wales for people born on 1 of 4 anonymous dates since 1971. Life event data includes information on migrations, births and deaths. Migration data is taken from National Health Service (NHS) registration systems; births and deaths are taken from the civil register data. A comparison of all-cause mortality with the Human Mortality Database finds mortality in the LS to be representative of national mortality (Wallace and Kulu, 2014). Moreover, for the larger migrant populations living in England and Wales, cause-specific mortality among South Asians and Caribbeans in the 1971 cohort has been shown to be similar to mortality in the 100 per cent cross-sectional data (Harding and Balarajan, 2001).

Migrants are defined using country of birth, a question asked at each census from 1971 to 2011. The post-war New Commonwealth migrant populations (India, Pakistan, Bangladesh, and Jamaica) are the focus of the analyses, alongside regional groupings of other countries. Descendants of migrants are defined somewhat differently using a combination of country of birth and ethnicity to differentiate ethnic minority groups by those born in England and Wales (descendants of migrants) from those born abroad (migrants). Descendants are therefore a combination of the second, and subsequent, generations (G2+).

METHODS

Each section uses event history analysis. Three of the four analyses estimate continuous event history models (a Gompertz distribution of the hazard function is assumed), with the exception being the analysis on health-motivated remigration which uses a discrete-time event history model. This is because the precise date of emigration is often missing and only the decade of exit is known. This discrete-time model is a multinomial logistic regression model which analyses the likelihood of an individual moving or dying in the ten-year period between two census points. For more detailed information on the data setup and the methods used, please refer to the relevant articles (Wallace and Kulu, 2014, 2015; Wallace, 2016a, 2016b).

CENSORING BIAS

In this section, the first of the two factors which can introduce bias into migrant mortality rates is addressed: censoring bias. A migrant population is a highly changeable one which is difficult to accurately capture in data sources as people enter and leave the host country over variable periods of time (Anson, 2004). Crucially, if migrants decide to leave the host country permanently, but do not inform the relevant authorities of their return or onward migration, they will continue to 'age' in host country databases after having left the country, even if they later die elsewhere (Abraido-Lanza et al., 1999). This leads to an overestimation of exposure in the denominator and an underestimation of the number of deaths in the numerator of calculations (Kibele et al., 2008), questioning the reliability of migrant mortality rates.

In previous studies, the magnitude of mortality underestimation among migrants has been found to vary. In Sweden, one of the first studies to investigate the impact of censoring bias on migrant mortality rates concluded that said errors largely explained the advantage, though low mortality persisted among some groups (Weitoft et al., 1999). In a direct response to this study, Razum et al. (2000) used data robust to denominator inaccuracies to demonstrate that low mortality among migrants in Germany could not be explained away by censoring bias alone. However, subsequent studies in Germany have observed substantial mortality underestimation among migrants, particularly those older than 65 years (Kibele et al., 2008; Kohls, 2010). Studies in France (Khlat and Courbage, 1996; Darmon and Khlat, 2001) and Belgium (Anson, 2004) find, like Razum et al. (2000), that the advantage cannot be explained away by censoring bias.

Capturing Migration in the LS Data

An immigration is recorded when a migrant registers with the NHS or completes a census form for the first time. However, while the date of arrival is asked for on the NHS form, it is not cross-checked against other sources (Hattersley, 1999). Emigration is recorded when an LS member de-registers from the NHS, but it is known that not many people de-register. Hattersley (1999) has compared the LS data with International Passenger Survey data from 1987 to 1989 and concluded that emigrations were under-recorded by as much as 75 per cent. Those who do not report their emigration are lost to follow-up when they are not enumerated at census and no longer record life events. For this analysis, the assumption is made that loss to follow-up is unrecorded emigration (Razum, 2006).

When an LS member records an emigration, death, or is censored, risk-time can be calculated by subtracting age of entry from the age of death, emigration, or end of observation. However, if an LS member becomes lost to follow-up, there is no date from which to subtract. Thankfully, because the LS data contains multiple census points, even if an emigration is not recorded it is possible to identify the decade in which it took place. The LS member can be exited from the analysis before the census from which they are missing. This ensures that individuals will only contribute risk-time while they are known to be alive and likely still in the country (Hattersley, 1999).

However, this still leaves a ten-year period where the emigration could have taken place. So, in order to determine how robust migrant mortality rates are to this period of uncertainty a sensitivity analysis was performed. Three emigration scenarios were projected (early – two years after final census appearance; middle – four years; and late – seven years) based on the empirical distribution of recorded emigrations. Given the uncertainty surrounding the accuracy of the entry date provided to the NHS when LS members enter between censuses, a scenario was also specified where the date of immigration was limited to the first census appearance (migrants could not enter between censuses). A final 'conservative' scenario was projected where entry was limited to first census appearance alongside an early emigration for those lost to follow-up. Table 10.1 presents the results from Wallace and Kulu (2014).

As one might expect, the hazard ratios decrease across the models (from left to right) as risk-time contributions increase and the denominators in the calculations of mortality rates are inflated. However, while the hazard ratios decrease and the confidence intervals narrow (giving rise to the possibility of a 'false positive'), the hazard ratios are not biased to the extent that migrant mortality advantage is systematically and artificially created across migrant groups. Consequently, while censoring bias contributes to the under-estimation of migrant mortality, it cannot be considered a primary explanation of the migrant mortality advantage.

THE SALMON BIAS EFFECT

While the previous section has demonstrated migrant mortality rates to be robust after adjusting for censoring bias, little is known about the health status of migrants who remigrate from England and Wales (Wallace, 2016b). In this section, the second of the two factors which can introduce bias into migrant mortality rates is addressed. The 'salmon bias effect' posits that migrants who start to suffer from a limiting long-term illness return to their country of origin (Valles, 2016), reflecting a cultural desire

Table 10.1 Sensitivity analysis of censoring bias: all-cause mortality among migrants in England and Wales, 1971–2001

Country or region of birth	Conservative		Immigration		Emigration					
					2-years		4-years		7-years	
	Hazard Ratio	95% CIs	Hazard Ratio	95% CIs	Hazard Ratio	95% CIs	Hazard Ratio	95% CIs	Hazard Ratio	95% CIs
England and Wales	1		1		1		1		1	
Ireland	1.26***	1.16–1.36	1.24***	1.15–1.34	1.24***	1.14–1.33	1.22***	1.13–1.31	1.18***	1.09–1.28
India	1.06	0.97–1.15	1.04	0.95–1.13	1.00	0.91–1.09	0.98	0.90–1.07	0.95	0.87–1.04
Pakistan	0.94	0.80–1.08	0.92	0.79–1.06	0.87*	0.75–1.01	0.85**	0.73–0.99	0.81***	0.70–0.94
Bangladesh	0.97	0.75–1.20	0.94	0.75–1.19	0.85	0.68–1.08	0.83	0.66–1.05	0.79**	0.62–0.99
Jamaica	1.14*	0.99–1.29	1.11	0.97–1.26	1.13*	0.98–1.29	1.09	0.96–1.25	1.04	0.91–1.19
Other Caribbean	0.96	0.78–1.14	0.93	0.77–1.12	0.93	0.77–1.13	0.90	0.75–1.09	0.86	0.71–1.03
ES Africa	1.01	0.83–1.20	1.00	0.83–1.20	0.90	0.75–1.08	0.89	0.74–1.07	0.87	0.72–1.04
WC Africa	1.16	0.84–1.48	1.10	0.84–1.45	0.99	0.75–1.30	0.95	0.72–1.25	0.88	0.67–1.16
W Europe	0.74***	0.65–0.84	0.73***	0.64–0.83	0.72***	0.63–0.82	0.70***	0.62–0.80	0.68***	0.60–0.78
E Europe	1.08	0.93–1.23	1.07	0.93–1.23	1.05	0.91–1.20	1.03	0.90–1.19	1.01	0.88–1.17
China	0.95	0.68–1.22	0.92	0.69–1.22	0.86	0.64–1.14	0.83	0.63–1.11	0.80	0.60–1.06
Other Asia	0.85	0.65–1.05	0.82	0.65–1.04	0.74**	0.58–0.94	0.72 ***	0.57–0.91	0.69***	0.55–0.88
Rest of World	1.07	0.96–1.18	1.04	0.94–1.15	0.98	0.89–1.09	0.96	0.87–1.06	0.91	0.83–1.01

Notes:
Models adjusted for age, sex and census period.
Values significant to 99 per cent (***), 95 per cent (**) and 90 per cent (*).

Source: Wallace and Kulu (2014), authors' calculations based on ONS LS.

to die in their birthplace in familiar surroundings and under the care of relatives (Razum and Twardella, 2002). If large numbers of migrants remigrate from the host country as their health deteriorates, their deaths will not be counted in the calculations, leading to an underestimation of mortality, particularly at older ages.

In the literature, evidence supporting a salmon bias effect is mixed. In the US, while low mortality has been attributed to a salmon bias effect among Mexicans (Palloni and Arias, 2004), others confirm its existence but believe it is of too small a magnitude to fully explain the advantage (Turra and Elo, 2008), or cannot find any evidence for a salmon bias effect (Abraido-Lanza et al., 1999). In Denmark a trend towards fewer returns among ill migrants has been observed (Norredam et al., 2015). In Belgium, a study calculated the mortality rate required to offset the advantage and found mortality among returnees would need to be very high (Vandenheede et al., 2015).

The aim of this section is to examine whether migrants are more likely to remigrate from England and Wales in poor health (measured using limiting long-term illness [LLTI]). Although the primary focus is remigration, deaths are modelled as a competing-risk because, if a salmon bias effect is operating, migrants are likely to die shortly after arriving in their next destination (which should be the country of origin). Unfortunately, while the remigration can be observed, the impending death cannot. However, by modelling the likelihood of mortality contingent on LLTI status (a reliable predictor of mortality which is often used as a proxy for it in the absence of mortality information) of migrant populations, one can infer an approximate mortality risk for migrant leavers who remigrate having reported an LLTI from the mortality risk of the migrant stayers who die in England and Wales having reported an LLTI.

Figure 10.1 shows the results from the multinomial logistic regression model in Wallace (2016b). As having the largest population, India is selected as the reference group. Only migrants who originate from South Asia are more likely to emigrate in ill health. Among South Asian stayers, those who report an LLTI at the start of the census period are 2–2.5 times more likely to die before the next census than South Asian stayers who do not report an LLTI. This indicates that mortality *could* also be higher among South Asian leavers who report an LLTI and that their remigration *might* contribute to an undercount of deaths in their mortality calculations. An additional interaction in the model between country/region of birth, LLTI and duration of stay (<10 years; ≥ 10 years; not shown) indicates that this salmon bias effect among South Asians is limited to those who have lived in England and Wales for less than 10 years.

Overall, for nearly all of the migrant groups, no evidence was observed

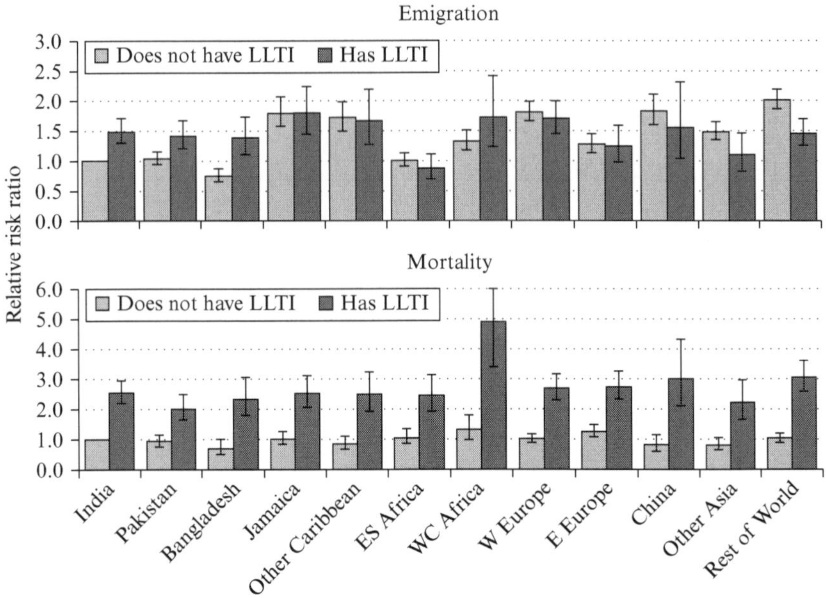

Note: Adjusted for age, census period, sex, duration of stay, occupation type, education level, area of residence type and marital status.

Source: Wallace (2016b), authors' calculations based on ONS LS.

Figure 10.1 Likelihood of remigration or death relative to health status, 1991–2011

of a salmon bias effect. United Kingdom residents have (almost) free access to universal health care (Nazroo, 2014). So, if a migrant develops an LLTI which by definition requires long-term care, it would make sense for them to remain in England and Wales to receive treatment, especially for migrants from developing countries who may have limited access to less advanced health care in the country of origin (Norredam et al., 2015). While this is certainly true, health care decisions are not based solely on cost and it is important to acknowledge other factors such as uncertainty surrounding the entitlement to health care and how the care system works, language, waiting times for various treatments, and the location of immediate family.

Among migrants from South Asia, the findings were consistent with a salmon bias effect. Perhaps this could relate to the relatively early onset of chronic conditions among South Asians (Lee and Garg, 2015). South

Asians who develop chronic conditions earlier on in life, and require treatment for said conditions, are likely to have shorter durations of stay upon diagnosis. As such, they may still retain strong ties to family in the country of origin (their spouse may not yet have moved) and be unfamiliar with how to access and use the health care system in England and Wales, all of which may prove more important in the decision to remigrate than cost. However, while this may introduce some bias into their mortality rates, the size of the advantage that will later be observed suggests that the salmon bias effect is, like censoring bias, contributing to an under-estimation, rather than explaining away the advantage.

MIGRANT MORTALITY RATES ARE FACTS, NOT ARTEFACTS

In the first section, migrant mortality rates are shown to be robust to biases associated with censoring and the salmon bias effect. Resultantly, the two factors can be ruled out as major causes of an artificial migrant mortality advantage and mortality differences between migrants and non-migrants can be considered reliable. In this section, the three remaining explanations (selection, cultural factors, and a rapid health transition) are outlined and then the results from the analyses by sex, age, and cause of death are presented and discussed with reference to said explanations.

Selection Effects

Central to the migrant mortality advantage is the presumed selection of healthy people at the time of migration from the country of origin (Razum, 2008). The theory posits that migrants select directly for health and indirectly for observable (e.g. education level) and unobservable (e.g. being forward-looking) characteristics positively correlated with health. The strength of selection is proposed to vary depending upon the motives for moving (stronger for economic reasons, weaker for family reasons) (Boulogne et al., 2012), gender (with selection said to be stronger among males) (Khlat and Courbage, 1996), and age (with selection being most pronounced during early adulthood, but weaker in childhood and later adult life) (Vang et al., 2016).

Cultural Factors

This explanation proposes that migrants practise more favourable health behaviours related to the prevailing cultural norms and values in the country of origin, such as healthier dietary habits or greater levels of family support (Abraido-Lanza et al., 1999; Darmon and Khlat, 2001). Upon arrival, these behaviours create a cultural buffer which protects their health from diseases related to developed populations and generates an advantage (Jasso et al., 2004). Over time, as migrants acculturate to the unhealthier behaviours and norms of the host society (Abraido-Lanza et al., 2005; Beiser, 2005), migrant health converges towards that of the host population (Jasso et al., 2004).

The Rapid Health Transition

The rapid health transition posits that migrants from developing countries undergo a rapid health transition which, upon arrival, is instantaneous in the reduced risk for infectious, maternal and childhood diseases (the main causes of death in the country of origin) owing to access to better health care, hygiene and environmental conditions, and only gradual in the accumulation of risk for chronic diseases (the main causes of death in the developed host country) (Razum and Twardella, 2002). Eventually, chronic diseases will become the main cause of death and mortality converges to that of the host population, but only after a considerable lag period (Spallek et al., 2011).

Results

Consider the findings on all-cause mortality among migrants by gender (Table 10.2) from Wallace and Kulu (2015). In the baseline model, an advantage can already be observed in many of the migrant populations. Only female migrants from Jamaica have higher mortality than the England and Wales-born. After adjusting socioeconomic position an advantage becomes apparent in nearly all groups (it is further emphasized in the groups in which it has already presented) and mortality among Jamaican females becomes similar to the England and Wales-born. Contrary to the literature, the magnitude of the mortality advantage among females tends to be comparable to, if not stronger than, the magnitude of the advantage among males.

Next, given the three explanations specifically make reference to age (either directly or through duration of stay) it is important to investigate age variation in the advantage. Figure 10.2 presents findings from the age interaction models (age is used as a proxy for duration of stay) in Wallace and Kulu (2014). The cumulative percentage of migrants who have entered by each five-year age group is plotted in the background to demonstrate the suitability of age as a proxy. Mortality differences are most pronounced

Table 10.2 All-cause mortality among migrants in England and Wales, 1971–2012

Country or region of birth	Males				Females			
	Basic		SEP-adjusted		Basic		SEP-adjusted	
	Hazard Ratio	95% CIs	Hazard Ratio	95% CIs	Hazard Ratio	95% CIs	Hazard Ratio	95% CIs
England and Wales	1		1		1		1	
Ireland	1.29***	1.20–1.38	0.99	0.92–1.06	1.25***	1.15–1.35	1.09**	1.01–1.18
India	0.89***	0.83–0.95	0.83***	0.78–0.90	0.91**	0.82–1.00	0.74***	0.68–0.82
Pakistan	0.73***	0.65–0.82	0.63***	0.56–0.71	0.93	0.80–1.09	0.62***	0.53–0.73
Bangladesh	0.89	0.75–1.05	0.72***	0.61–0.85	0.66***	0.50–0.89	0.41***	0.30–0.54
Jamaica	0.97	0.86–1.10	0.66***	0.58–0.74	1.18**	1.03–1.34	0.90	0.78–1.03
Other Caribbean	0.88	0.75–1.03	0.69***	0.59–0.81	0.82*	0.67–1.01	0.69***	0.56–0.84
ES Africa	0.70***	0.60–0.82	0.67***	0.57–0.78	0.88	0.74–1.04	0.74***	0.62–0.87
WC Africa	1.00	0.83–1.21	0.81**	0.67–0.97	0.64***	0.46–0.88	0.52***	0.38–0.71
W Europe	0.77***	0.70–0.86	0.72***	0.65–0.80	0.77***	0.70–0.85	0.70***	0.63–0.77
E Europe	0.98	0.86–1.10	0.79**	0.70–0.90	0.82**	0.70–0.96	0.74***	0.63–0.86
China	0.87	0.71–1.08	0.85	0.69–1.05	0.61***	0.42–0.88	0.51***	0.36–0.74
Other Asia	0.57***	0.47–0.71	0.56***	0.45–0.69	0.60***	0.48–0.75	0.54***	0.43–0.67
Rest of World	0.84***	0.76–0.93	0.80***	0.73–0.89	0.82***	0.73–0.92	0.76***	0.68–0.86

Notes:
Basic model adjusted for age and census period.
SEP model further adjusted for occupation type, education level, area of residence type and marital status.
Values significant to 99 per cent (***), 95 per cent (**) and 90 per cent (*).

Source. Wallace and Kulu (2015), authors' calculations based on ONS LS.

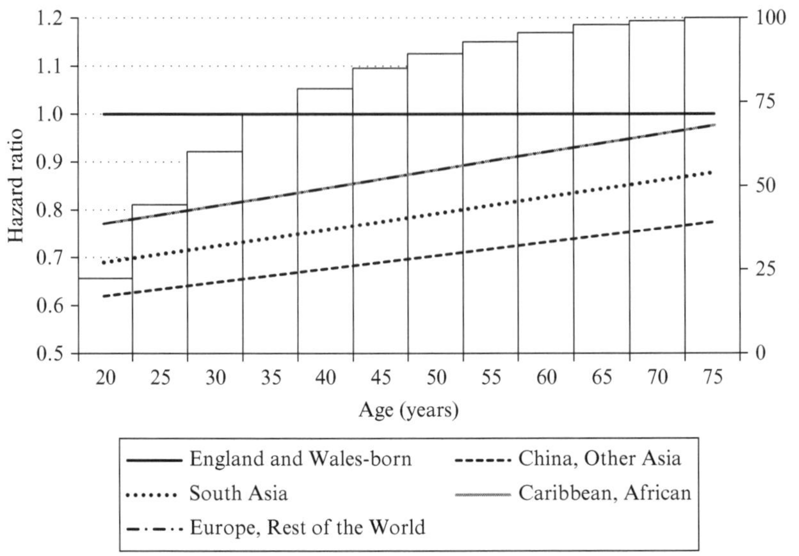

Source: Wallace and Kulu (2014), authors' calculations based on ONS LS.

Figure 10.2 Age variation in all-cause mortality among migrants, 1971–2001

at age 20. The size of mortality differences between migrants and non-migrants then decreases over time, converging fully among Caribbean and African migrants and partially for South Asian and other Asian migrants.

To determine which causes of death drive this mortality advantage among migrants, and provide some insight into cultural factors and the rapid health transition, Figure 10.3 presents findings on cause-specific mortality among migrants. Male and female migrants have systematically low mortality from respiratory diseases and cancer. Greater variation is observed in mortality from cardiovascular diseases, with some groups experiencing similar levels (Pakistan and Eastern Europe), lower levels (Western Europe, East and South Africa, and Other Asia), and higher levels (males from India and females from Jamaica) relative to the England and Wales-born. For infectious diseases, higher mortality is predominantly observed in migrants from developing countries.

Figure 10.4 places these results in context of their contribution to overall mortality. Among male migrants, the influence of cardiovascular diseases and cancer on overall mortality tends to be similar. However, among South Asian males cardiovascular diseases are the main cause of death while mortality from cancers is very low. Among female migrants, mortality from

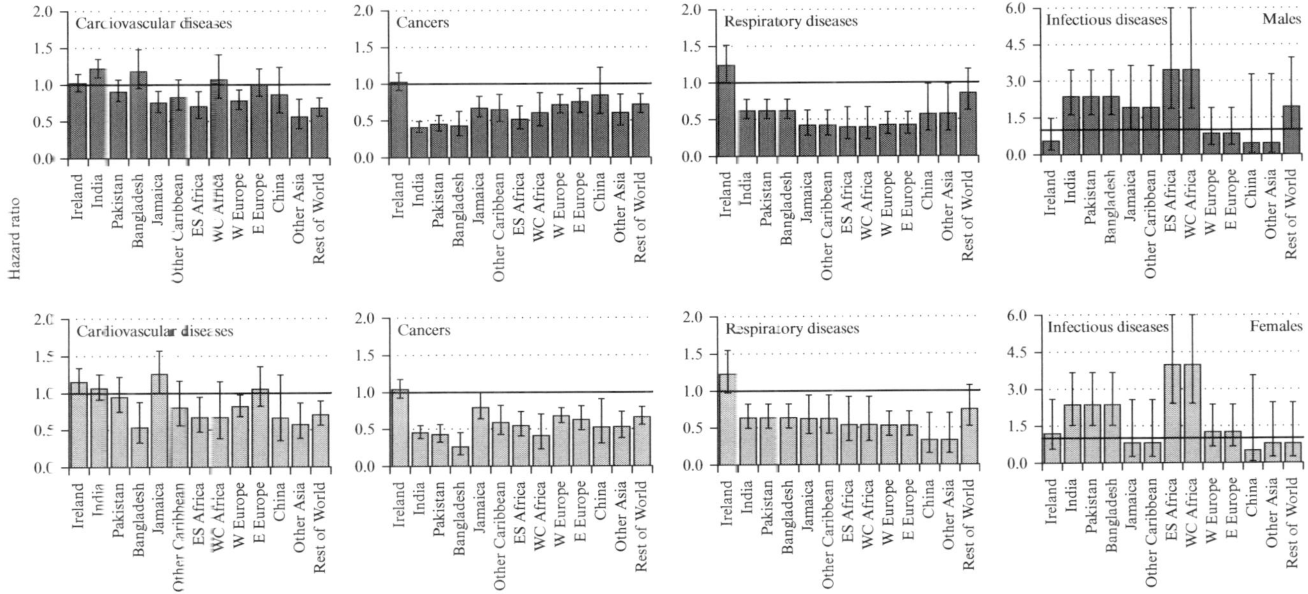

Notes:
Adjusted for age, census period, occupation type, education level, area of residence type and marital status.
Owing to low number of death events in respiratory and infectious diseases, the following groups are combined in the analysis of these two disease groups: India, Pakistan and Bangladesh (South Asia), Jamaica and Other Caribbean (Caribbean), East and South and West and Central Africa (Africa), China and Other Asia (Asia) and Western and Eastern Europe (Europe).

Source: Wallace and Kulu (2015), authors' calculations based on ONS LS.

Figure 10.3 Cause-specific mortality among migrants, 1971–2012

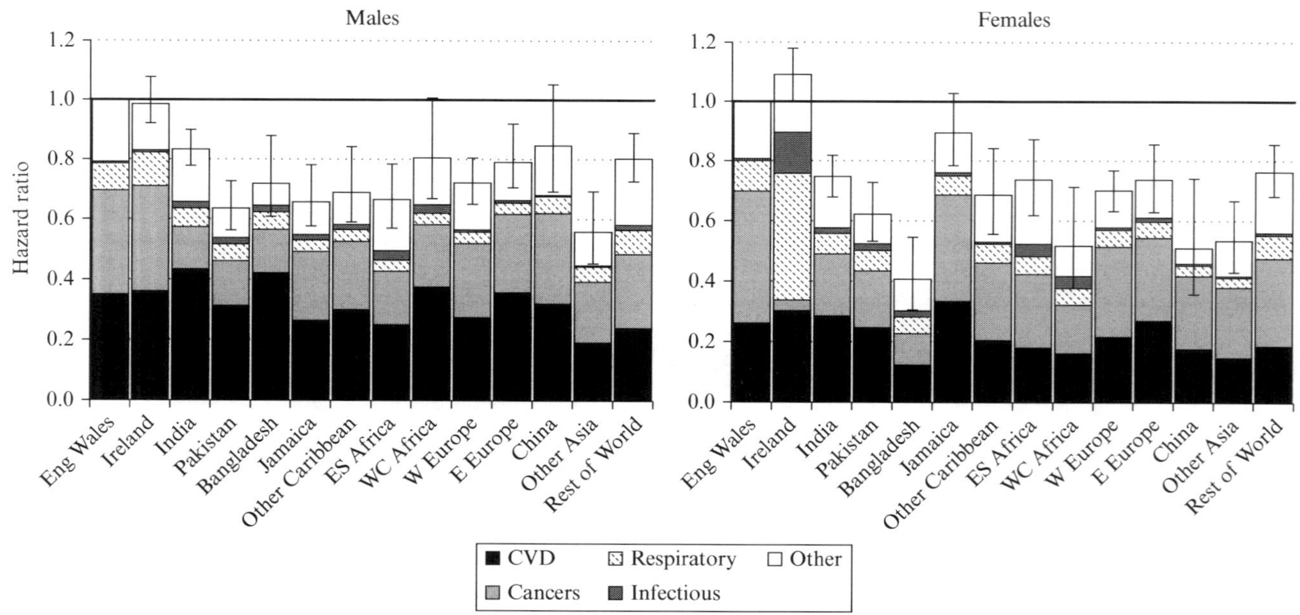

Note: Adjusted for age, census period, occupation type, education level, area of residence type and marital status (mortality from all other causes of death is plotted so the sum of the bars will equal the value for the all-cause mortality hazard ratio).

Source: Wallace and Kulu (2015), authors' calculations based on ONS LS.

Figure 10.4 Contribution of specific causes of death to all-cause mortality, 1971–2012

cancer is often the more influential of the two diseases. Again however, among South Asian females cardiovascular diseases are the main cause of death. For both males and females, respiratory and infectious diseases only make small contributions to overall mortality rates.

Finally, Figure 10.5 from Wallace and Kulu (2015) provides further insight into cultural factors and the rapid health transition by investigating whether cancer and cardiovascular diseases become more prominent causes of death over age. A partial attenuation is observed in cancer mortality, but mortality differences in cardiovascular diseases remain stable over time.

Discussion

The above findings are consistent with a selection narrative. First, for migrants originating from countries/regions where the overall health situation is much worse relative to the host country (e.g. East and South Africa and West and Central Africa), those experiencing a mortality advantage relative to the England and Wales-born can be considered atypically healthy relative to non-migrants in the country of origin. Second, the advantage was largest at ages where selection is posited to be most pronounced due to the influx of young adult migrants largely moving for economic reasons. The approximation of mortality differences over age is consistent with a decrease in the number of migrants arriving at older ages, older migrants arriving for non-economic reasons (such as family reunification), and an increase in duration of stay (and with it an increase in exposure to the local environment in terms of socioeconomic conditions and prevailing cultural and social norms) among those who arrived at younger ages. However, the findings do not support the notion of gender differences in selection.

In relation to the cultural factors hypothesis, the findings showed that the advantage was driven by low mortality from cancers and cardiovascular diseases. The two diseases are strongly influenced by modifiable risk factors in diet, smoking, and exercise. Thus lower mortality from cardiovascular diseases and cancers among migrants could indicate that migrant behaviours (perhaps positively influenced by the prevailing culture in the origin society) initially protect migrants from chronic diseases. The attenuation of the advantage over time would then be consistent with a gradual acculturation to the prevailing cultural norms of the host society which increases the risk for diseases within these two broad disease groups.

Finally, the analyses support a rapid health transition among non-western migrants. This is because mortality from infectious diseases is no longer a major cause of death which is consistent with a decrease in the risk of death from said diseases owing to access to advanced health

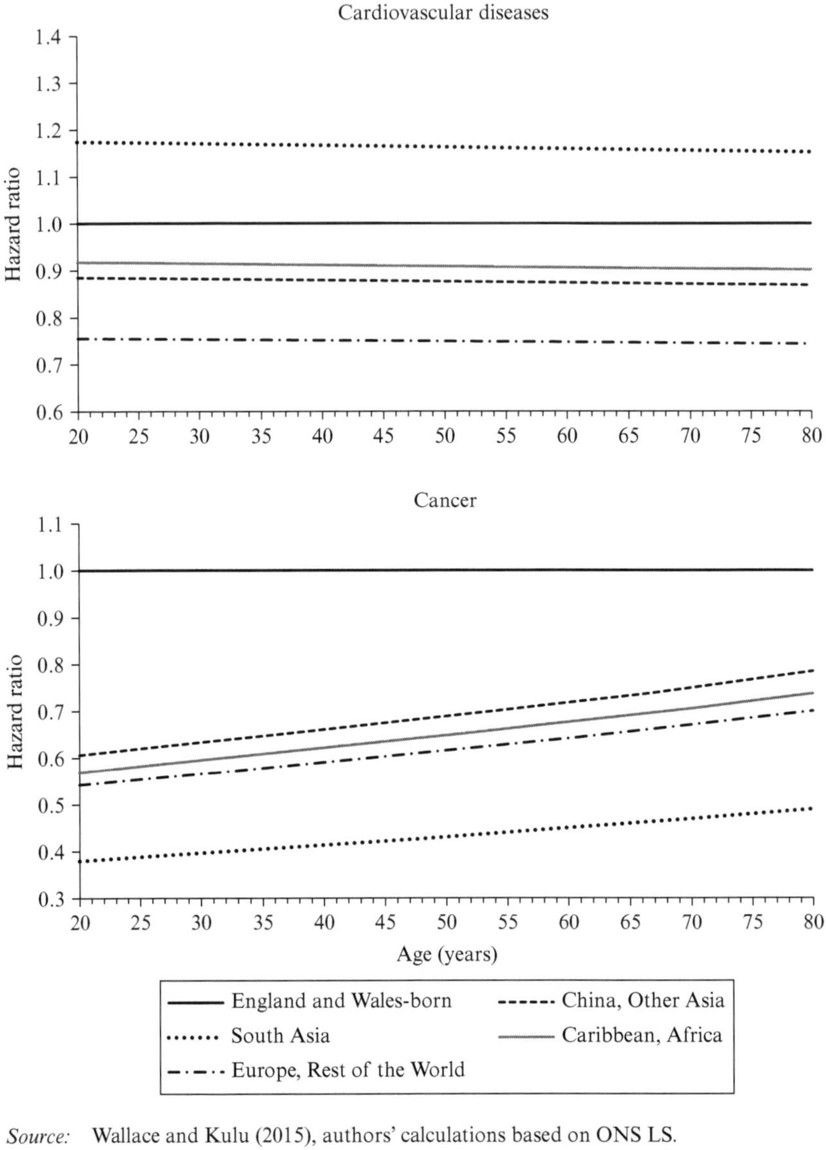

Source: Wallace and Kulu (2015), authors' calculations based on ONS LS.

Figure 10.5 Effect of duration of stay on cardiovascular and cancer mortality among migrants, 1971–2012

care and more hygienic and sanitary conditions. Additionally, at young ages (upon arrival) mortality from cancers and cardiovascular diseases was low among migrants from developing countries. This may reflect a lack of early life exposure to chronic disease risk factors. Lastly, all-cause and cancer mortality approximated to the England and Wales-born over time. As with the cultural factors hypothesis, this can be interpreted as acculturation to the health lifestyle in developed countries which causes an accumulation of chronic disease risk.

Overall, it is difficult to say which explanation is most relevant in determining the migrant mortality advantage. For selection, mortality comparisons are only made relative to the England and Wales-born. So, while the case can be made that migrants from, say, East and South Africa are atypically healthy relative to non-migrants in the origin countries, it is difficult to say the same thing about migrants from, say, Western Europe, particularly when this group originates from countries with similar to better health situations than in England and Wales.

Additionally, for cultural factors it is difficult to conclude whether migrants simply originate from countries with healthier prevailing cultural norms, or that people who practise healthier behaviours migrate (itself a selection effect). However, it is interesting that the migrant groups in this study originate from countries where the prevailing cultural and social norms are as different from one another as they are from England and Wales. Perhaps this weakens the cultural factors argument and strengthens the idea of selection as a general mechanism acting in migration.

Finally, a rapid health transition may well be operating among migrants from developing countries, but it cannot explain why migrants from Western Europe, who would not undergo any kind of health transition, would experience a mortality advantage over the England and Wales-born. With that in mind, it cannot be the sole explanation of the migrant mortality advantage. In all likelihood, aspects of all three mechanisms are operating to generate an advantage.

DESCENDANTS OF MIGRANTS

In developed countries, although the descendants of migrants represent an increasing share of the population, little is known about their mortality. In particular, it is of interest whether the mortality advantage observed among migrants persists among their descendants. This is because descendants who do not migrate to the host country are not subject to health selection. Moreover, their health behaviours may be more closely aligned with the majority population in England and Wales than the majority population in the country of origin. The acculturation process among migrants is believed to be crucial to inter-generational changes in health behaviours (Spallek et al., 2011).

Initially, the study used a broader categorization of three groups: the reference (White born in England and Wales), descendants of migrants (not White born in England and Wales), and migrants (not White born abroad) in order to investigate whether the advantage persists among descendants (see table 2 in Wallace, 2016a, for hazard ratios). In the baseline model, mortality was higher among descendants relative to both migrants and the White England and Wales-born. After adjusting socioeconomic position, mortality among descendants remained higher than among migrants, but became similar to the White England and Wales-born.

The broader groups were then divided into lower level ethnic groups to observe whether the identified pattern of high, socioeconomic-driven mortality was consistent across groups. Owing to the small size of many of the subgroups, the model was only able to adjust for sex. While this is not ideal for a mortality study, the broader model showed that mortality patterns among male and female descendants were consistent in the size of the excess mortality and the scale of attenuation. In the baseline model, excess mortality was observed among the descendants of migrants with the ethnic backgrounds Pakistani, Bangladeshi, Black Caribbean, Black Other, and group Other. After adjusting socioeconomic position, only the excess mortality among the descendants of Black Caribbeans persisted (see table 3 in Wallace, 2016a, for hazard ratios).

The above findings corroborate the small number of existing studies which observe an excess mortality in descendants which approximates upon adjusting socioeconomic position (Tarnutzer and Bopp, 2012; Scott and Timaeus, 2013; De Grande et al., 2014; Vandenheede et al., 2015).

This loss of the advantage between migrants and their descendants may relate to the fact that descendants of migrants do not move and are not subject to any health selection. The patterns could also relate to changes in health behaviours between generations. An increase in smoking prevalence has been documented (particularly among descendants of Black Caribbeans which may go some way to explaining their excess mortality) (Smith et al., 2009; Aspinall and Mitton, 2014), alongside an increase in alcohol consumption and decrease in diet quality (Smith et al., 2009). These changes in behaviour may also contribute to the loss of the advantage.

It was interesting that the effect of adjusting socioeconomic position was more profound among descendants, despite their socioeconomic position being similar to (or better than) migrants. A tentative explanation is that migrants often hold higher socioeconomic positions in the origin society than the position they currently hold in the host society (Deboosere and Gadeyne, 2005). Their previously high position in the origin society may have allowed them to generate a higher level of health, generating an advantage. However, descendants' health during their formative years is determined solely by their parent's socioeconomic position in the host country. If their parents occupy a lower position, then the mortality risk of their descendants may reflect the higher risk associated with worse conditions.

CONCLUSIONS

In summary, a migrant mortality advantage has been observed among nearly all migrant groups living in England and Wales (for both sexes) with variation in its magnitude across country and region of origin. The advantage was most pronounced at young adult ages and approximated towards the mortality of the England and Wales-born with age. For some migrant groups an advantage was apparent before adjusting for differences in socioeconomic position; in other groups a mortality advantage only became apparent after. The advantage was driven by lower mortality from cancers and in some migrant groups from cardiovascular diseases. Finally, a mortality advantage did not persist among the descendants of migrants.

It is fascinating that a migrant mortality advantage has presented across migrant groups with such diversity in terms of their country of origin and cultural and social norms. The key contribution of this research is the confirmation that the advantage cannot be explained away by censoring bias. Further, with the exception of South Asians, migrants who become ill do not leave England and Wales, suggesting the salmon bias effect cannot explain away the advantage either. Resultantly, the migrant mortality advantage is shown to be real and generated, to varying degrees of influence, by selection, cultural factors, and rapid health transition.

NOTE

* The permission of the Office for National Statistics (ONS) to use the Longitudinal Study is gratefully acknowledged, as is the help provided by staff of the Centre for Longitudinal Study Information & User Support (CeLSIUS). CeLSIUS is supported by the ESRC Census of Population Programme (Award Ref: ES/K000365/1). The author alone is responsible for the interpretation of the data.

This research was supported by the Economic and Social Research Council (ES/J500094/1) ('Mortality among Migrants and their Descendants in England and Wales') through the North West Doctoral Training Centre. The author would like to thank Hill Kulu, Paul Williamson and Gemma Catney for their collaboration and feedback in this research. The author would also like to thank Domantas Jasilionis for his advice on modelling cause-specific mortality.

REFERENCES

Abraido-Lanza, A.F., M.T. Chao and K.R. Florez (2005), 'Do healthy behaviors decline with greater acculturation? Implications for the Latino mortality paradox', *Social Science & Medicine*, **61** (6), 1243–55.

Abraido-Lanza, A.F., B.P. Dohrenwend, D.S. Ng-Mak and J.B. Turner (1999), 'The Latino mortality paradox: a test of the "salmon bias" and healthy migrant hypotheses', *American Journal of Public Health*, **89** (10), 1543–8.

Anson, J. (2004), 'The migrant mortality advantage: a 70 month follow-up of the Brussels population', *European Journal of Population*, **20** (3), 191–218.

Aspinall, P.J. and L. Mitton (2014), 'Smoking prevalence and the changing risk profiles in the UK ethnic and migrant minority populations: implications for stop smoking services', *Public Health*, **128** (3), 297–306.

Beiser, M. (2005), 'The health of immigrants and refugees in Canada', *Revue Canadienne de Santé Publique*, **96** (2), 530–44.

Boulogne, R., E. Jougla, Y. Breem, A.E. Kunst and G. Rey (2012), 'Mortality differences between the foreign-born and locally born population in France (2004–2007)', *Social Science and Medicine*, **74** (8), 1213–23.

Darmon, N. and M. Khlat (2001), 'An overview of the health status of migrants in France, in relation to their dietary practices', *Public Health Nutrition*, **4** (2), 163–72.

De Grande, H., H. Vandenheede, S. Gadeyne and P. Deboosere (2014), 'Health status and mortality rates of adolescents and young adults in the Brussels-Capital Region: differences according to region of origin and migration history', *Ethnicity & Health*, **19** (2), 122–43.

Deboosere, P. and S. Gadeyne (2005), 'Adult migrant mortality advantage in Belgium: evidence using census and register data', *Population*, **60** (5), 655–98.

Hajat, A., T. Blakely, S. Dayal and S. Jatrana (2010), 'Do New Zealand's immigrants have a mortality advantage? Evidence from the New Zealand Census-Mortality Study', *Ethnicity & Health*, **15** (5), 531–47.

Harding, S. and R. Balarajan (2001), 'Mortality data on migrant groups living in England and Wales: issues of adequacy and of interpretation of death rates', in J. Haskey and S. Huxstep (eds), *Population Projections by Ethnic Group: A Feasibility Study*, London: The Stationery Office, pp. 115–27.

Hattersley, L. (1999), *International Migration Data in the Longitudinal Study*, London: Office for National Statistics.

Jasso, G., D.S. Massey, M.R. Rosenzweig and J.P. Smith (2004), 'Immigrant health: selectivity and acculturation', in N.B. Anderson, R.A. Bulatao and B. Cohen (eds), *Critical Perspectives on Racial and Ethnic Differences in Health in Late Life*, Washington, DC: National Research Council, pp. 29–46.

Khlat, M. and Y. Courbage (1996), 'Mortality and causes of death of Moroccans in France, 1979–1991', *Population*, **8** (January), 59–94.

Kibele, E., R. Scholz and V.M. Shkolnikov (2008), 'Low migrant mortality in Germany for men aged 65 and older: fact or artifact?', *European Journal of Epidemiology*, **23** (6), 389–93.
Kohls, M. (2010), 'Selection, social status or data artefact – what determines the mortality of migrants in Germany?', in T. Salzmann, B. Edmonston and J. Raymer (eds), *Demographic Aspects of Migration*, Wiesbaden: VS Verlag für Sozialwissenschaften, pp. 153–77.
Lee, V. and A. Garg (2015), *South Asian Health Report*, Surrey, BC, Fraser Health Authority.
Nazroo, J.Y. (2014), *Ethnic Inequalities in Health: Addressing a Significant Gap in Current Evidence and Policy*, London: The British Academy.
Norredam, M., O.H. Hansen, J.H. Petersen, A.E. Kunst, M. Kristiansen, A. Krasnik and C. Agyemang (2015), 'Remigration of migrants with severe disease: myth or reality? A register-based cohort study', *European Journal of Public Health*, **25** (1), 84–9.
Palloni, A. and E. Arias (2004), 'Paradox lost: explaining the Hispanic adult mortality advantage', *Demography*, **41** (3), 385–415.
Razum, O. (2006), 'Commentary: of salmon and time travellers – musing on the mystery of migrant mortality', *International Journal of Epidemiology*, **35** (4), 919–21.
Razum, O. (2008), 'Migrant mortality, healthy migrant effect', in W. Kirch (ed.), *Encyclopedia of Public Health*, New York: Springer, pp. 932–5.
Razum, O. and D. Twardella (2002), 'Time travel with Oliver Twist – towards an explanation for a paradoxically low mortality among recent immigrants', *Tropical Medicine & International Health*, **7** (1), 4–10.
Razum, O., H. Zeeb and S. Rohrmann (2000), 'The "healthy migrant effect" – not merely a fallacy of inaccurate denominator figures', *International Journal of Epidemiology*, **29** (1), 191–2.
Razum, O., H. Zeeb, H.S. Akgun and S. Yilmaz (1998), 'Low overall mortality of Turkish residents in Germany persists and extends into a second generation: merely a healthy migrant effect?', *Tropical Medicine & International Health*, **3** (4), 297–303.
Scott, A.P., and I.M. Timaeus (2013), 'Mortality differentials 1991–2005 by self-reported ethnicity: findings from the ONS Longitudinal Study', *Journal of Epidemiology & Community Health*, **67** (9), 743–50.
Smith, N.R., Y.J. Kelly and J.Y. Nazroo (2009), 'Intergenerational continuities of ethnic inequalities in general health in England', *Journal of Epidemiology and Community Health*, **63** (3), 253–8.
Spallek, J., H. Zeeb and O. Razum (2011), 'What do we have to know from migrants' past exposures to understand their health status? A life course approach', *Emerging Themes in Epidemiology*, **8** (1), 6.
Tarnutzer, S. and M. Bopp (2012), 'Healthy migrants but unhealthy offspring? A retrospective cohort study among Italians in Switzerland', *BMC Public Health*, **12** (1), 1104–11.
Turra, C.M. and I.T. Elo (2008), 'The impact of salmon bias on the Hispanic mortality advantage: new evidence from social security data', *Population Research and Policy Review*, **27** (5), 515–30.
Valles, S.A. (2016), 'The challenges of choosing and explaining a phenomenon in epidemiological research on the "Hispanic paradox"', *Theoretical Medicine and Bioethics*, **37** (2), 129–48.

Vandenheede, H., D. Willaert, H. De Grande, S. Simoens and C. Vanroelen (2015), 'Mortality in adult immigrants in the 2000s in Belgium: a test of the "healthy-migrant" and the "migration-as-rapid-health-transition" hypotheses', *Tropical Medicine & International Health*, **20** (12), 1832–45.

Vang, Z.M., J. Sigouin, A. Flenon and A. Gagnon (2016), 'Are immigrants healthier than native-born Canadians? A systematic review of the healthy immigrant effect in Canada', *Ethnicity & Health*, **3** (6), 1–33.

Wallace, M. (2016a), 'Adult mortality among the descendants of immigrants in England and Wales: does a migrant mortality advantage persist beyond the first generation', *Journal of Ethnic and Migration Studies*, **42** (9) 1558–77.

Wallace, M. (2016b), 'Mortality among immigrants and their descendants in England and Wales', PhD thesis, University of Liverpool, Liverpool.

Wallace, M. and H. Kulu (2014), 'Low immigrant mortality in England and Wales: a data artefact?', *Social Science & Medicine*, **120** (November), 100–109.

Wallace, M. and H. Kulu (2015), 'Mortality among immigrants in England and Wales by major causes of death, 1971–2012: a longitudinal analysis of register-based data', *Social Science & Medicine*, **147** (December), 209–21.

Weitoft, G.R., A. Gullberg, A. Hjern and M. Rosen (1999), 'Mortality statistics in immigrant research: method for adjusting underestimation of mortality', *International Journal of Epidemiology*, **28** (4), 756–63.

11. Health and mortality patterns among migrants in France

Myriam Khlat and Michel Guillot

INTRODUCTION

In France, epidemiological research on migrant health and mortality has developed relatively slowly. The first publications on the mortality of foreigners date back to the 1980s. They were followed in the 1990s by a coordinated series on cancer mortality in migrants, which were all authored by a team of researchers working with the World Health Organization's International Agency for Research on Cancer (IARC). Those belonged to a long tradition in cancer epidemiology, which values migrant studies for their potential insights on the relative importance of environmental factors in disease aetiology (Parkin and Khlat, 1996).

Very few national-level studies can be found in the literature between the late 1990s and the mid-2000s. The latter date was a turning point, with the publication in close succession of a series of uncoordinated papers on migrants' health. Most of the studies were based on nationally representative surveys: health surveys (*Enquête Décennale Santé*, *Enquête santé et Protection Sociale*, *Enquête Santé Mentale en Population Générale* and *Etude Longitudinale Française depuis l'Enfance*); broader surveys containing pieces of information on health, among which were biographical surveys (*Enquête Histoire de Vie*); European cross-national surveys (*Survey of Ageing, Health and Retirement in Europe*, *European Union Survey on Income and Living Conditions*); or surveys specifically targeting migrant populations (*Enquête Passage à la Retraite des Immigrés* and *Enquête Trajectoires et Origines*). Other studies relied on disease or hospital registers, particularly for the description of infectious diseases or perinatal morbidity. The rationale of this batch of studies was quite different from that prevailing in cancer epidemiology, as the main focus was on social inequalities related to migration.

From the early 2010s, several papers on migrants' mortality in Europe were also published in a comparative perspective, within the framework of the European Union-funded project Migrant and Ethnic Minority

Health Observatory (MEHO). France was one immigration country among others in this project, which aimed at considering inequalities related to migration for different countries of origin, generating hypotheses about the causes of diseases and ultimately investigating the association between integration policies in different countries and migrants' mortality.

A literature review on health of migrants in France in relation to their dietary practices was published in 2001 (Darmon and Khlat, 2001), and another on their health and health-care use in 2012 (Berchet and Jusot, 2012). In this chapter, we update and complete these reviews, with a particular focus on studies dealing with specific diseases, which shed new light on the situation of migrants with regard to the 'accelerated health transition' framework.

THEORETICAL BACKGROUND

Several hypotheses and theories have been developed within this area of research on migrants' health and mortality. The 'migrant mortality paradox' concept emphasizes the contradiction between the advantaged mortality level and disadvantaged socio-economic condition of migrants. The predominant hypothesis for this paradox is that of the 'healthy migrant effect', according to which individuals who migrate are among the healthiest of their population of origin. An alternative explanation is the 'salmon-bias' hypothesis, which assumes that migrants tend to return to their home country whenever they become seriously ill, leaving behind the healthiest members of the community. Recently, a framework has been developed that views migration through the lens of the theory of health transition. According to this theory, migrants moving from less-developed to more-developed countries experience an 'accelerated health transition' (Spallek et al., 2011). Upon arrival, they benefit from better environmental conditions and health care, which permits a fast reduction of their mortality from infectious diseases. In parallel, they are progressively exposed to the western lifestyle and the related traditional risk factors of chronic diseases, resulting after a lag period in a rise of those diseases. Shortly, the hypothesis of migration as 'accelerated health transition' predicts a fast decline of the initially high infectious-disease mortality of migrants and a progressive reduction of their advantage in terms of chronic disease mortality over time. Very few studies have investigated this hypothesis to date (Vandenheede et al., 2015; Wallace and Kulu, 2015).

HISTORY OF IMMIGRATION TO FRANCE

France stands out in Europe as the oldest country of immigration and as having received the largest numbers of immigrants over time (Noiriel, 1988; Weil, 2005). The first wave of immigration to France arose during the Second Empire (1852–70) with neighbouring countries providing the bulk of immigrant workers. A second wave during the 1920s originated mainly from eastern European countries. During the Second World War, France suffered the destruction of much of its infrastructure, and there was again a great need of foreign workers for the reconstruction and modernization of the country. The most important flows of this third immigration wave arrived during the economic boom of the 1950s and 1960s. They originated primarily from former colonies undergoing the process of decolonization, and particularly from Algeria, which became independent in 1962. In parallel, the country once again recruited workers from neighbouring countries, and especially from Portugal. The 1973 oil crisis altered the labour market and led to a major shift in immigration policies in Western Europe, with the end of labour migration in France (Therborn, 1987). Since that date, family reunification and asylum have represented the principal channels for immigration (Wihtol de Wenden, 2012), and the population of migrants has become increasingly diverse, with larger proportions from sub-Saharan Africa and Asia. The creation of the borderless Schengen area in 1995 and the 2004 and 2007 enlargements of the European Union also led to increases in immigration from other European Union countries.

Overall, migrants with the longest duration of stay are from Southern Europe (with Portuguese more recently arrived than Spaniards and Italians), followed by those from North Africa (Algeria, Tunisia and, later, Morocco), then by those from sub-Saharan Africa, Turkey and Eastern Europe (Breuil-Genier et al., 2011). Migration from Southeast Asia (Cambodia, Laos and Vietnam) was very concentrated in time, with half of the arrivals occurring between 1976 and 1982. The size of the migrant communities from the earlier waves is gradually shrinking, owing to deaths and returns to the home country.

METHODS

Search Strategy

We searched PubMed, Cairn and the French bibliographic databases from the health or social sciences field (BDSP, library of the national public health agency Santé Publique France, library of the Institut National d'Etudes Démographiques, library of Migrinter laboratory and ProQuest tool). Our search algorithms in PubMed were: ((France[MeSH Terms]) AND ('transients and migrants') OR ('emigrants and immigrants')) AND health[MeSH Terms]) OR mortality[MeSH Terms]) OR causes of death[MeSH Terms]) OR aging[MeSH Terms]. For the French databases, we used the terms: (Immigré or Immigration) and France and (Santé or Morbidité or Mortalité or Causes de décès or Vieillissement).

Our review concerned publications reporting country of birth or nationality-based mortality or health differences from empirical quantitative nationally representative studies. Only book chapters and articles in peer-reviewed journals were included.

SUMMARY OF THE FINDINGS

National-level studies specifically targeting mortality, health or health-related behaviours of migrants are presented in tabular form. Other studies more limited in scale or with a different focus are referred to in the interpretation and discussion. The selected studies differed in their definition of migrant status: some considered country of birth, others current nationality and others a combination of the two. Only a few applied the official definition combining country of birth and nationality at birth.

Mortality Studies

Our selection consisted of 17 articles in peer-reviewed journals and one book chapter (Table 11.1). All studies had an un-linked design, relating aggregate deaths collected from the national register of deaths to the corresponding person-years at risk calculated from the census. Altogether a large time period was covered, extending from the mid-1970s to the mid-2000s.

Within this set of mortality studies, two subsets of coordinated papers each based on a common dataset made up in total about two-thirds of the papers. The first subset is related to a large collaborative project on cancer in Italian migrant populations coordinated by the International Agency for Research on Cancer (IARC). This project, which dates back to the end of the 1980s, was sponsored jointly by the IARC and the Italian League against Cancer, and its originality consisted in the follow-up of a single source population (Italians) in ten of its destination countries, including France.

The change in cancer risk after migration and the speed with which

Table 11.1 Studies of mortality among migrants in France

Study period	Mortality outcome	Study group(s)	First author, year
1974–75	Total and cause-specific	Algerians, Moroccans, Portuguese, Spaniards, Italians, Poles	Brahimi, 1980
1980–82	Total and cause-specific	Foreigners	Bouvier-Colle, 1985
1979–85	Cancer	Born in Algeria, Morocco, Tunisia, Western sub-Saharan Africa, Eastern sub-Saharan Africa, Vietnam/Cambodia/Laos, China/Taiwan	Bouchardy, 1992[a]
		Born in Italy	Bouchardy, 1993[a]
		Born in Vietnam/Cambodia/Laos, China/Taiwan/Hong Kong	Bouchardy, 1994[a]
		Born in West/East/Central/Other Africa	Bouchardy, 1995[a]
		Born in Switzerland	Wanner et al., 1995a[a]
		Born in Algeria, Morocco, Tunisia, Egypt	Bouchardy, 1996[a]
1979–85	Total and cause-specific	Country of birth or groups of countries	Wanner et al., 1997[a]
1979–91	Total and cause-specific	Moroccans born abroad	Courbage, 1996
2005–07	Cancer	Born in Turkey	Spallek, 2012[b]
	Diabetes mellitus	Born in North Africa, Other Africa, Turkey, Other	Vandenheede, 2012[b]
	Circulatory diseases	Born in China, Poland, Turkey, Yugoslavia	Bhopal, 2011[b]
	Circulatory diseases	Born in Asia, Caribbean, Europe, Latin America, Middle East, North Africa, sub-Saharan Africa	Rafnsson, 2013[b]
	Total and cause-specific	North Africa, sub-Saharan Africa, Caribbean, Other Latin America, South Asia, east Asia, eastern Europe, Turkey	Ikram, 2015[b]
		Born in Turkey, Morocco	Ikram, 2015[b]
2004–07	Total and cause-specific	Born in Algeria, Morocco, Tunisia, Turkey + groups of countries	Boulogne, 2012[b]
1998–2007	Maternal deaths	Citizenship by continent or sub-continent	Saurel-Cubizolles, 2012

Notes:
[a] From IARC project on Cancer in Italian migrant populations.
[b] From MEHO project.

it developed was the main outcome of interest, and was interpreted as a clue (or lack thereof) of the relative importance of specific environmental factors in the aetiology of different cancers. Seven publications belong to this subset (Bouchardy et al., 1992, 1994, 1996, 1998; Bouchardy, 1993; Wanner et al., 1995a, 1997).

The second subset of studies relates to the MEHO, which aimed at comparing and monitoring the health status of immigrants in Western Europe with a public health perspective. This large-scale European cooperation project was funded by the European Union Commission at the end of the 2000s, and included a large number of host countries and migrant groups. Six publications belong to this subset (Bhopal et al., 2011; Spallek et al., 2012; Vandenheede et al., 2012 Rafnsson et al., 2013; Ikram et al., 2015a, 2015b).

The remaining publications had a national focus, with an interest in either younger age groups (Bouvier-Colle et al., 1985), pregnancy and the perinatal period (Saurel-Cubizolles et al., 2012) or one specific migrant group (Courbage and Khlat, 1996). Two publications were more comprehensive in scope (Brahimi, 1980; Boulogne et al., 2012).

The study on Moroccans (Courbage and Khlat, 1996) had the longest observation period (13 years). It is also more elaborate methodologically, as the authors evaluated the completeness of death registration coverage by using an indirect method originally designed for developing countries suffering from incomplete registration of deaths. This approach allowed the authors to uncover that the proportion of missing deaths was negligible for women (2 per cent) and more significant for men (23 per cent), and to confirm that the findings were robust to corrections for under-registration of deaths.

Considering all-cause mortality, the existence, direction and width of the foreign-born versus native-born difference varied according to age, gender and origin. A mortality advantage was visible from the early adult ages, much more so for men than for women (Courbage and Khlat, 1996; Boulogne et al. 2012), and at the opposite younger migrants suffered from higher mortality (Bouvier-Colle et al., 1985). The latter disadvantage early in life accords with a study of social inequalities in infant mortality, in which social categories were found to converge, while the increased mortality of children born to foreign parents (second generation) remained (Dinh, 1998). Among adult men, the under-mortality was particularly marked for migrants from North Africa and sub-Saharan Africa, while those from Eastern Europe had higher mortality (Ikram et al., 2015a). In the latter study, a striking gender contrast was found for migrants from sub-Saharan Africa, as females suffered from higher mortality in comparison with the local-born, unlike males. No adjustment for socio-economic confounders was made, except in Wanner et al. (1997). Since migrants tend to have lower socio-economic status than the native-born population, lack of adjustment is unlikely to explain observed mortality advantages, but may have contributed to mortality disadvantages for certain groups.

Overall, migrants had higher mortality from deaths caused by infectious diseases (particularly tuberculosis) and diabetes, and lower mortality from cancers and violent deaths (Courbage and Khlat, 1996; Boulogne et al., 2012). Regarding cancers, very distinctive patterns were found for migrants from North Africa, sub-Saharan Africa and Southeast Asia, with lower risks than the host population for most cancer sites together with higher risks for a few cancers (Bouchardy et al., 1992, 1994, 1995, 1996). A review of cancer risks in non-western migrants to Europe including this set of studies (Arnold et al., 2010) confirmed the importance of exposures experienced before, during and after migration, and concluded that migrants were more prone to cancers related to early life infections, such as liver, cervical and stomach cancer, and less prone to cancers related to a western lifestyle, such as colorectal, breast and prostate cancers. A similar conclusion was reached in a review of cancer in Mediterranean migrants (Khlat, 1995).

In terms of circulatory disease mortality, migrants from China, Poland, Turkey or Yugoslavia had in France higher death rates than the local-born, but lower death rates compared to their counterparts in other immigration countries (Bhopal et al., 2011; Rafnsson et al., 2013). This pattern was discussed in the context of the so-called 'French paradox', according to which circulatory diseases are relatively low in France despite high prevalence of traditional risk factors (for example, smoking, high-fat diet), with the suggestion that this paradox may also apply to some extent to France's foreign-born population. For diabetes mortality, a general pattern of disadvantage was visible in migrants, and the lower the gross domestic product of the country of origin, the larger the disadvantage, which led to the suggestion of a major role of socio-economic change, and in particular lifestyle changes including diet and exercise (Vandenheede et al., 2012).

Finally, specific risks were attached to pregnancy and childbirth for foreign women, whose maternal mortality rate over the period 1998–2007 was as high as 12.5 per 100000 live births, versus 7.9 among French women (Saurel-Cubizolles et al., 2012). In another study, Moroccan women were also shown to be disproportionately affected by maternal deaths (Courbage and Khlat, 1996).

Health Studies

Studies were of two types. First, 19 articles were based on nationally representative large-scale interview surveys, with relevant information on global indicators of health and on reported morbidity and health behaviours (Table 11.2). Second, four articles were based on data from registries for diseases subject to compulsory reporting, such as HIV, tuberculosis or hepatitis B, or hospital registries for perinatal conditions (Table 11.3). The chronology of the publications in Tables 11.2 and 11.3 reflects the expansion of research on migrants' health in France starting from the mid-2000s.

Global Indicators of Health

Based on data from the early 1990s (Khlat et al., 1998), respondents of North African origin enjoyed a health advantage. Later findings were mixed. In the *Enquête Passage à la Retraite des Immigrés* (2002–03), migrants turned out to have worse health outcomes than the local-born, but their disadvantage was largely explained by their work conditions (Attias-Donfut and Tessier, 2005). Also, not all migrant groups experienced a disadvantage. Males originating from Asia and southern Africa, and females originating from northern Europe, were advantaged in comparison with the local population (Vaillant and Wolff, 2010). In the *Enquête Histoire de Vie*, male migrants from non-European countries, and particularly those from North Africa, reported functional limitations less frequently than the native-born, while no significant difference was found for female migrants, regardless of their region of origin (Lert et al., 2007). On the contrary, analysis of the *Enquête Trajectoires et Origines* did lead to the conclusion of a definite health disadvantage, with however better health among the newly arrived male migrants (Cognet et al., 2012; Hamel and Moisy, 2012, 2015). In-depth analyses by health economists of the *Enquête Décennale Santé* and of the *Enquête Santé et Protection Sociale* either provided no salient difference after adjustment for socio-economic confounders (Mizrahi and Mizrahi, 2008), or provided heterogeneous findings, with no significant difference remaining after adjustment for socio-economic conditions, dietary habits and tobacco and alcohol consumption (Berchet and Jusot, 2009, 2010; Jusot et al., 2009). In a cross-national study of populations aged 50 years in 11 European countries, migrants in France generally had worse health than the local-born (Solé-Auro and Crimmins, 2008). Another study of the same type showed an interesting North–South gradient in Europe, with better health status among migrants in Italy and Spain than in France and Belgium (Moullan and Jusot, 2014).

Specific Diseases or Conditions

A few studies documented specific diseases or conditions which disproportionately affected migrants. For instance, the prevalence of

Table 11.2 Studies of health, health behaviours and health care use of migrants in France based on national health interview surveys

Survey	Outcome variable	Study groups	First author, year
Enquête Conditions de Vie des Ménages, 1987	Preventive health care utilization, nutritional habits, tobacco, alcohol	Migrants from Italy, Spain/Portugal, North Africa	Wanner et al., 1995b
Enquête Décennale de Santé (EDS), 1991–92	Reported health and morbidity, tobacco, body mass index	Household head of Moroccan, Algerian or Tunisian nationality	Khlat, 1998
Enquête Passage à la Retraite des Immigrés (*PRI*), 2002–03	Self-rated health, work-related injuries, occupational diseases, disabilities, health-care utilization	Migrants from Southern Europe, Northern Europe, Eastern Europe, Northern Africa, sub-Saharan Africa, America, Middle East, Asia	Attias-Donfut, 2005
	Self-rated health	Same as above	Vaillant, 2010
Enquête Histoire de Vie, 2003	Functional limitations, overweight	Migrants	Lert, 2007
EDS, 2002–03 *Enquête Santé et Protection Sociale (ESPS)*, 2000-2002 *Enquête sur les Hospitalisés*, 1991	Self-rated health, health-care expenditures	Foreigners	Mizrahi, 2008
EDS, 2002–03	Self-rated health	Foreign-born by sub-continent	Jusot, 2009
EDS, 2002–03, *Enquête Entred*, 2007	Diabetes	Migrants from North Africa	Fosse, 2012
Enquête Santé Mentale en Population Générale (*SMPG*), 1999–2003	Psychotic disorders	First, second and third generation migrants	Amad, 2013
Survey of Health, Ageing and Retirement in Europe (SHARE), 2004–05	Self-rated health, chronic diseases, disabilities, smoking, overweight	Migrants	Solé-Auro, 2008

Table 11.2 (continued)

Survey	Outcome variable	Study groups	First author, year
ESPS, 2006, 2008	Self-rated health	First and second generation migrants	Berchet, 2009
ESPS, 2006	Self-rated health, nutritional habits, tobacco, alcohol	Foreign-born by sub-continent	Berchet, 2010
Enquête Trajectoires et Origines (*TEO*), 2008	Self-rated health	Migrants from Turkey, South-East Asia, Portugal, Morocco/Tunisia/ Algeria, sub-Saharan Africa, Spain/Italy	Cognet, 2012 Hamel, 2012 Hamel, 2015
ESPS, 2006, 2008	Health-care utilization	Migrants	Berchet, 2013
ESPS, 2004, 2006, 2010	Self-rated health	Migrants	Moullan, 2014
European Union Survey on Income and Living Conditions (SILC), 2011	Self-rated health	Foreign-born	Malmusi, 2014
Etude Longitudinale depuis l'Enfance (*ELFE*), 2011	Alcohol, tobacco use in pregnancy	Foreign-born	Melchior, 2015

Table 11.3 Studies of specific disease or conditions in migrants based on national disease or hospital registers

Data source	Outcome variable	Study groups	First author, year
National AIDS register, 1978–98	New AIDS cases	Foreigners by country	Savignoni, 1999
National tuberculosis register, 2006	New tuberculosis cases	Migrants	Che, 2009
National registers for: HIV infection, 2009 Tuberculosis, 2008, 2009 Hepatitis B, 2008, 2009	New HIV diagnoses, tuberculosis cases and chronic HBV infection cases	Foreign-born by continent or sub-continent	Lot, 2012
Enquête Nationale Périnatale, 1998, 2003, 2010	Premature births, low birthweight	Foreigners by continent or sub-continent	Saurel-Cubizolles, 2012

diabetes was more elevated among migrants from North Africa than among the French-born population. Women were particularly affected, and their vulnerability was not entirely explained by a higher prevalence of obesity, which led to the suggestion of a genetic predisposition to diabetes (Fosse and Fagot-Campagna, 2012). In addition, diabetic persons from North Africa were not as closely monitored as the native-born population, and more frequently suffered from ophthalmologic complications. The pattern of disadvantage found for women is consistent with the higher mortality from diabetes in female migrants from Morocco compared with the French population (Courbage and Khlat, 1996).

Migration and particularly forced migration are associated with painful life events and the stress of adaptation to a new environment, and in the most extreme cases with psycho-traumatism. In a general health survey, there was no indication of a higher prevalence of reported mental morbidity among migrants from North Africa (Khlat et al., 1998). However, migrants were found to have an elevated prevalence of psychotic disorders in a more targeted mental health survey (Amad et al., 2013).

Migrant mortality was higher overall for deaths caused by infectious diseases (Boulogne et al., 2012). Conditions such as HIV infection, tuberculosis and hepatitis B indeed have high prevalence in some regions of the world, in particular in sub-Saharan Africa, which puts migrants from these regions at greater risk for these diseases. Information on the situation of migrants was based on the analysis of data collected through compulsory registration systems (for HIV and tuberculosis) or disease reference centres based in hospitals (for hepatitis B). During the first ten years of the AIDS epidemic, the cumulative incidence rate was twice as high among foreigners as among the French population, with highest risks among sub-Saharan Africans and Haitians (Savignoni et al., 1999). In 2009, nearly half of the reported cases of HIV infection and of tuberculosis were migrants, and so were three-quarters of the patients newly referred for hepatitis B treatment (Lot et al., 2012). From those figures, the authors estimated that rates of new HIV diagnoses and tuberculosis cases were respectively ten and eight times higher among migrants than among persons born in France, with late diagnosis compounding the problem.

Sexual and reproductive health is considered an area of concern for migrant women. Analysis of data from perinatal surveys led to the conclusion that foreign women, and particularly those originating from sub-Saharan countries, had a higher rate of stillbirths, pre-term births and low birthweight babies (Saurel-Cubizolles et al., 2012). A higher prevalence of perinatal conditions among women from North Africa was also reported from a population-based survey (Khlat et al., 1998). This is consistent with the finding of an excess mortality from maternal causes among foreign women in France (Saurel-Cubizolles et al., 2012), and especially among women of Moroccan origin (Courbage and Khlat, 1996).

Health-related Behaviours

The relative advantage or disadvantage of migrants for overweight, tobacco and alcohol consumption is strongly patterned by gender. Considering migrants aged 50 years and older, no excess prevalence of overweight was found, based on age and sex-adjusted estimates (Solé-Auro and Crimmins, 2008). There seems to be a specific pattern among female migrants, as a higher prevalence was found for foreign women (Lert et al., 2007). This concerns particularly women of North African origin (Khlat et al., 1998), which is consistent with their higher mortality from diabetes and circulatory diseases. On the contrary, female migrants from North Africa had a lower level of tobacco consumption than French nationals, while males had a higher consumption (Khlat et al., 1998; Saurel-Cubizolles et al., 2012; Wanner et al., 1995b). Both genders had a lower consumption of alcohol (Wanner et al., 1995b). Paradoxically, Moroccan men have a much lower mortality from lung cancer than nationals, in spite of their higher level of smoking (Courbage and Khlat, 1996), but this may be due to a more recent diffusion of smoking in this population. In the ELFE cohort study of children born in France in 2011, migrant women as a whole had lower consumption of alcohol and tobacco than native-born women during pregnancy (Melchior et al., 2015).

DISCUSSION

As research on migrants' health only started to expand in France in the 2000s, there is to date a limited number of studies in comparison to other large immigration countries. Yet, an overview of this set of national population-based studies yields a coherent picture and raises important questions and avenues for future research.

Healthy Migrant Effect or Vulnerable Populations?

The so-called 'healthy migrant effect' universally reported in the international literature is only visible in a subset of studies: (1) mortality studies, in which differences are predominantly in favour of male migrants starting from the early adult ages (and irregularly in favour of female migrants), and (2) the first health study, based on data from the early 1990s. Most health surveys from the 2000s provided mixed findings, which were to some extent more in line with the traditional representation of migrants as 'vulnerable populations'.

There was more evidence of a disadvantage for self-rated health than for the declaration of chronic diseases or functional limitations. It has been suggested that a subjective notion such as poor self-rated health may be enhanced by social isolation and hardship, while the notions of chronic diseases or functional limitations may be more difficult to understand by some or be under-reported owing to less demanding expectations or norms in terms of health (Berchet and Jusot, 2012).

Studies based on medical diagnoses provided strong evidence of a specific vulnerability of migrants to infectious diseases and perinatal conditions. Regarding HIV, a recent study challenged the common-held belief that HIV-positive migrants contracted HIV prior to migration. Using cross-sectional survey data, the authors showed that a third to a half of sub-Saharan migrants receiving HIV care in France have been infected post-migration (Desgrées-du-Loû et al., 2015), particularly during periods of social hardship (Desgrées-du-Loû et al., 2016), and called for more targeted efforts in terms of prevention and early care. The epidemiological profile of tuberculosis cases in migrants in France is also more in favour of recent infections than of post-migration reactivations (Che and Antoine, 2009), as opposed to what has been hypothesized in Canada (De Maio, 2010).

Regarding access to health care, health economists have demonstrated that, for the same level of need, migrants present lower access to general practitioners and to specialists, partly owing to lower health care coverage (Mizrahi and Mizrahi, 2008; Berchet, 2013). Migrants were also found to more frequently give up health-care seeking for financial reasons (Boisguerin and Haury, 2008), and their disadvantage was compounded by less frequent recourse to preventive medicine, including vaccination and screening (Wanner et al., 1995b; Grillo et al., 2012; Rondet et al., 2014). Quality of health care provided to migrants has also been questioned (Bhopal, 2007), and a call has recently been issued to support more inclusive and migrant-sensitive approaches in routine health care and prevention campaigns, as opposed to migrant-specific more exclusive approaches (Razum and Spallek, 2014).

In the light of those findings, the mortality advantage of migrants appears as doubly paradoxical: first, in relation to their socio-economic profile; second, in relation to their health profile. Some authors have pinpointed that the health-mortality paradox had been identified from separate studies and could therefore be attributed to differences in the selection of study populations. Yet, it is worth noting that the immigrants living in workers' hostels and illegal immigrants, likely to be in poorer health, are under-represented, if represented at all, in population-based health surveys, while they contribute to mortality statistics. Other explanations have been suggested by the same authors, namely, that migrants would be suffering more from disabling illnesses than from life-threatening illnesses, or be dying from causes not related to perceived health (Stirbu et al., 2006).

The mortality data may be questioned in the same way as the health data, as it may be subject to artefact from inadequate recording of deaths. Indeed, deaths occurring abroad are not part of the numerator count, which inevitably leads to an under-estimation of mortality for the foreign-born, as they constitute an internationally mobile population. Further to that, the preferential return of unhealthy migrants to their home country ('salmon bias') is likely to compound the positive health selection at entry (Khlat and Darmon, 2003). It is worth noting also that the 'salmon bias' is more likely to be a factor in Western Europe, given the geographical proximity of most migrants to their host countries, than in Canada, Australia or the USA.

Overall, there is a very specific and coherent pattern of cancer mortality, with an under-mortality for cancers related to western lifestyles and an over-mortality for cancers related to predispositions or known early exposures in countries of origin. Differential mortality by broad groups of causes of death also provided a coherent set of findings, with migrants enjoying under-mortality from cancers and circulatory diseases. External consistency with the body of knowledge on the risk factors for individual cancers and with the health transition framework strengthens the mortality findings.

Temporal Factors: Duration of Stay Effects

Several specific findings emphasize duration of stay as a determinant of migrant health. Longer duration of stay was associated with worse self-rated health, after adjustment for confounders (Attias-Donfut and Tessier, 2005), and women who had immigrated during adolescence had more activity of daily living (ADL) limitations (Lert et al., 2007). Also, male migrants who had arrived within the past five years had significantly better health than the local-born, regardless of their age at arrival and educational level, but this was not found among females (Hamel and Moisy, 2012, 2015). Lastly, the disadvantage in terms of chronic diseases and disabilities only pertained to naturalized immigrants, whereas non-naturalized immigrants had a better health profile than the native-born population (Jusot et al., 2009). The latter finding was interpreted as reflecting the wear of the health-selection effects over time, as naturalized migrants have been living in France for longer, on average, than non-naturalized migrants.

The absence of evidence of a health advantage among migrants aged 50 in France accords with this pattern (Solé-Auro and Crimmins, 2008).

The faster deterioration of health has to be related to the disproportionate exposure of migrants to hardship in terms of their work and employment conditions in comparison with the local-born, notwithstanding unemployment and discrimination on the labour and housing market (Mizrahi and Mizrahi, 2008; Jusot et al., 2009; Berchet and Jusot, 2010). As an outcome of isolation, higher risk of suicide for migrants would be expected, and yet, mortality from this cause was consistently found to be lower among migrants in Europe (Ikram, 2015a). In the survey *Trajectoires et origins*, the discriminations the migrants were particularly subjected to were found to have a negative influence on their health self-report (Cognet et al., 2012; Hamel and Moisy, 2012). On the other hand, it has been suggested that 'immigrants who experience discrimination may be more likely to report worsening health' (De Maio, 2010).

Temporal Factors: Time Period Effects

In addition to the worsening of health with increasing duration of stay, there may be a deterioration of migrants' health over historical time. Indeed, the advantage found in the early 1990s study contrasts with the more mitigated situation found in the 2000s (Mizrahi and Mizrahi, 2008). An important factor may be the labour market crisis prevailing in France for several decades, which is likely to have aggravated the situation of migrants. The changing profiles of migrants to the European Union and of their health situation has been pinpointed, and it has been suggested that economic crises may disproportionately exacerbate the risk of infectious diseases in migrants (Villalonga-Olives and Kawachi, 2014), and perhaps even lead to the loss of the healthy migrant effect (Gotsens et al., 2015).

Age and Gender Patterns

Younger migrants clearly are disadvantaged healthwise, and this may be related to the circumstances of their migration as children or adolescents accompanying their parents, and therefore not subjected to health selection. Another striking feature emerging from this collection of studies is the contrast between the relative advantage enjoyed by male migrants and the disadvantage observed for female migrants. Traditionally, females arrive for family reunification rather than for work, and are, like their children, less subjected to health selection of the 'healthy worker effect' type. Females form an increasing part of the migrant population in France (more than half according to the latest statistics; Beauchemin et al., 2013), and those originating from North Africa seem to carry a specific pattern of disadvantage characterized by insufficient recourse to prevention and screening, associated with diabetes, metabolic diseases, overweight and perinatal problems. This is in contrast with the sizeable advantage conferred to men originating from North Africa by their comparatively lower level of alcohol consumption, given that in France the prevalence of alcohol-related diseases is quite high. However, male migrants have a comparatively high level of smoking, which is not the case with female migrants. Recently, the added value of integrating a gender perspective to understand migrants' health in epidemiological studies has been emphasized (Llacer et al., 2007).

Health Transition

After the 'migration as a natural experiment' framework of cancer epidemiologists, and the public health perspective of migrants as 'vulnerable populations', the health transition framework views migration as an 'accelerated health transition' (Spallek et al., 2011). Within the health transition framework, migrants are expected to arrive in the host countries with a higher prevalence of infectious diseases, and they were indeed shown in France to disproportionately suffer from such diseases (Alba and Silberman, 2002; Che and Antoine, 2009; Lot et al., 2012). However, the study on HIV infection demonstrates their vulnerability to contracting those diseases after arrival (Desgrées-du-Loû et al., 2015). It is worth noting also that the most recent waves of migrants originate from countries well advanced in the health transition process, and in which chronic diseases are on the rise.

CONCLUSION

Although evidence on migrants' health and mortality in France is relatively limited, this review brings up several important issues, many of which overlap with what has been found in other receiving countries. A double paradox surrounding migrants' mortality advantage emerges: first, in the face of socio-economic disadvantage; and second, in the face of deteriorating health and unmet health needs. Other questions relate to the factors underlying the initial health capital of migrants and the eventual reversal of their advantage. In order to better understand the health needs and processes at play in different migrant groups and generations, more detailed questions should be included in survey questionnaires, relating to date of arrival, nationality at birth, parental country of birth and reason for migration. Temporal trends should be carefully explored, and the influence on the 'healthy migrant effect' of the economic crises and the hardship to which migrants are disproportionately exposed needs to be investigated. Health trajectories of migrants should be explored with special attention to specific conditions or diseases, to differences according to reason for migration and country of origin, and to compositional factors over time. More attention should also be given to mental health, to lifestyle factors underlying chronic diseases and to the designing of preventive interventions and campaigns for the benefits of all. An ideal study design would be the cohort type, whereby both health and mortality would be observed over time within and across different immigration cohorts. Although issues relating to migrants' health and health transitions in their host country are methodologically challenging, they are of great relevance to theoretical debates on the social determinants of health, particularly in the context of the political upheavals in many parts of the world and the ensuing refugees' crises.

REFERENCES

Alba, R., and R. Silberman (2002), 'Decolonization immigrations and the social origins of the second generation: the case of North Africans in France', *International Migration Review*, **36** (4), 1169–93.

Amad, A., D. Guardia, J. Salleron, P. Thomas, J.-L. Roelandt and G. Vaiva (2013), 'Increased prevalence of psychotic disorders among third-generation migrants: results from the French Mental Health in General Population Survey', *Schizophrenia Research*, **147** (1), 193–5.

Arnold, M., Razum, O. and J.-W. Coebergh (2010), 'Cancer risk diversity in non-western migrants to Europe: an overview of the literature', *European Journal of Cancer*, **46** (14), 2647–59.

Attias-Donfut, C. and P. Tessier (2005), 'Santé et vieillissement des immigrés' ('Health and ageing of immigrants'), *Retraite et société*, **46** (3), 90–129.

Beauchemin, C., C. Borrel and C. Régnard (2013), 'Les immigrés en France: en majorité des femmes', *Population & Sociétés*, **502** (July–August), 1–4.

Berchet, C. (2013), 'Le recours aux soins en France: une analyse des mécanismes qui génèrent les inégalités de recours aux soins liées à l'immigration' ('Health care utilisation in France: An analysis of the main drivers of health care use inequalities related to migration'), *Revue d'épidémiologie et de santé publique*, **61** (supplement 2), S69–S79.

Berchet, C. and F. Jusot (2009), 'Inégalités de santé liées à l'immigration et capital social: une analyse en décomposition' ('Health inequalities related to immigration and social capital: a decomposition analysis'), *Economie Publique*, **24–5** (1–2), 73–100.

Berchet, C. and F. Jusot (2010), 'L'état de santé des migrants de première et de seconde génération en France' ('Health status of first- and second-generation migrants in France'), *Revue Economique*, **61** (6), 1075–98.

Berchet, C. and F. Jusot (2012), 'Etat de santé et recours aux soins des immigrés en France: une revue de la littérature' ('Health status and health care use of immigrants in France: a literature review'), *Bulletin épidémiologique hebdomadaire*, **172**, 17 January (BEH No. 2–3–4) 17–21.

Bhopal, R.S. (2007), 'Racism in health and health care in Europe: reality or mirage?', *European Journal of Public Health*, **17** (3), 238–41.

Bhopal, R.S., S.B. Rafnsson, C. Agyemang, A. Fagot-Campagna, S. Gianpaoli, N. Hammar et al. (2011), 'Mortality from circulatory diseases by specific country of birth across six European countries: a test of concept', *European Journal of Public Health*, **22** (3), 353–9, doi:http://dx.doi.org/10.1093/eurpub/ckr062.

Boisguerin, B. and B. Haury (2008), 'Les bénéficiares de l'AME au contact avec le système de soins' ('Beneficiaries of state medical aid in contact with the health care system'), *Etudes et Résultats*, **645** (July), 1–8.

Bouchardy, C. (1993), 'France', in M. Geddes, D.M. Parkin, M. Khlat, D. Balzi and E. Buiatti (eds), *Cancer in Italian Migrant Populations*, Lyon: IARC, pp. 149–59.

Bouchardy, C., M. Khlat and D.M. Parkin (1992), 'Mortalité par cancer chez les immigrés du Maghreb, d'Afrique Noire et d'Asie du Sud-Est en France: quelques résultats préliminaires' ('Cancer mortality among migrants from Maghreb, sub-saharan Africa and south-east Asia in France: some preliminary results'), *Bulletin du Cancer*, **6** (September), 90–94.

Bouchardy, C., M. Khlat, P. Wanner and M. Parkin (1998), 'Mortalité par cancer des migrants en France, 1979–1985' ('Cancer mortality among migrants in France, 1979–1985'), Centre International de Recherche sur le Cancer, Lyon.

Bouchardy, C., D.M. Parkin and M. Khlat (1994), 'Cancer mortality among Chinese and Southeast Asian migrants in France', *International Journal of Cancer*, **58** (5), 638–43.

Bouchardy, C., D.M. Parkin, P. Wanner and M. Khlat (1996), 'Cancer mortality among North African migrants in France', *International Journal of Epidemiology*, **25** (1), 5–13.

Bouchardy, C., P. Wanner and D. Parkin (1995), 'Cancer mortality among sub-Saharan African migrants in France', *Cancer Causes and Control*, **6** (6), 539–44.

Boulogne, R., E. Jougla, Y. Breem, A. Kunst and G. Rey (2012), 'Mortality differences between the foreign-born and locally born population in France (2004–2007)', *Social Science and Medicine*, **74** (8), 1213–23.

Bouvier-Colle, M.-H., J.B. Magescas and F. Hatton (1985), 'Causes de décès et jeunes étrangers en France' ('Causes of death of young foreigners in France'), *Revue d'Epidémiologie et de Santé Publique*, **33** (6), 409–16.

Brahimi, M. (1980), 'La mortalité des étrangers en France' ('Mortality of foreigners in France'), *Population*, **35** (3), 603–22.

Breuil-Genier, P., C. Borrel and B. Lhommeau (2011), 'Les immigrés, les descendants d'immigrés et leurs enfants' ('Immigrants, descendants of immigrants and their children'), in INSEE (ed.), *France, portrait social*, Paris: INSEE, pp. 33–9.

Che, D. and D. Antoine (2009), 'Immigrants et tuberculose: données épidémiologiques récentes' ('Immigrants and tuberculosis: recent epidemiological data'), *Médecine et maladies infectieuses*, **39** (3), 187–90.

Cognet, M., C. Hamel and M. Moisy (2012), 'Santé des migrants en France: l'effet des discriminations liées à l'origine et au sexe' ('Health of migrants in France: effect of discriminations related to origin and to gender'), *Revue Européenne des Migrations Internationales*, **28** (2), 11–34.

Courbage, Y. and M. Khlat (1996), 'Mortality and causes of death of Moroccans in France, 1979–91', *Population*, **8**, 59–94.

Darmon, N. and M. Khlat (2001), 'An overview of the health status of migrants in France in relation to their dietary practices', *Public Health Nutrition*, **4** (2), 163–72.

De Maio, F. (2010), 'Immigration as pathogenic: a systematic review of the health of immigrants to Canada', *International Journal for Equity in Health*, **9** (1), 27.

Desgrées-du-Loû, A., J. Pannetier, A. Ravalihasy, A. Gosselin, V. Supervie, H. Panjo et al. (2015), 'Sub-Saharan African migrants living with HIV acquired after migration, France, ANRS Parcours Study, 2012 to 2013', *Euro Surveillance*, **20** (46), pii=30065, doi:http://dx.doi.org/10.2807/1560-7917.ES.2015.20.46.30065.

Desgrées-du-Loû, A., J. Pannetier, A. Ravalihasy, M. Le Guen, A. Gosselin, H. Panjo et al. (2016), 'Is hardship during migration a determinant of HIV infection? Results from the ANRS PARCOURS study of sub-Saharan African migrants in France', *AIDS*, **30** (4), 645–56.

Dinh, Q. (1998), 'Les inégalités sociales de mortalité s'estompent' ('Social inequalities in mortality are shrinking'), *Economie et Statistique*, **314** (June), 89–106.

Fosse, S. and A. Fagot-Campagna (2012), 'Prévalence du diabète, état de santé et recours aux soins des personnes diabétiques originaires d'un pays du Maghreb et résidant en France métropolitaine' ('Prevalence of diabetes, health status and health care seeking of diabetic persons from Maghreb countries residing in metropolitan France'), *Bulletin épidémiologique hebdomadaire*, 17 January (BEH no. 2–3–4), 35–6.

Gotsens, M., D. Malmusi, N. Villaroel, C. Vives-Cases, I. Garcia-Subirats, C. Hernando and C. Borrell (2015), 'Health inequality between immigrants and natives in Spain: the loss of the healthy immigrant effect in times of economic crisis', *European Journal of Public Health*, **25** (6), 923–9.

Grillo, F., M. Soler and P. Chauvin (2012), 'L'absence de dépistage du cancer du col de l'utérus en fonction des caractéristiques migratoires chez les femmes de l'agglomération parisienne en 2010' ('Absence of cervical cancer screening for women in Paris metropolitan area according to their migration characteristics in 2010'), *Bulletin épidémiologique hebdomadaire*, 17 January (BEH no. 2–3–4), 45–7.

Hamel, C. and M. Moisy (2012), 'Migrations, conditions de vie et santé en France à partir de l'enquête Trajectoires et origines, 2008' ('Migrations, life conditions and health in France based on the Trajectories and Origins Survey in 2008'), *Bulletin épidémiologique hebdomadaire*, 17 January (BEH no. 2–3–4), 21–4.

Hamel, C. and M. Moisy (2015), 'Migration et conditions de vie: leur impact sur la santé' ('Migration and life conditions: their impact on health'), in C. Beauchemin, C. Hamel and P. Simon (eds), *Trajectoires et origines*, Paris, INED, pp. 263–87.

Ikram, U., J. Mackenbach, S. Harding, G. Rey, R.S. Bhopal, E. Regidor et al. (2015a), 'All-cause and cause-specific mortality of different migrant populations in Europe', *European Journal of Epidemiology*, **31** (7), 655–65, doi:10.1007/s10654-015-0083-9.

Ikram, U., D. Malmusi, K. Juel, G. Regy and A. Kunst (2015b), 'Association between integration policies and immigrants' mortality: an explorative study across three European countries', *PLOS ONE*, **10** (6), e0129916, doi:10.1371/journal.pone.0129916.

Jusot, F., J. Silva, P. Dourgnon and C. Sermet (2009), 'Inégalités de santé liées à l'immigration en France' ('Health inequalities related to immigration in France'), *Revue Economique*, **60** (2), 385–411.

Khlat, M. (1995), 'Cancer in Mediterranean migrants – based on studies in France and Australia', *Cancer Causes and Control*, **6** (6), 525–31.

Khlat, M. and N. Darmon (2003), 'Is there a Mediterranean migrants mortality paradox in Europe?', *International Journal of Epidemiology*, **32** (6), 1115–18.
Khlat, M., C. Sermet and D. Laurier (1998), 'La morbidité dans les ménages originaires du Maghreb – sur la base de l'enquête santé de l'INSEE, 1991–92' ('Morbidity in households originating from the Maghreb – based on the INSEE health survey, 1991–92'), *Population*, **53** (6), 1155–84.
Lert, F., M. Melchior and I. Ville (2007), 'Functional limitations and overweight among migrants in the Histoire de Vie study', *Revue d'Epidémiologie et de Santé Publique*, **55** (6), 391–400.
Llacer, A., M.V. Zunzunegui, J. del Amo, L. Mazarrasa and F. Bolumar (2007), 'The contribution of a gender perspective to the understanding of migrants' health', *Journal of Epidemiology and Community Health*, **61** (supplement 2), 4–10.
Lot, F., D. Antoine, C. Pioche, C. Larsen, D. Che, F. Cazein et al. (2012), 'Trois pathologies infectieuses fréquemment rencontrées chez les migrants en France: le VIH, la tuberculose et l'hépatite B' ('Three frequent infectious diseases in migrants in France: HIV infection, tuberculosis and hepatitis B'), *Bulletin épidémiologique hebdomadaire*, 17 January (BEH no. 2–3–4), 25–30.
Malmusi, D. (2014), 'Immigrants' health and health inequality by type of integration policies in European countries', *European Journal of Public Health*, **25** (2), 293–9.
Melchior, M., A. Chollet, N. Glangeaud-Freudenthal, M.J. Saurel-Cubizolles, M.N. Dufourg, J. van der Waerden and A.L. Sutter-Dallay (2015), 'Tobacco and alcohol use in pregnancy in France: the role of migrant status in the nationally representative ELFE study', *Addictive Behaviors*, **51** (December), 65–71.
Mizrahi, A. and A. Mizrahi (2008), 'Morbidité et soins médicaux aux personnes nées à l'étranger' ('Morbidity and medical care provided to the foreign-born'), *Journal d'Economie Médicale*, **26** (3), 159–76.
Moullan, Y. and F. Jusot (2014), 'Why is the "healthy immigrant effect" different between European countries?', *European Journal of Public Health*, **24** (supplement 1), 80–86.
Noiriel, G. (1988), *Le creuset français, histoire de l'immigration (19ème, 20ème siècle) (The French Melting-pot, History of Immigration (19th Century, 20th Century))*, Paris: Le Seuil.
Parkin, D.M. and M. Khlat (1996), 'Studies of cancer in migrants: rationale and methodology', *European Journal of Cancer*, **32A** (5), 761–71.
Rafnsson, S.B., R.S. Bhopal, C. Agyemang, A. Fagot-Campagna, S. Harding, N. Hammar et al. (2013), 'Sizeable variations in circulatory disease mortality by region and country of birth in six European countries', *European Journal of Public Health*, **23** (4), 594–605.
Razum, O. and J. Spallek (2014), 'Addressing health-related interventions to immigrants: migrant-specific or diversity sensitive?', *International Journal of Public Health*, **59** (6), 893–5.
Rondet, C., A. Lapostolle, M. Soler, F. Grillo, I. Parizot and P. Chauvin (2014), 'Are immigrants and nationals born to immigrants at higher risk for delayed or no lifetime breast and cervical cancer screening? The results from a population-based survey in Paris metropolitan area in 2010', *PLOS ONE*, **9** (1), e87046.
Saurel-Cubizolles, M.-J., M. Saucedo, N. Drewniak, B. Blondel and M.-H. Bouvier-Colle (2012), 'Santé périnatale des femmes étrangères en France' ('Perinatal health of foreign-born women in France'), *Bulletin épidémiologique hebdomadaire*, 17 January (BEH no. 2–3–4), 30–34.
Savignoni, A., F. Lot, J. Pillonel and A. Laporte (1999), 'Situation du Sida dans

la population étrangère domiciliée en France depuis le début de l'épidémie jusqu'en juin 1998' ('The AIDS situation in the foreign-born population resident in France, from the onset of the epidemics until June 1998'), *Bulletin épidémiologique hebdomadaire*, **27**, 113–14.

Solé-Auro, A. and E.M. Crimmins (2008), 'Health of immigrants in European countries', *International Migration Review*, **42** (4), 861–76.

Spallek, J., M. Arnold, O. Razum, K. Juel, G. Rey, P. Deboosere et al. (2012), 'Cancer mortality patterns among Turkish immigrants in four European countries and in Turkey', *European Journal of Epidemiology*, **27** (12), 915–21.

Spallek, J., H. Zeeb and O. Razum (2011), 'What do we have to know from migrants' past exposures to understand their health status? A life course approach', *Emerging Themes in Epidemiology*, **8** (1), 6, doi:10.1186/1742-7622-8-6.

Stirbu, I., A. Kunst, V. Bos and J. Mackenbach (2006), 'Differences in avoidable mortality between migrants and the native Dutch in The Netherlands', *BMC Public Health*, **6** (1), 78, doi:10.1186/1471-2458-6-78.

Therborn, G. (1987), 'Migration and Western Europe: the Old World turning new', *Science*, **237** (4819), 1183–8.

Vaillant, N. and F.C. Wolff (2010), 'Origin differences in self-reported health among older migrants living in France', *Public Health*, **124** (2), 90–98.

Vandenheede, H., P. Deboosere, I. Stirbu, C. Agyemang, S. Harding, K. Juel et al. (2012), 'Migrant mortality from diabetes mellitus across Europe: the importance of socio-economic change', *European Journal of Epidemiology*, **27** (2), 109–17, doi:10.1007/s10654-011-9638-6.

Vandenheede, H., D. Willaert, H. De Grande, S. Simoens and C. Vanroelen (2015), 'Mortality in adult immigrants in the 2000s in Belgium: a test of the "healthy-migrant" and the "migration-as-rapid-health-transition" hypotheses', *Tropical Medicine and International Health*, **20** (12), 1832–45.

Villalonga-Olives, E. and I. Kawachi (2014), 'The changing health status of economic migrants to the European Union in the aftermath of the economic crisis', *Journal of Epidemiology and Community Health*, **68** (9), 801–3.

Wallace, M. and H. Kulu (2015), 'Mortality among immigrants in England and Wales by major causes of death, 1971–2012: a longitudinal analysis of register-based data', *Social Science & Medicine*, **147** (December), 209–21.

Wanner, P., C. Bouchardy and M. Khlat (1997), 'Causes de décès des immigrés en France, 1979–1985' ('Causes of death of immigrants in France, 1979–1985'), *Migrations-Santé*, **91** (4), 9–38.

Wanner, P., C. Bouchardy and D.M. Parkin (1995a), 'La mortalité par cancer chez les migrants suisses en France' ('Cancer mortality among Swiss migrants in France'), *Revue d'Epidémiologie et de Santé Publique*, **43** (1), 26–36.

Wanner, P., M. Khlat, and C. Bouchardy (1995b), 'Habitudes de vie et comportements en matière de santé des immigrés méditerranéens en France – Enquête Conditions de Vie, 1987' ('Life habits and health-related behaviours among Mediterranean migrants in France – Survey on Life Conditions 1987'), *Revue d'épidémiologie et de santé publique*, **43**, 548–59.

Weil, P. (2005), *La France et ses étrangers* (*France and Its Foreigners*) Paris: Gallimard.

Wihtol de Wenden, C. (2012), 'Tendances récentes des migrations en France' ('Recent trends in migration to France'), *Bulletin épidémiologique hebdomadaire*, 17 January (BEH no. 2–3–4), 15.

12. Mortality and morbidity patterns among immigrants residing in Germany

Patrick Brzoska and Oliver Razum

INTRODUCTION

One-fifth of the population residing in Germany are individuals with a so-called 'migration background' (16.4 million out of 80.9 million persons). This term has been coined by the Federal Statistical Office of Germany (Statistisches Bundesamt) and comprises all individuals 'who have immigrated into the territory of today's Federal Republic of Germany after 1949, and . . . all foreigners born in Germany and all persons born in Germany who have at least one parent who immigrated into the country or was born as a foreigner in Germany' (Statistisches Bundesamt, 2013, para. 3). People with a migration background thus either immigrated themselves from another country or are direct descendants of immigrants. (For better legibility, we will nevertheless use the term 'immigrants' for all persons with a migrant background in this chapter.) While 56 percent of immigrants in Germany have German citizenship, 44 percent are non-German nationals. With each about 3 million, Turkish immigrants and ethnic German 'resettlers' (return migrants from Eastern European countries) are the largest immigrant groups residing in the country (Table 12.1).

Many immigrants in Germany were originally recruited as labor migrants *(Gastarbeiter)* by the government during the 1950s, 1960s and early 1970s in a time of economic growth and labor shortage. Many of them decided to stay in the country and brought their families. Labor migration today again plays an increasingly important role following the Eastern enlargement of the European Union in the beginning of the twenty-first century and the free movement of people (including those seeking jobs) as one of its fundamental principles. Ethnic German resettlers *(Aussiedler* and *Spätaussiedler)*, predominantly from the former Soviet Union and Poland, return-migrated to Germany in large numbers since the late

Table 12.1 Population in Germany by migration background

Groups	Number (million)	Proportion of total population (%)
People without migration background ('non-immigrants')	64.5	79.7
People with a migration background ('immigrants')	16.4	20.3
Sub-populations (type of migration background):		
Turkish	2.9	3.6
Former Soviet Union	2.9	3.6
Polish	1.6	2.0
Former Yugoslavian	1.5	1.9
Italian	0.8	1.0
South and Southeast Asian	0.8	1.0

Source: Statistisches Bundesamt (2015b).

1980s following the collapse of the Soviet Union. Finally, Germany has always been a destination for refugees and asylum seekers who flee war, violence, extreme poverty and natural disasters, many of whom try to start a new life in Germany (Bommes, 2014). In 2015, with civil wars or strife in countries such as Syria, over a million people seeking refuge arrived in Germany.

Immigrants differ from non-immigrants in many aspects of their health, comprising differences in the prevalence and incidence of diseases as well as in mortality patterns. These differences result from positive and negative factors immigrants are exposed to throughout their lives. We give an overview of data on the social and health situation of immigrants in Germany, and describe limitations of existing evidence. We further illustrate that aside from a lower socioeconomic status, immigrants also encounter barriers in health care that limit their access to health services and that may also affect health care quality and outcomes.

LIFE-COURSE EXPOSURES AND SOCIAL SITUATION OF IMMIGRANTS

Immigrants are exposed to different positive and negative factors throughout their lifetimes which influence their mortality and morbidity (Razum and Twardella, 2002). This comprises exposures in the host country and – in case they immigrated themselves – factors they were exposed to in the country of origin as well as during the migratory process (Spallek et al., 2011).

Directly upon arrival, immigrants tend to have a better health status than the majority population of the host countries they immigrate to. This can be explained by the 'healthy migrant effect'; since migration is a potentially risky and often a lengthy process, those that decide to leave their home countries are predominantly young and healthy and are better able to handle the stress of migration. This implies a health advantage over the population of the country of origin, and often also over the population of the host country. Immigrants from lower-income countries, in addition, are at a lower risk for certain chronic conditions such as cancer and cardiovascular disease, corresponding to the population of the countries they originate from. Many immigrants can also benefit from solid and reliable social and family networks. The risk of infectious diseases, additionally, quickly decreases to the respective levels of the host country as a result of better hygiene and medical treatment resulting in a further health benefit. Over the time that immigrants spend in the host country, they adapt to the lifestyle of the majority population. As a result, their risk of chronic diseases increases. In combination with a partially higher prevalence of genetic predispositions for type-II diabetes and stroke, their health may deteriorate over time and may result in a higher disease burden despite initial health benefits (Razum and Twardella, 2002; Razum 2009; Kohls 2010).

Aside from adopting an unfavorable lifestyle, such as a higher smoking prevalence among men, some immigrant groups in Germany are exposed to negative social determinants which contribute to health disparities. One of these is an, on average, lower socioeconomic status. This shows, for example, in a higher proportion of unskilled blue-collar workers as well as in a lower net equivalized income among immigrants as compared to non-immigrants (Statistisches Bundesamt, 2015b). Since immigrants more often work in the production industry, they are also more frequently exposed to negative physical, mental and social factors at work (Oldenburg et al., 2010). Many immigrants also have a low proficiency in the German language (Haug, 2008) as well as a low health literacy (Horn et al., 2015), both of which can make it difficult to use health information according to their needs and preferences. In addition, some immigrants experience discrimination which may have negative health consequences (Salentin, 2008; Williams and Mohammed, 2013; Schunck et al., 2015).

Immigrants, on average, are younger than non-immigrants, which also applies to the sub-population of non-Germans (Figure 12.1). As this population ages demographically, its risk for age-associated diseases

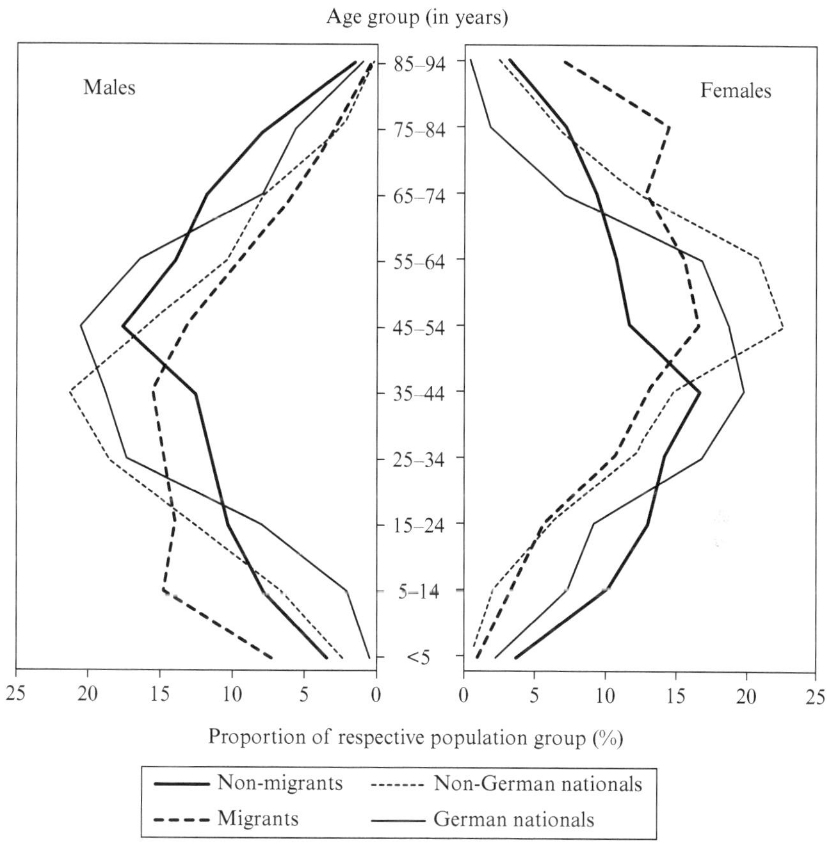

Source: Statistisches Bundesamt (2015b).

Figure 12.1 Age structure of males and females in Germany by migration status and nationality

increases steadily, as does the absolute number of individuals suffering from chronic diseases. The same is true for the number of immigrants who need health care services because of such conditions. This will further increase challenges facing the health care system with respect to the provision of services meeting the needs of its increasingly diverse clients. As outlined in this chapter, currently, many health care providers do not sufficiently cater to the needs of immigrants. This affects the access to and the quality of health services for this population group.

EMPIRICAL DATA ON THE HEALTH OF IMMIGRANTS

Data on the health of immigrants in Germany is limited. Only a few health surveys, such as the German Health Interview and Examination Survey for Children and Adolescents (KiGGS), enable us to also identify immigrants with German citizenship. Routine data of social security organizations and official statistics only allow to stratify by nationality (Razum et al., 2008; Brzoska et al., 2012). Since information such as the birthplace of parents and individuals' first language spoken is not collected, immigrants with a German citizenship usually cannot be identified in these data sources (Schenk et al., 2006; Brzoska et al., 2012). Occasionally, methods such as name-based algorithms can be applied to identify certain groups of immigrants, for example, immigrants of Turkish descent (Razum et al., 2000, 2001). Available findings, therefore, have to be interpreted with caution and are not necessarily representative for the entire population of immigrants residing in Germany.

Mortality

Analyses of mortality data show a multifaceted and partially contradicting picture. Official causes of death statistics reveal that at younger ages, the all-cause mortality among non-Germans is higher than among German nationals. The mortality ratio is up to 2.0 for females in the age group of 5 to under 10 years. Starting with the age group of 10 to below 15 years, the pattern is reversed (Figure 12.2).

The higher mortality in younger ages is considered to result from congenital disorders, infectious diseases and a higher incidence of accidents (Kohls, 2011). Overall, the age-standardized mortality for non-German nationals is 22 percent lower than for German nationals (Statistisches Bundesamt, 2015a). An overall lower mortality has also been reported for the sub-groups of immigrants of Turkish and ethnic German descent (Razum et al., 1998b; Zeeb et al., 2002; Kyobutungi et al., 2006b). Such subgroup-specific analyses, however, cannot routinely be conducted as they require the collation of data from all individual federal states.

Despite being on a lower level, the mortality of non-Germans has remained almost stagnant over the years while a steep mortality decline among German nationals can be observed (the increase in mortality rates for non-Germans in 2011 is due to a downwards correction of the total number of non-Germans living in Germany based on the census conducted in the same year) (Figure 12.3) (Razum et al., 2008; Kohls, 2011). Thus a convergence occurs which, however, does not benefit the immigrant population.

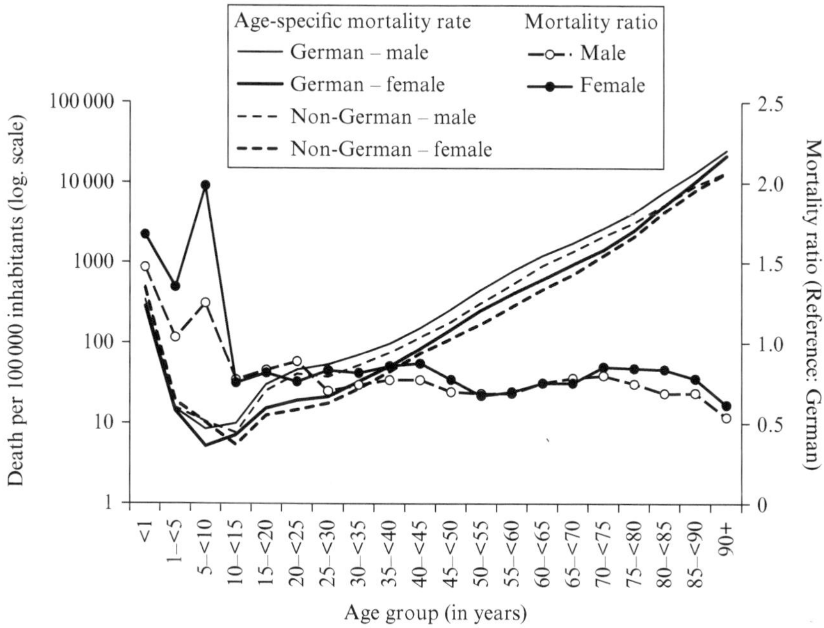

Sources: Official mortality statistics, Federal Statistical Office of Germany; Statistisches Bundesamt (2015a).

Figure 12.2 Age-specific mortality rates among Germans and non-Germans and respective mortality ratio, 2014, stratified by sex

The pattern of causes of death is broadly similar between German and non-German nationals. With respect to almost all ICD-10 diagnostic groups non-Germans have a lower overall mortality than Germans. Exceptions are perinatal conditions (P00–P96) and symptoms, signs and abnormal clinical and laboratory findings (R00–R99), where the mortality is higher for non-Germans than for Germans. Differentials in perinatal deaths are often interpreted as an indicator of social and health inequalities; whereas the coding of 'signs and symptoms' may reflect inaccuracies in the assignment of causes of death. In addition, a higher mortality from chronic hepatitis infection and HIV contributes to an overall higher mortality from infectious and parasitic diseases (A00–B99) among non-German women (Table 12.2).

The lower mortality of immigrants may result from a healthy migrant effect owing to self-selection as described above, that is, predominantly those who are fit and healthy consider immigrating into a new country. In the 1950s through to the 1970s, the immigration of healthy individuals was

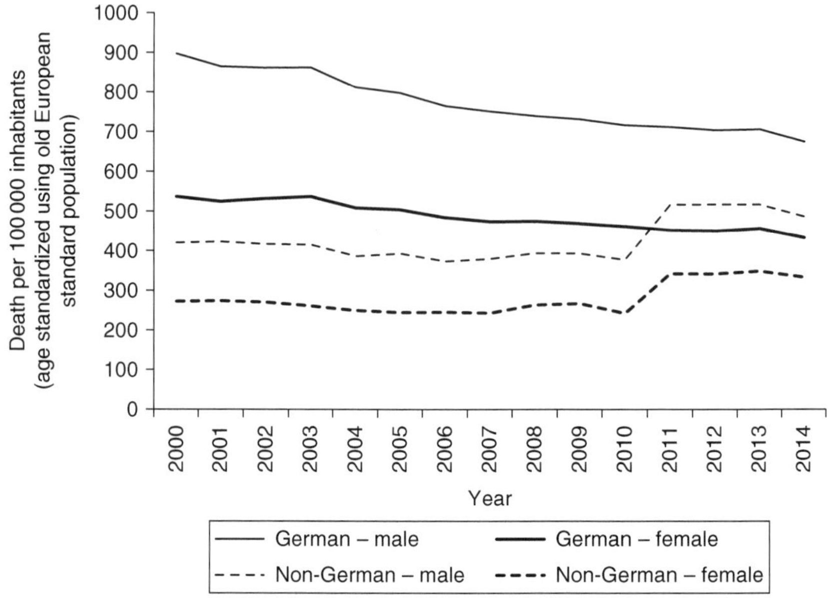

Sources: Official mortality statistics, Federal Statistical Office of Germany; Statistisches Bundesamt (1998–2015).

Figure 12.3 Age-standardized mortality rates among Germans and non-Germans, 2000–2014, stratified by sex

also fostered by the German government; only individuals who had passed health checks and thus were more likely to cope with physical strains at work were recruited as labor migrants (Miller, 2012). However, it also has to be considered that particularly older immigrants are highly transnational, that is, they spend several months a year in their country of origin. Those who die abroad (or move back to their country of origin for good without de-registering in Germany) are not registered by official mortality statistics in Germany. This may lead to an underestimation of the true number of deaths among non-Germans (Kohls, 2010). This underestimation is also indicated by routine data of the German Statutory Pension Insurance Scheme, which, in contrast to official statistics, shows that non-Germans aged 65 years or older have an up to 24 percent higher mortality than the German population, which is true for both men and women. Since the vital status of individuals is directly linked to pension benefits, data from the German Statutory Pension Insurance Scheme is considered to better reflect the true mortality of immigrants than official mortality statistics. However, it is limited by the fact that certain occupational groups such as

Table 12.2 Age-standardized mortality rates among Germans and non-Germans, 2014, stratified by sex and ICD-10 diagnostic group

ICD-10 diagnostic group		German		Non-German	
		Male	Female	Male	Female
A00–B99	Certain infectious and parasitic diseases	12.5	15.6	12.0	17.3
C00–D48	Neoplasms	194.5	199.3	150.6	151.8
D50–D90	Diseases of the blood and blood-forming organs and certain disorders involving the immune mechanism	1.8	2.8	1.3	2.1
E00–E90	Endocrine, nutritional and metabolic diseases	19.2	26.2	13.1	22.0
F00–F99	Mental and behavioral disorders	21.5	30.3	14.2	22.1
G00–H95	Diseases of the nervous system, eye, adnexa, ear, mastoid process	19.5	22.8	13.3	16.0
I00–I99	Diseases of the circulatory system	210.9	275.8	136.1	202.1
J00–J99	Diseases of the respiratory system	45.0	43.7	35.5	40.5
K00–K93	Diseases of the digestive system	33.3	31.8	21.6	21.4
L00–L99	Diseases of the skin and subcutaneous tissue	0.8	1.4	0.4	1.4
M00–M99	Diseases of the musculoskeletal system and connective tissue	1.8	3.5	0.9	2.9
N00–N99	Diseases of the genitourinary system	13.1	18.6	10.2	14.5
O00–O99	Pregnancy, childbirth and the puerperium	–	0.1	–	0.1
P00–P96	Certain conditions originating in the perinatal period	2.2	1.5	3.1	2.5
Q00–Q99	Congenital malformations, deformations and chromosomal abnormalities	2.3	2.1	2.3	2.0
R00–R99	Symptoms, signs and abnormal clinical and laboratory findings, not elsewhere classified	24.4	19.3	26.1	25.0
S00–T98	Injury, poisoning and certain other consequences of external causes	41.2	24	26	18.0
V01–Y98	External causes of morbidity and mortality	40.9	16.5	25.6	12.4

Sources: Official mortality statistics, Federal Statistical Office of Germany; Statistisches Bundesamt (2015a).

civil servants as well as those self-employed or unemployed are not covered by this insurance scheme (Kohls, 2015).

Cause-specific Mortality Data for Selected Immigrant Groups

Most official statistics and many registries in Germany differentiate only between German and non-German nationals. There are only a few studies that allow assessing cause-specific mortality among particular immigrant groups. One approach taken was to ask a state-level statistical office to collate mortality information by selected cause and nationality from all federal states into one dataset. Such analyses have been done in the late 1990s and early 2000s for Turkish nationals in Germany; besides total mortality, they investigated mortality from cardiovascular diseases and from suicide. Total mortality as well as mortality from CVD were considerably lower than in the German population (the analyses had to be restricted to age groups below 65 years owing to the lack of a reliable and appropriately stratified denominator population in the higher age groups; Razum et al., 1998a). The only exception was suicide in girls and young women. While suicide mortality was also lower among men below 65 years and among middle-aged women, Turkish girls and young women below age 18 years experienced a significantly higher suicide mortality than their German peers (relative risk RR = 1.8 [95%-CI = 1.4–2.3]) (Razum and Zeeb, 2004). This could be owing to intergenerational conflicts in families where the parents are more traditional than their daughters.

A second approach was to set up a cohort in order to assess mortality of resettlers mostly from the former Soviet Union. The cohort comprised n = 34393 resettlers who return-migrated to Germany from 1990 and were initially followed-up for up to 13 years (until 2002). The authors hypothesized that this group would experience a higher mortality in particular for cardiovascular diseases compared with the autochthonous German population, given the comparatively high mortality in many Eastern European countries and the stress of migrating. Furthermore, as whole communities migrated, a positive selection (healthy migrant effect) was not expected (Ronellenfitsch et al., 2006; Becher et al., 2007). However, standardized mortality ratios (SMRs) were significantly lower compared to autochthonous Germans for all causes of death (SMR for the whole cohort 0.85 [95%-CI = 0.81–0.89]). This mortality advantage was particularly pronounced for older resettlers but not for younger resettlers (SMR > 1). Duration of stay showed no clear effect on SMRs. In larger families, SMRs were significantly lower than in smaller families, indicating a possible positive role of social support on mortality. Regarding cardiovascular diseases, SMR for both sexes was 0.79 [95%-CI = 0.73–0.85] (Ronellenfitsch et al., 2006; Becher et al., 2007).

Total cancer mortality, as well as mortality from lung and breast cancer, was lower in resettler women than in autochthonous women (SMR 0.76 [95%-CI = 0.67–0.89], 0.61 [95%-CI = 0.34–1.01] and 0.47 [95%-CI = 0.29–0.70], respectively). Male resettlers experienced similar all-cancer mortality as autochthonous men (SMR 0.97 [95%-CI = 0.86–1.10]); a breakdown by cancer site showed higher mortality from lung and stomach cancers while mortality from prostate cancer was lower (SMR 0.48 [95%-CI = 0.25–0.84]) (Kyobutungi et al., 2006a).

Among male resettlers, mortality due to all external causes of death was 39 percent higher than among autochthonous men; for suicides, it was 30 percent higher. Among women, no major differences for these causes were found (Kyobutungi et al., 2006b; Becher et al., 2007).

Currently, a large 'national cohort' is being set up in Germany. In the long run, it may provide more detailed mortality data for immigrants and their descendants than is currently available. However, immigrants are not oversampled, and continuous efforts are required to ensure adequate participation of this group (Reiss et al., 2014).

Morbidity

Data on the morbidity of immigrants is available from surveys and from routine data of social security organizations. Evidence based on official statistics suggests that especially older non-Germans have a higher prevalence and incidence of certain communicable and non-communicable diseases than Germans of the same age (and there is little evidence to suggest that this could not be extended to immigrants). In terms of infectious diseases, the incidence of tuberculosis among non-Germans is 12 times as high as the respective incidence among Germans (Brodhun et al., 2014). Turkish immigrants have also been reported to have a higher prevalence of hepatitis B and *Helicobacter pylori* infections. *Helicobacter pylori* infection presumably also contributes to a higher incidence of gastritis and stomach cancer in this population group (Zeeb et al., 2002). The incidence of other types of cancer such as breast or skin cancer, however, is lower among immigrants than among the majority population (Spallek et al., 2009).

Surveys also reported a higher prevalence of certain chronic conditions such as diabetes mellitus type 2, chronic pain and mental disorders (Razum et al., 2008; Bermejo et al., 2010; Icks et al., 2011; Rommel et al., 2015; Schouler-Ocak et al., 2015).

As regards work-related morbidity, non-German nationals are at a higher risk of occupational accidents and diseases as well as of early retirement due to disability. Differences in disability-related retirement rates increase with age and are particularly pronounced between older German nationals and individuals of Turkish origin (Brzoska et al., 2013; Brzoska and Razum, 2015b).

Information on the health of children and adolescents is provided by the longitudinal KiGGS study. The baseline survey was conducted between 2003 and 2006 on 17 641 children and adolescents of which 17.1 percent were of immigrant descent. Similar to the health status of the adult immigrant population, the KiGGS survey reveals inconsistent differences in the health of immigrants below the age of 18 years compared with non-immigrants. Children and adolescents whose both parents are immigrants have a higher prevalence of overweight and obesity, which is particularly true for boys and girls of Turkish descent, for boys of Polish descent and girls of South European descent. This is attributed to an unfavorable diet mediated by culturally related body images among parents, who consider their children too thin even if they are of normal weight. Immigrant children and adolescents also have a higher prevalence of mental disorders and of anemia as well as a higher lifetime prevalence for measles infection. They also more frequently report injuries related to accidents. The prevalence for conditions such as scoliosis and atopic dermatitis and the lifetime prevalence for chickenpox and scarlet fever, in contrast, are significantly lower than among non-immigrant children. The health status of children who have only one parent of immigrant background is comparable to non-immigrant children with respect to most conditions (Robert Koch-Institut, 2008).

Little is known about the health of refugees and asylum seekers. Experience of violence and repression in the country of origin as well as difficult living conditions in the destination countries of refugees such as overcrowded shelters almost certainly affect their well-being (Hadgkiss and Renzaho, 2014; Schwienhorst and Stich, 2015). In spite of the recent influx of large numbers of refugees and asylum seekers, there is only insufficient data on their physical and mental health (Nicolai et al., 2015; Bozorgmehr et al., 2016; Razum et al., 2016). A small study conducted on the long-term consequences of war experiences among 50 refugees in Germany who fled the Balkan war in the early 1993 revealed that almost 80 percent have one or more psychiatric disorders, with post-traumatic stress disorders and depression being the most common conditions (von Lersner et al., 2008).

Utilization and Effectiveness of Health Care Services

In addition to risk factors that immigrants have been exposed to in their country of origin, an unfavorable lifestyle and a lower socioeconomic status, health disparities can be explained by inequities in terms of the utilization and effectiveness of health care services (Razum et al., 2008; Solé-Auró and Crimmins, 2008; Derose et al., 2009; Brzoska et al., 2010b). In many European countries, including Germany, immigrants have a higher utilization of general practitioners, but also of hospital and emergency outpatient ward care than the non-immigrant population (Norredam et al., 2009; Solé-Auró et al., 2012). The situation is different for preventive services, which immigrants utilize less frequently than non-immigrants (Keller and Baune, 2005; Zeeb et al., 2004). As outlined in the following, this also applies to tertiary preventive services such as rehabilitation, where, in addition, a lower effectiveness for immigrants as compared to non-immigrants has been observed. Rehabilitative services are of particular relevance for non-German nationals considering their overall higher burden of chronic disease and higher rates of work-related disability. As a measure of tertiary prevention, rehabilitation can mitigate the consequences of acute and chronic diseases and can restore a deteriorated health status (World Health Organization, 2011). In Germany immigrants with a residence status are entitled to use measures of prevention as well as health care services in general free of charge as part of their social insurance. The situation is different for refugees and asylum seekers, who currently are only allowed to utilize basic health care while staying in Germany (Bozorgmehr and Razum, 2015; Norredam et al., 2006).

Data from the German Socio-economic Panel (SOEP), a large-scale representative household survey and routine data from the German Statutory Pension Insurance Scheme show that non-German nationals utilize medical rehabilitation less often than Germans (crude odds ratio [OR] for utilization = 0.68; 95%-CI = 0.51–0.92). This observation cannot be explained by differences in the distribution of demographic, socioeconomic and health characteristics between both populations (adjusted OR for utilization = 0.66; 95%-CI = 0.49–0.90); Brzoska et al., 2010b). A further analysis, in which also immigrants with a German citizenship could be considered, led to similar findings (Voigtländer et al., 2013).

Routine data of the German Statutory Pension Insurance Scheme on about 275 000 individuals surveyed during 2007–11 shows that particularly Turkish nationals in Germany are less satisfied than Germans with different aspects of rehabilitative services. While only 58 percent of all Turkish patients are reported to be satisfied with the services they received in general, the respective proportion was 77 percent among German nationals. Similar differences were identified with regard to aspects such as nursing or medical care (Brzoska and Razum, 2015a) (Table 12.3). Differences are independent of socioeconomic and socio-demographic factors as multivariate analyses reveal (Brzoska et al., 2017).

Table 12.3 Proportion of individuals who are highly satisfied with their rehabilitative treatment, stratified by domains of rehabilitation and nationality

Domain of rehabilitation	Nationality			
	German	Turkish	Former Yugoslavian	Portuguese/ Spanish/ Italian/Greek
Medical care	68.3	62.6	69.8	70.3
Psychological care	73.8	68.3	80.0	79.2
Nursing care	81.9	75.0	83.5	83.4
Health education during rehabilitation	64.5	48.9	65.8	62.2
Treatments during the rehabilitation	76.0	58.8	71.0	68.7
Counseling during rehabilitation	60.0	47.7	57.4	57.1
Agreement on treatment goals	41.4	43.2	51.2	46.9
Overall satisfaction	76.7	57.9	69.6	69.6

Note: n = 274513.

Sources: Rehabilitation patient survey conducted by the German Statutory Pension Insurance Scheme (2007–11); Brzoska and Razum (2015a).

Those non-German nationals who do utilize rehabilitative services benefit less than their German counterparts, which becomes evident in a number of different outcomes. For example, while 54.2 percent of all Germans who underwent rehabilitation during 2007–11 reported an improvement of their health/performance after rehabilitation, the respective proportions were considerably lower for non-German nationals, being 28.1 percent for Turkish nationals, 34.5 percent for Former Yugoslavian nationals and 38.0 percent for nationals from Portugal, Spain, Italy or Greece. Just like the differences regarding utilization and satisfaction, the differential is independent of demographic and socioeconomic covariates. After controlling for these factors, Turkish and Former Yugoslavian nationals had a 62 percent and 68 percent higher chance, respectively, of an unfavorable perceived treatment outcome than Germans (adjusted OR = 1.62; 95%-CI = 1.45–1.80 and adjusted OR = 1.68; 95%-CI = 1.52–1.85, respectively). The respective chance among nationals from Portugal, Spain, Italy or Greece was 24 percent higher (adjusted OR = 1.24; 95%-CI = 1.12–1.37) (Brzoska et al., 2016). Similar differences were observed for other outcomes such as the occupational performance and the risk for disability

Table 12.4 Overview of findings on rehabilitative outcomes among Germans and non-German patients

	Outcome		
Nationality	Poor self-rated treatment outcome OR[a] (95%-CI)	Poor occupational performance OR[b] (95%-CI)	Disability retirement after rehabilitation HR[c] (95%-CI)
German (Reference)	1	1	1
Turkish	1.62 (1.45; 1.80)	1.23 (1.16; 1.30)	1.70 (1.49; 1.95)
Former Yugoslavian	1.68 (1.52; 1.85)	1.47 (1.38; 1.56)	1.41 (1.22; 1.64)
Portuguese/Spanish/Italian/ Greek	1.24 (1.12; 1.37)	1.06 (0.98; 1.14)	1.17 (0.97; 1.40)

Notes:
[a] Odds ratio adjusted for age, sex, marital status, educational level, occupational position, self-rated performance before rehabilitation, time absent from work before rehabilitation owing to illness, diagnosis, satisfaction with rehabilitation.
[b] Odds ratio adjusted for age, sex, marital status, occupational status, occupation, occupational position, time absent from work before rehabilitation owing to illness, diagnosis.
[c] Hazard ratio adjusted for age, sex, marital status, occupational status, occupation, occupational position, time absent from work before rehabilitation owing to illness, diagnosis, additional rehabilitative treatments received.

Sources: Brzoska et al. (2010b); Brzoska and Razum (2012); Brzoska et al. (2016).

retirement after rehabilitation (Brzoska et al., 2010b; Brzoska and Razum, 2012) (Table 12.4).

Barriers in Health Care

Immigrants in Germany experience several barriers in the health care system (Bermejo et al., 2012; Yilmaz-Aslan et al., 2014), which may also explain reduced utilization and effectiveness of medical rehabilitation among this population group. Qualitative investigations in rehabilitative care revealed that these barriers may arise from problems in communication with health care providers resulting from insufficient information about rehabilitative services, poor German language proficiency and poor health literacy. They interfere with an adequate provision of rehabilitative care by, for example, hindering health professionals from instructing patients about therapies and exercises. They may also reduce access to health care by making it difficult for patients to file an application for rehabilitation with their health insurance organization or to find institutions that suit their needs and expectations best. Aside from language-related communication problems, beliefs and expectations not sufficiently accounted for by health care providers may result in a reduced patient satisfaction and may limit the effectiveness of health care (Brzoska et al., 2010a, 2010b; Brzoska and Razum, 2015a). Interestingly, though, access barriers and differences in outcomes could not be found in pregnancy-related health services in Berlin, a city with a high proportion of immigrants. In a study enrolling 7100 consecutive deliveries in three Berlin hospitals, participation in antenatal care was only slightly (and to a clinically non-relevant degree) lower among Turkish immigrant women than among autochthonous women; their birth outcomes even tended to be better (David et al., 2014). There were similar findings for other indicators and for the whole subgroup of immigrant women (David et al., 2015). These findings suggest that barriers towards access to, and differences in outcome of, health services can be overcome when health services are willing to adapt to the needs and expectations of an increasingly heterogeneous population.

CONCLUSION

Immigrants constitute an increasing share of the population in Germany. In some aspects their health differs from that of the majority population. Whether immigrants have a higher or lower mortality than non-immigrants is difficult to generalize. Moreover, available evidence is contradictory and limited in several respects. In terms of morbidity, immigrants have a higher incidence of certain infectious diseases and a higher prevalence of some chronic conditions. Unfavorable social determinants as well as access barriers to, and a limited effectiveness of, health services contribute to this differential. Not all health care services sufficiently cater for the needs of immigrants and lack appropriate diversity awareness. As a consequence, this population group encounters substantial barriers in the health system. In order to improve their health status, these barriers need to be removed. This can be accomplished through the implementation of diversity-sensitive concepts of health care.

REFERENCES

Becher, H., O. Razum, C. Kyobutungi, J. Laki, J.J. Ott, U. Ronellenfitsch and V. Winkler (2007), 'Mortalität von Aussiedlern aus der ehemaligen Sowjetunion', *Deutsches Ärzteblatt*, **104** (23), 1655–61.

Bermejo, I., L.P. Hölzel, L. Kriston and M. Härter (2012), 'Subjektiv erlebte

Barrieren von Personen mit Migrationshintergrund bei der Inanspruchnahme von Gesundheitsmaßnahmen', *Bundesgesundheitsblatt – Gesundheitsforschung – Gesundheitsschutz*, **55** (8) 944–53.
Bermejo, I., E. Mayninger, L. Kriston and M. Härter (2010), 'Psychische Störungen bei Menschen mit Migrationshintergrund im Vergleich zur deutschen Allgemeinbevölkerung', *Psychiatrische Praxis*, **37** (5), 225–32.
Bommes, M. (2014), 'Migration and migration research in Germany', in E. Vesta and V. Vuddamalay (eds), *International Migration and the Social Sciences. Confronting National Experiences in Australia, France and Germany*, Basingstoke: Palgrave Macmillan, pp. 143–221.
Bozorgmehr, K. and O. Razum (2015), 'Effect of restricting access to health care on health expenditures among asylum-seekers and refugees: a quasi-experimental study in Germany, 1994–2013', *PLOS ONE*, **10** (7), e0131483, accessed 26 June 2017 at http://journals.plos.org/plosone/article?id=10.1371/journal.pone.0131483.
Bozorgmehr, K., S. Noest, H.M. Thaiss and O. Razum (2016), 'Die gesundheitliche Versorgungssituation von Asylsuchenden: bundesweite Bestandsaufnahme über die Gesundheitsämter', *Bundesgesundheitsblatt – Gesundheitsforschung – Gesundheitsschutz*, **59** (5), 545–55.
Brodhun, B., D. Altmann, B. Hauer, L. Fiebig and W. Haas (2014), *Bericht zur Epidemiologie der Tuberkulose in Deutschland für 2014*, Berlin: Robert Koch-Institut.
Brzoska, P. (2012), 'Die Nutzung von Routinedaten in der rehabilitationswissenschaftlichen Versorgungsforschung bei Menschen mit Migrationshintergrund: Möglichkeiten und Grenzen', *Gesundheitswesen*, **74** (6), 371–8.
Brzoska, P. and O. Razum (2012), 'Das Risiko einer Erwerbsminderung nach Abschluss der medizinischen Rehabilitation. Ein Vergleich von Rehabilitanden deutscher und ausländischer Staatsangehörigkeit im Längsschnitt', paper presented at the seventh anniversary of the German Society for Epidemiology, Regensburg, 26–29 September.
Brzoska, P. and O. Razum (2015a), 'Erreichbarkeit und Ergebnisqualität rehabilitativer Versorgung bei Menschen mit Migrationshintergrund', *Bundesgesundheitsblatt – Gesundheitsforschung – Gesundheitsschutz*, **58** (6), 553–9.
Brzoska, P. and O. Razum (2015b), 'Migration and occupational health: high work-related burden', *Public Health Forum*, **23** (2), 113–35.
Brzoska P., O. Sauzet, Y. Yilmaz-Aslan, T. Widera and O. Razum (2016), 'Self-rated treatment outcomes in medical rehabilitation among German and non-German nationals residing in Germany: cross-sectional study', *BMC Health Services Research*, **16** (March), 105, doi:10.1186/s12913-016-1348-z.
Brzoska, P., O. Sauzet, Y. Yilmaz-Aslan, T. Widera, and O. Razum (2017), 'Satisfaction with rehabilitative health care services among German and non-German nationals residing in Germany: a cross-sectional study', *BMJ Open*, http://dx.doi.org/10.1136/bmjopen-2016-015520.
Brzoska, P., S. Voigtländer, B. Reutin, Y. Yilmaz-Aslan, I. Barz, K. Starikow et al. (2010a), 'Rehabilitative Versorgung und gesundheitsbedingte Frühberentung von Personen mit Migrationshintergrund in Deutschland', Research Report 402, Bundesministerium für Arbeit und Soziales, Berlin.
Brzoska, P., S. Voigtländer, J. Spallek and O. Razum (2010b), 'Utilization and effectiveness of medical rehabilitation in foreign nationals residing in Germany', *European Journal of Epidemiology*, **25** (9), 651–60.
Brzoska, P., S. Voigtländer, J. Spallek and O. Razum (2012), 'Die Nutzung von

Routinedaten in der rehabilitationswissenschaftlichen Versorgungsforschung bei Menschen mit Migrationshintergrund: Möglichkeiten und Grenzen', *Gesundheitswesen*, **74** (6), 371–8.

Brzoska, P., S. Voigtländer, J. Spallek and O. Razum (2013), 'Arbeitsunfälle, Berufskrankheiten und Erwerbsminderung bei Menschen mit Migrationshintergrund', in T. Schott and O. Razum(eds), *Migration und gesundheitliche Ungleichheit in der Rehabilitation*, Weinheim: Beltz Juventa, pp. 49–61.

David, M., T. Borde, S. Brenne, W. Henrich, J. Breckenkamp and O. Razum (2015), 'Caesarean section frequency among immigrants, second- and third-generation women, and non-immigrants: prospective study in Berlin/Germany', *PLOS ONE*, **10** (5), e0127489.

David, M., T. Borde, S. Brenne, B. Ramsauer, W. Henrich, J. Breckenkamp and O. Razum (2014), 'Comparison of perinatal data of immigrant women of Turkish origin and German women – results of a prospective study in Berlin', *Geburtshilfe und Frauenheilkunde*, **74** (5), 441–8.

Derose, K.P., B.W. Bahney, N. Lurie and J.L. Escarce (2009), 'Review: immigrants and health care access, quality, and cost', *Medical Care Research and Review*, **66** (4) 355–408.

Hadgkiss, E.J. and A.M. Renzaho (2014), 'The physical health status, service utilisation and barriers to accessing care for asylum seekers residing in the community: a systematic review of the literature', *Australian Health Review*, **38** (2), 142–59.

Haug, S. (2008), 'Sprachliche Integration von Migranten in Deutschland', Working Paper 14, series integration report, part 2, Bundesamt für Migration und Flüchtlinge, Nuremburg.

Horn, A., D. Vogt, M. Messer and D. Schaeffer (2015), 'Health Literacy von Menschen mit Migrationshintergrund in der Patientenberatung stärken', *Bundesgesundheitsblatt – Gesundheitsforschung – Gesundheitsschutz*, **58** (6), 577–83.

Icks A., B. Kulzer and O. Razum (2011), 'Diabetes bei Migranten', in diabetesDE (ed.), *Deutscher Gesundheitsbericht Diabetes 2011*, Berlin: diabetesDE, pp. 48–154.

Keller, A. and B. Baune (2005), 'Impact of social factors on health status and help seeking behavior among migrants and Germans', *Journal of Public Health*, **13** (1), 22–9.

Kohls, M. (2010), 'Selection, social status or data artefact – what determines the mortality of migrants in Germany?', in T. Salzmann, B. Edmonston and J. Raymer (eds.), *Demographic Aspects of Migration*, Wiesbaden: VS Verlag, pp. 153–7.

Kohls, M. (2011), *Morbidität und Mortalität von Migranten in Deutschland*, Nuremberg: Bundesamt für Migration und Flüchtlinge.

Kohls, M. (2015), 'Sterberisiken von Migranten. Analysen zum Healthy-Migrant-Effekt nach dem Zensus 2011', *Bundesgesundheitsblatt – Gesundheitsforschung – Gesundheitsschutz*, **58** (6), 519–26.

Kyobutungi, C., U. Ronellenfitsch, O. Razum and H. Becher (2006a), 'Mortality from cancer among ethnic German immigrants from the former Soviet Union, in Germany', *European Journal of Cancer*, **42** (15), 2577–84.

Kyobutungi, C., U. Ronellenfitsch, O. Razum and H. Becher (2006b), 'Mortality from external causes among ethnic German immigrants from former Soviet Union countries, in Germany', *European Journal of Public Health*, **16** (4), 376–82.

Miller, J.A. (2012), 'On track for West Germany: Turkish "guest-worker" rail transportation to West Germany in the postwar period', *German History*, **30** (4), 550–73.
Nicolai, T., O. Fuchs and E. von Mutius (2015), 'Caring for the wave of refugees in Munich', *New England Journal of Medicine*, **373** (17), 1593–5.
Norredam, M., A. Mygind and A. Krasnik (2006), 'Access to health care for asylum seekers in the European Union – a comparative study of country policies', *European Journal of Public Health*, **16** (3), 285–9.
Norredam, M., S.S. Nielson and A. Krasnik (2009), 'Migrants' utilization of somatic healthcare services in Europe – a systematic review', *European Journal of Public Health*, **20** (5), 555–63.
Oldenburg, C., A. Siefer and B. Beermann (2010), 'Migration als Prädiktor für Belastung und Beanspruchung?', in B. Badura, H Schröder, J Klose, and K. Macco (eds), *Fehlzeiten-Report 2010*, Berlin: Springer, pp. 141–51.
Razum, O. (2009), 'Migration, Mortalität und der Healthy-migrant-Effekt', in M. Richter and K. Hurrelmann (eds), *Gesundheitliche Ungleichheit*, Wiesbaden: Verlag für Sozialwissenschaften, pp. 267–82.
Razum, O. and D. Twardella (2002), 'Time travel with Oliver Twist – towards an explanation for a paradoxically low mortality among recent immigrants', *Tropical Medicine and International Health*, **7** (1), 4–10.
Razum, O. and H. Zeeb (2004), English translation: 'Suicide mortality among Turks in Germany', *Der Nervenarzt*, **75** (11), 1092–8.
Razum, O., A. Bunte, A. Gillsdorf, T. Ziese and K. Bozorgmehr (2016), 'Gesundheitsversorgung von Geflüchteten: Zu gesicherten Daten kommen', *Deutsches Ärzteblatt*, **113** (4), A-130/B-111/C-111.
Razum, O., H. Zeeb and S. Akgün (2001), 'How useful is a name-based algorithm in health research among Turkish migrants in Germany?', *Tropical Medicine and International Health*, **6** (8), 654–61.
Razum, O., H. Zeeb and A. Gerhardus (1998a), 'Cardiovascular mortality of Turkish nationals residing in West Germany', *Annals of Epidemiology*, **8** (5), 334–41.
Razum, O., H. Zeeb, H.S. Akgün and S. Yilmaz (1998b), 'Low overall mortality of Turkish residents in Germany persists and extends into second generation: merely a healthy migrant effect?', *Tropical Medicine and International Health*, **3** (4), 297–303.
Razum, O., H. Zeeb, K. Beck, H. Becher, H. Ziegler and C. Stegmaier (2000), 'Combining a name algorithm with a capture-recapture method to retrieve cases of Turkish descent from a German population-based cancer registry', *European Journal of Cancer*, **36** (18), 2380–84.
Razum O., H. Zeeb, U. Meesmann, L. Schenk, M. Bredehorst, P. Brzoska et al. (2008), *Migration und Gesundheit*, Berlin: Robert Koch-Institut.
Reiss, K., N. Dragano, U. Ellert, J. Fricke, K.H. Greiser, T. Keil et al. (2014), 'Comparing sampling strategies to recruit migrants for an epidemiological study. Results from a German feasibility study', *European Journal of Public Health*, **24** (5), 721–6.
Robert Koch-Institut (2008), *Kinder- und Jugendgesundheitssurvey (KiGGS) 2003–2006: Kinder und Jugendliche mit Migrationshintergrund in Deutschland*, Berlin: Robert Koch-Institut.
Rommel, A., A.C. Saß, S. Born and U. Ellert (2015), 'Die gesundheitliche Lage von Menschen mit Migrationshintergrund und die Bedeutung des sozioökonomischen Status', *Bundesgesundheitsblatt – Gesundheitsforschung – Gesundheitsschutz*, **58** (6), 543–52.

Ronellenfitsch, U., C. Kyobutungi, H. Becher and O. Razum (2006), 'All-cause and cardiovascular mortality among ethnic German immigrants from the Former Soviet Union: a cohort study', *BMC Public Health*, **6** (1), 1.
Salentin, K. (2008), 'Diskriminierungserfahrungen ethnischer Minderheiten in der Bundesrepublik', in A. Groenemeyer and S Wieseler (eds), *Soziologie sozialer Probleme und sozialer Kontrolle: Realitäten, Repräsentationen und Politik*, Wiesbaden: VS Verlag für Sozialwissenschaften, pp. 515–26.
Schenk, L., A.M. Bau, T. Borde, J. Butler, T. Lampert, H. Neuhauser et al. (2006), 'Mindestindikatorensatz zur Erfassung des Migrationsstatus. Empfehlungen für die epidemiologische Praxis', *Bundesgesundheitsblatt-Gesundheitsforschung-Gesundheitsschutz*, **49** (9), 853–60.
Schouler-Ocak, M., M.C. Aichberger, S. Penka, U. Kluge and A. Heinz (2015), 'Psychische Störungen bei Menschen mit Migrationshintergrund in Deutschland', *Bundesgesundheitsblatt – Gesundheitsforschung – Gesundheitsschutz*, **58** (6), 527–32.
Schunck, R., K. Reiss and O. Razum (2015), 'Pathways between perceived discrimination and health among immigrants: evidence from a large national panel survey in Germany', *Ethnicity and Health*, **20** (5), 493–510.
Schwienhorst, E.M. and A. Stich (2015), 'Medizinische Versorgung von Flüchtlingen und Asylbewerbern. Erfahrungen aus dem Würzburger Modell', *Flugmedizin, Tropenmedizin, Reisemedizin*, **22** (3), 116–21.
Solé-Auró, A. and E.M. Crimmins (2008), 'Health of immigrants in European countries', *International Migration Review*, **42** (8), 861–76.
Solé-Auró, A., M. Guillén and E.M. Crimmins (2012), 'Health care usage among immigrants and native-born elderly populations in eleven European countries: results from SHARE', *European Journal of Health Economics*, **13** (6), 741–54.
Spallek, J., M. Arnold, S. Hentschel and O. Razum (2009), 'Cancer incidence rate ratios of Turkish immigrants in Hamburg, Germany: a registry based study', *Cancer Epidemiology*, **33** (6), 413–18.
Spallek, J., H. Zeeb and O. Razum (2011), 'What do we have to know from migrants' past exposures to understand their health status? A life course approach', *Emerging Themes in Epidemiology*, **8** (1), 6.
Statistisches Bundesamt (1998–2015), 'Todesursachenstatistik', series 12, line 4, Statistisches Bundesamt, Wiesbaden.
Statistisches Bundesamt (2013), 'Persons with a migration background', Statistisches Bundesamt, Wiesbaden.
Statistisches Bundesamt (2015a), 'Todesursachenstatistik', series 12, line 4, Statistisches Bundesamt, Wiesbaden.
Statistisches Bundesamt (2015b), 'Bevölkerung und Erwerbstätigkeit. Bevölkerung mit Migrationshintergrund, Ergebnisse des Mikrozensus 2014', series 1, line 2.2, Statistisches Bundesamt, Wiesbaden.
Voigtländer, S., P. Brzoska, J. Spallek, A. Exner and O. Razum (2013), 'Die Inanspruchnahme medizinischer Rehabilitation bei Menschen mit Migrationshintergrund, in T. Schott and O. Razum (eds), *Migration und gesundheitliche Ungleichheit in der Rehabilitation*, Weinheim: Beltz Juventa, pp. 92–104.
Von Lersner, U., H. Rieder and T. Elbert (2008), 'Psychische Gesundheit und Rückkehrvorstellungen am Beispiel von Flüchtlingen aus dem ehemaligen Jugoslawien', *Zeitschrift für Klinische Psychologie und Psychotherapie*, **37** (2), 112–21.

Williams, D.R. and S.A. Mohammed (2013), 'Racism and health I: Pathways and scientific evidence', *American Behavioral Scientist*, **57** (8), doi:0002764213487340.
World Health Organization (2011), *World Report on Disability*, Geneva: World Health Organization.
Yilmaz-Aslan, Y., P. Brzoska, M. Bluhm, A. Aslan and O. Razum (2014), 'Illness perceptions in Turkish migrants with diabetes: a qualitative study', *Chronic Illness*, **10** (2), 107–21.
Zeeb, H., B.T. Baune, W. Vollmer, D. Cremer and A. Krämer (2004), 'Gesundheitliche Lage und Gesundheitsversorgung von erwachsenen Migranten – ein Survey bei der Schuleingangsuntersuchung', *Gesundheitswesen*, **66** (2), 76–84.
Zeeb, H., O. Razum, M. Blettner and C. Stegmaier (2002), 'Transition in cancer patterns among Turks residing in Germany', *European Journal of Cancer*, **38** (5), 705–11

13. Migration, health and mortality in Italy: an unfinished story

Graziella Caselli, Silvia Loi and Salvatore Strozza

INTRODUCTION

Since the late 1970s Italy has become a country of immigration after being one of the main European countries of emigration for more than a century, with around 27 million expatriates and 11–13 million repatriates (Birindelli, 1989; Golini, 1997; Bonifazi, 2013). Today, foreign residents number more than 5 million, and if we also take non-residents into account we arrive at almost 6 million – around 10 percent of the population. They are almost all citizens of developing countries and from Central and Eastern Europe, with a significant presence of those that joined the European Union (EU) during the past decade. It should be underlined, however, that the foreign population, which has gradually increased over time, has reached a really important number only in the past decade. For this reason, we do not yet have very full information and knowledge on the health conditions and mortality levels of immigrants.

Before analyzing the health and mortality of foreigners, it would be useful to provide a general picture on immigration and the characteristics of the foreign population in Italy. The next section of this chapter describes the development of the phenomenon of migration. The subsequent section discusses the health conditions of the foreign population, using the results that have emerged from literature on hospitalizations and perinatal outcomes, accidents and work-related health problems, by elaborating the micro-data of an important survey carried out in 2009 on self-rated health, activity limitations and chronic morbidity. A comparison of mortality levels of Italians and foreigners is dealt with in the following section on the basis of data elaborated by the National Institute of Statistics (Istat). It considers adult mortality by gender and cause of death, as well as infant mortality, considering both the neonatal and post-neonatal period.

Where possible, we have sought to distinguish foreigners by macro-areas of citizenship, following the hypothesis that some observable differences concerning morbidity and mortality are partly the result of different life histories, social and cultural behaviors and working conditions that characterize the individuals of different nationalities.

In general, the empirical information available for Italy, which is cited in this work, makes it possible to discuss and consider some hypotheses that have emerged in the international literature (for example, healthy immigrant effect, salmon bias, and the possible convergence of health and mortality levels of foreigners and the national population).

FOREIGN IMMIGRATION AND PRESENCE IN ITALY: A BRIEF OVERVIEW

For a long time a country of emigration for its own citizens, in the late 1970s Italy became the destination for migrants from other countries, both those nearby (for example, Tunisia and Yugoslavia) and geographically distant (for example, Cape Verde, the Philippines, Horn of Africa). The arrivals increased in the 1980s, and new areas of origin emerged for the immigrants. Their presence was further extended in the country, with an increase in those authorized, following the first regularization[1] of more than 100000 foreigners from diverse regions encompassing Latin America, Asia and Eastern Europe (Strozza and Zucchetti, 2006). The importance of the irregular component is a typical aspect of the first phase of immigration in Italy, as in other Southern European countries.

Immigration and foreign presences grew markedly in the 1990s and even new areas of origin emerged. Immigrants came from Albania, Romania, Yugoslavia and other countries in Eastern Europe, as well as Somalia, Morocco, the Philippines and as far away as Peru. At the dawn of the new millennium (2000) there were around 1400 million foreigners with a regular residence permit (minors following their parents are not included in the calculation), while the irregular ones were estimated at around 200000 (Blangiardo and Tanturri, 2006).

The Extraordinary Immigration of the Past 15 Years

In the first decade of the new millennium, immigration took on absolutely exceptional and unforeseeable dimensions. As well as an increase of the flows that were already numerically large (particularly from Romania, Albania, Morocco and China), there were new, substantial migrations from some of the former Soviet republics (above all, Ukraine and Moldova), as well as from the Indian subcontinent and Ecuador. In the 2001 census, regular foreign residents numbered something like one and a half million, around 2.6 percent of the total population. Just ten years after, the 2011 census registered more than 4 million foreigners as resident in Italy, with a coverage error higher than 11 percent (Mazziotta, 2014). If we take into account those missed by the census, the total number of foreign residents must have been around 4.5 million, which was more than 7.5 percent of the total population. This is a truly exceptional increase, due mainly to a net immigration of almost 3 million persons in just ten years (Impicciatore and Strozza, 2015).

The face of immigration changed in the years of the most recent economic crisis, with fewer arrivals for labor reasons and family reunification becoming the main cause of regular immigration (Impicciatore and Strozza, 2015). In addition, there was also increasing immigration of refugees and asylum seekers. Following the Arab Spring in 2011, those saved at sea and brought into Italian territory numbered over 63 000 (more than 37 000 of whom were asylum seekers), coming mainly from Tunisia. The greatest humanitarian emergency was registered in 2014–15, with around 324 000 foreigners (mainly from Syria and Eritrea) saved from the sea and brought to ports in Sicily and other southern Italian regions, without counting the thousands of persons who did not survive and died in the Mediterranean (over 7000 according to the United Nations High Commissioner for Refugees).

The Foreign Population: A Kaleidoscope of Origins and Characteristics

Immigration was displaying an increasing trend until 2008 and, though less substantial and with different characteristics, remained significant in the years of the last economic crisis. It showed a real upswing in the resident foreign population, which moved from fewer than 500 000 persons in the early 1990s to over 5 million by 2015 (Figure 13.1). The figure is higher than 5.8 million if we also consider non-residents, who are in the country both in regular and irregular condition of stay. If we also include those who have acquired Italian citizenship and those born in Italy from mixed couples (who are Italian from birth), then we reach around 7 million persons of foreign origin, almost 12 percent of the total population (Strozza, 2015).

Among foreign residents, women are slightly more numerous than men (52 percent), and the structure by age appears still very young, markedly younger than the Italian population (Figure 13.2). In 2013 the average age of foreigners was no more than 32 years, 12 years less than the average for Italians. Among foreigners, the young (under 18) number more than 22 percent, while among Italians, they hardly reach 16 percent of the population. This situation is reversed with the old (65 and above) who account for

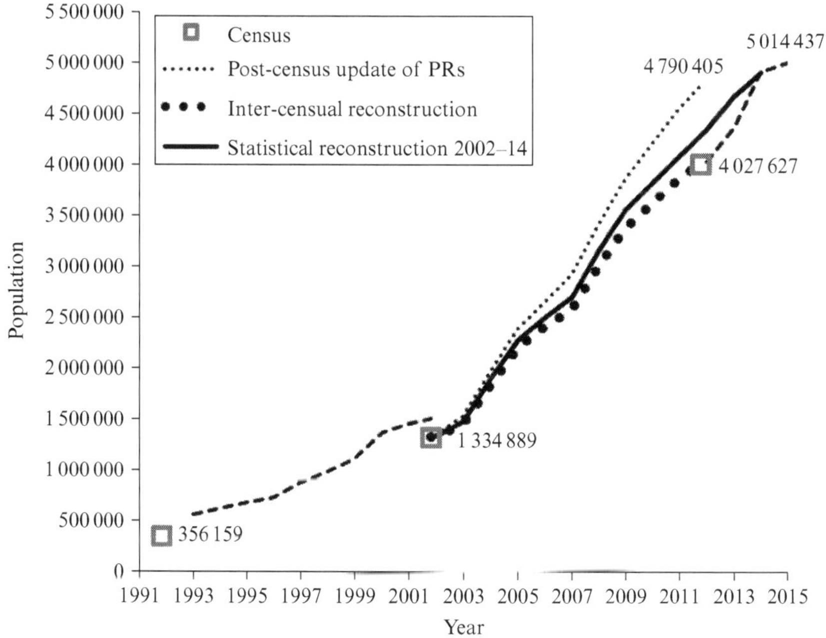

Note: PRs = Population Registers.

Source: Authors' elaboration on Istat data (Istat, 2015).

Figure 13.1 *Trends of foreign resident population according to available sources and elaborations: Italy, 1991–2015 (absolute values generally at the beginning of year)*

almost 23 percent of Italians, while among foreigners, they are less than 3 percent. Not only are the two structures by age notably different, but the low number of old foreigners makes it impossible to examine health conditions and survival in this important age group.

Although these are the average overall figures, it should be noted that the foreign population is much more complex and varied than in other host countries (Strozza, 2010; Peixoto et al., 2012). Romanians, Albanians and Moroccans form the most numerous national groups (respectively, near 23, just under 10 and 9 percent of the total of foreigners) in early 2015. The overwhelming majority of foreigners are from the so-called countries of strong migratory pressure (CSMP)[2] (96 percent), above all from Central and Eastern Europe (more than 49 percent), almost equally divided between those inside and outside the EU (respectively, 26.7 and

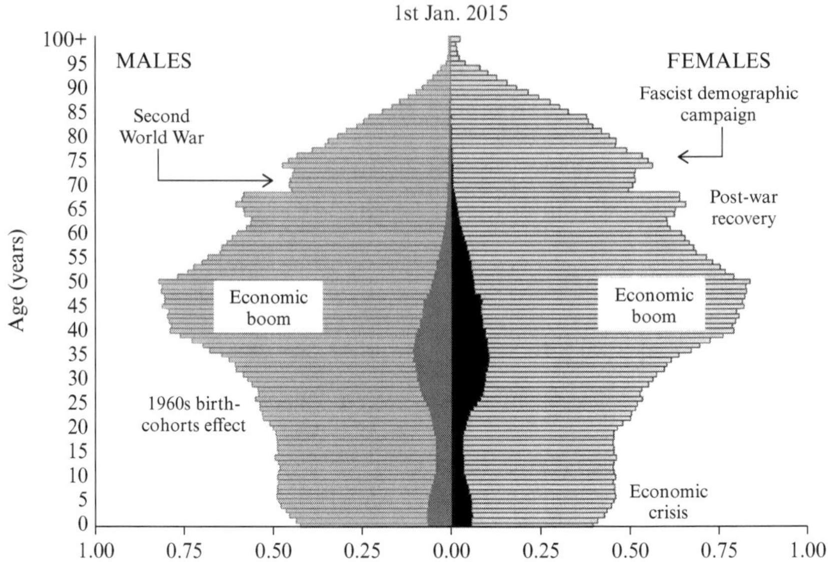

Note: The foreign population is highlighted in dark grey and black.

Source: Authors' elaboration on Istat data, accessed December 2015 at http://www.istat.it.

Figure 13.2 Age pyramid of resident population distinguished between nationals and foreigners: Italy, 1 January 2015 (percentage values)

22.5 percent). But there are also significant shares of Africans (less than 21 percent), Asians (more than 19 percent) and Latin-Americans (more than 7 percent). This wide range of nationalities often corresponds to different demographic, social and/or migratory characteristics, as well as settlement models, levels of assimilation and/or specific socio-economic behaviors (Rossi and Strozza, 2007; Strozza, 2015).

These are the aspects that impact on health conditions and survival. For example, we might note that there is still a strong imbalance in the gender structure of some of the more numerous nationalities: men are clearly in the majority among the Senegalese (women accounting for barely 27 percent), as well as in national groups of the Indian subcontinent and North Africa (Egypt and Tunisia in particular); while the reverse is true among the Ukrainians, Poles, Moldovans, Peruvians and Ecuadorians. Gender and country of origin are significantly associated with job opportunities for immigrants, to the point of determining an ethnicization of the labor market (Zanfrini, 2002).

According to the figures of the Italian labor force survey, there is a high level of segregation by sector of employment and a strong concentration of foreign individuals in the lower levels of the occupations (they make up a third of unskilled workers). Often they are workers in the so-called 3D jobs – dirty, dangerous and demanding (Abella et al., 1995) – a category that has been further extended in the Italian literature in its negative connotation with the expression '*lavori delle 5 P*' (*pesanti, pericolosi, precari, poco pagati* and *penalizzati socialmente* – 5P jobs, that is, heavy, dangerous, precarious, ill-paid and socially disadvantageous) (Ambrosini, 2005). Access to unqualified and semi-qualified manual work proved to be fairly easy for immigrants before the economic crisis, and a little less in recent years. Self-employment and non-manual jobs were and remain extremely difficult, with very little possibility of upward occupational mobility.

In summary, after almost 40 years of immigration, the foreign population today is composed of persons who have arrived recently for work or in search of protection, intending to stay only a short time in the country; immigrants who arrived some time ago and who have decided to remain permanently or for some years; their children, who either arrived with their parents, were reunited with them later, or were born in Italy, and who are about to enter or have already entered the school system, or who have finished their studies and are looking for or are already in employment (Dalla Zuanna et al., 2009; Strozza, 2009). As already mentioned, it is important to note that the new arrivals continue to be numerous, but fewer arrive for work and more for family reunification or for asylum. The second generation is growing, and the immigrants who arrived several decades ago are aging. If the foreign population consisted at first mainly of young adults, there are now more older adults than in the past, quite often close to retirement – although the old are still few – and, of course, the pre-school and school-age descendants of immigrants.

The different types of migration flows generate specific health needs, with a varying short-term impact on the national health system. The arrival of workers, most of them young, has a non-significant short-term impact on public health; family reunifications bring out needs connected with the reproductive health of women and the health of children; asylum seekers fleeing wars and persecution often require immediate psychological support, as well as immediate medical support for those in critical conditions after being saved from the sea.

These considerations suggest we examine the health conditions of immigrants, their use of the health services, as well as their mortality levels, in a comparative perspective. The study of the differences between Italians and foreigners that follows is inevitably incomplete, and no more than a first reading of a story that is still unfolding.

THE HEALTH OF IMMIGRANTS, USE OF AND ACCESS TO HEALTH SERVICES

In Italy, there is still little literature on the relation between migration and health. This lack of studies on the subject is due to migration being a very recent phenomenon in the country and the limited availability of useful data for studying migrants' health. Both at national and local level existing studies are extremely fragmentary, all of them analyzing cross-sectional data that do not allow us to observe and study the phenomenon in a longitudinal perspective. The limited availability of survey data has meant that administrative data have been mainly used, restricting the analyses to only some objective dimensions of health: hospitalization (Cacciani et al., 2006; Geraci et al., 2014) and perinatal outcomes (Cacciani et al., 2011). The studies carried out with the use of survey data concern accidents and work-related health problems (Rosano et al., 2012; Salvatore et al., 2013), and, more recently, activity limitations, chronic morbidity and self-rated health (Loi, 2016). In this connection, it is worth emphasizing that, since the dimensions of health under consideration are different and bring out different dimensions, by definition they are not comparable.

Hospitalizations, Reproductive Health and Perinatal Outcomes

Hospitalizations are a constant and reliable data source on objective health conditions. In Italy the national health system is universally guaranteed for a series of basic health services, even for irregular foreigners. This guarantee of universality contributes to the high use of hospital structures by foreigners, particularly irregular ones, who face obstacles to use other facilities.

Tables 13.1 and 13.2 show, respectively, the data on hospital discharges for hospitalization (H) and for day hospital (DH) of the foreign and Italian population from 2003 to 2011 (with the exception of 2010) (Geraci et al., 2014). As we can see from the two tables, the total number of foreign patients admitted, whether for H or DH, has increased over time. Observing the rates of hospitalization standardized by age, for all the population sub-groups and for both sexes, we can see a gradual reduction over time. Equally clear is the difference by gender: women account for higher rates than men. In addition, for the foreign population we observe lower rates compared with Italians for both sexes. However, in the case of women, the differences between foreigners and Italians are less marked. This can be explained by the greater recourse to hospitals by foreign women, particularly when hospital assistance is needed during pregnancy and at the moment of childbirth, or for the voluntary interruption of a pregnancy.

Table 13.1 Ordinary hospital discharges (absolute values, percentage values and standardized rates by age, per 1000), foreigners from CSMP and Italians by sex, 2003–09 and 2011

	Ordinary hospital discharges					
	Males			Females		
Year	Discharges CSMP	Std rate CSMP	Std rate Italians	Discharges CSMP	Std rate CSMP	Std rate Italians
2003	93069	122.7	154.3	152045	162.5	148.2
2004	98502	108.1	149.8	169062	145.6	146.1
2005	105278	101.5	146.3	189884	141.5	142.6
2006	114220	100.5	142.9	212942	141.4	141.1
2007	120192	94.3	137.0	227627	133.7	135.7
2008	126648	91.5	132.8	242862	126.6	132.9
2009	130340	86.9	129.8	255201	117.8	130.0
2011	132909	79.9	120.4	262619	101.1	124.3

Notes:
Values standardized with the direct method.
Standard population is the population resident in Italy, obtained from the 2001 Census (Geraci et al., 2014, p. 273).

Source: Geraci et al. (2014, p. 276).

This is also confirmed by the figures for hospitalizations by cause. In particular, we should note that hospitalizations for causes connected to reproductive health are the only ones to register higher rates for foreign women (Italian women often use the private sector). In particular, the figures published by Geraci and colleagues (2014, pp. 279–80) indicate a high rate of hospitalization for complications in pregnancy, childbirth and the puerperium (33.8 per thousand in H and 9.8 per thousand in DH for foreign women, and 26.9 per thousand in H and 4.9 per thousand in DH for Italians) and abortion-related disorders (8.4 per thousand in DH for foreign women and 3.3 per thousand for Italians).

Another very important objective dimension of health concerns perinatal health. A recent study on the subject had as its aim the analysis of the association between migrant status and adverse perinatal health outcomes in Lazio (Cacciani et al., 2011), the most populous region of Central Italy, which also contains the capital Rome. The figures on the hospital discharge database were analyzed in two different periods (1996–98 and 2006–08). Analysis of the indicators of perinatal health, including gestational age, Apgar score, neonatal respiratory disorders, need for special or intensive

Table 13.2 Hospital discharges after Day Hospital treatment (absolute values, percentage values and standardized rates by age, per 1000), foreigners from CSMP and Italians by sex, 2003–09 and 2011

	Hospital discharges after Day Hospital treatment					
	Males			Females		
Year	Discharges CSMP	Std rate CSMP	Std rate Italians	Dimissioni CSMP	Std rate CSMP	Std rate Italians
2003	25016	40.9	61.1	61253	62.4	64.5
2004	29781	43.5	64.5	72608	63.1	68.2
2005	33321	37.7	66.1	80408	57.7	69.6
2006	35519	32.7	64.4	87258	52.9	67.6
2007	36522	29.9	60.2	89788	47.1	62.2
2008	39543	28.6	58.6	93269	44.5	60.2
2009	38530	24.9	52.8	92443	39.1	55.2
2011	38952	22.5	47.8	91658	32.2	49.8

Notes:
Values standardized with the direct method.
Standard population is the population resident in Italy, obtained from the 2001 Census (Geraci et al., 2014, p.273).

Source: Geraci et al. (2014, p.276).

neonatal care, and in-hospital deaths, showed a general greater vulnerability for the children of foreign mothers compared with those with Italian mothers for all the indicators of perinatal health considered and in both periods (Cacciani et al., 2011, p.8). It also revealed important differences by nationality of the mother. In particular, the most disadvantaged group proved to be that of mothers from West and sub-Saharan Africa, who registered a very high likelihood of adverse perinatal outcomes for all the indicators considered in both periods. There was no difference in risk between children of Italian mothers and mothers from developed countries.

Accidents and Work-related Health Problems

Accidents at work and, more generally, work-related health problems are another of the health dimensions studied by the Italian literature on the subject. Foreigners are often responding to labor demand from destination countries that is not being satisfied by the native population. In addition, the sectors in which they are employed require low qualifications, often consist of manual labor, and are therefore physically demanding and characterized by high accident risks. The effects of this kind of strenuous jobs on health are well known in the literature (for a review see Berkman et al., 2014). In the light of these considerations, the relation between working conditions and the health of the foreign population is extremely important to study. A recent study on the subject has analyzed differences in the occurrence of accidents at work between Italians and foreigners, and the differences in the main risk factors between the two populations with figures for 2007 (Salvatore et al., 2013). The study showed that the risk of having an accident at work is higher among foreigners than for Italians (adjusted odds ratio – OR 1.82, 95% confidence interval – CI 1.53–2.16). The authors also observed an association between the risk of accidents for male workers and two occupational characteristics: the type of work and the number of years worked. With reference to the type of work, a greater risk for foreign males is observed, particularly in the construction sector (adjusted OR 2.05, 95% CI 1.56–2.69), a sector in which in 2007 foreigners were mainly employed. In the same sector, the risk for foreigners without a professional qualification was even higher (adjusted OR 8.64, 95% CI 2.85–26.20). The analysis has no figures for the irregular component of the foreign population, and it is reasonable to believe that the picture for irregular foreigners is even more alarming. In the same work, it has been observed that, compared with Italians with the same kind of job, the risk of accidents at work for foreigners increases as the time they have worked in the same job increases. The same relation does not apply to Italians, for whom there is no such association.

A second study on the subject compared work-related health problems for foreigners and nationals in two European countries: Italy and Spain (Rosano et al., 2012). The comparative study confirmed the vulnerability of immigrant workers in both contexts. In this study, too, a high share of low-qualified workers in strenuous manual jobs was found, particularly in the construction sector and in agriculture.

Self-rated Health, Activity Limitations and Chronic Morbidity

To complete the picture provided by the analysis of the literature, we present the original results of an analysis carried out on micro-data of the Italian Survey on Income and Living Conditions – IT-Silc (Istat, 2009a). In 2009, the Italian EU-Silc was accompanied by an ad-hoc module on the foreign population (Istat, 2009b). The module has a sampling system that allows us to obtain representative estimates of the foreign population resident in Italy by nationality. It contains a section on the health conditions of the interviewees, by means of the Minimum European

Table 13.3 Age-adjusted prevalence of MEHM indicators: at least one activity limitation (GALI); Chronic Morbidity; poor SRH; Italians and foreigners by area of origin, Italy, 2009; percentage values (ages 18–64)

	Poor SRH		GALI		Chronic Morbidity	
	M	F	M	F	M	F
Italians	4.6	5.3	14.8	17.6	13.9	15.3
Foreigners	5.1	4.8	11.2	11.8	11.1	11.5
CSMP	5.9	5.3	13.5	12.9	13.0	12.2
HDC	2.0	1.9	4.6	5.6	6.6	9.6
New EU countries	3.1	4.7	5.4	9.2	4.0	9.7

Notes:
The variables have been recoded as follows: poor SRH includes the responses poor and very poor; GALI identifies the presence of at least one limitation, severe or non-severe; chronic morbidity refers to the presence of at least one chronic health problem.
New EU refers to countries entering the EU in 2007.

Source: Authors' elaboration on EU-Silc data (Istat, 2009b).

Health Module (MEHM) – a combination of three indicators: Self-Rated Health (SRH), Global Activity Limitation Indicator (GALI) and Chronic Morbidity (Cox et al., 2009). The SRH indicator identifies the subjective perception of health status. The indicator refers both to the presence of objective symptoms and to the social and emotional dimension of health. The GALI refers to the presence of long-term activity limitations that impede daily activities, and the Chronic Morbidity refers to the presence of at least one longstanding health problem.

Table 13.3 shows the age-adjusted prevalence of the three indicators. Given the young age structure of the foreign population in Italy, the analyses are for the age span 18–64, as will also be done for the analysis of mortality. As we can see, the foreign population shows better overall health conditions than Italians, irrespective of sex. Only one exception is observed in the case of subjective health (SRH): foreign men seem to be in a slightly worse condition than Italian men (SRH age-adjusted prevalence 5.1 percent and 4.6 percent for foreigners and Italians respectively). The comparison by gender confirms the women's health disadvantage, both Italian and foreign, which is well known in the literature (Caselli and Egidi, 2011). A deeper analysis of the foreign population by macro area of nationality shows marked heterogeneity. Foreigners from the CSMP are the most disadvantaged group, always registering a higher prevalence than the other groups for all three indicators and for both sexes. It is very likely that this figure is due to the worse socio-economic and working conditions of the African population in Italy. On the contrary, foreigners from highly developed countries (HDCs) prove to be the group with the best health conditions. Their socio-economic status was most likely already better in their country of origin, compared with foreigners from CSMP. In addition, in the host country they represent a share of the foreign population employed in more qualified jobs, with a higher socio-economic status, all factors positively associated with health status.

A recent study on migrants' health in Italy not only confirmed the health advantage of immigrants over natives (foreign-born versus Italian-born), but also observed that there is a strong association between health status and time of permanence in the destination country (Loi, 2016). Controlling for age, sex, marital status, education, area of origin, area of residence in the destination country and material deprivation, the risk of having at least one activity limitation, or suffering from a chronic health problem and of reporting poor SRH increases as duration of permanence increases. Specifically, taking as reference the most recent arrivals (0–4 years before the interview), the OR progressively increases over time of permanence. Controlling for the changes in the composition of the migration flows entering Italy in recent decades by macro areas of origin, it was also observed that the immigrant/native differential weakens as duration of stay increases. That is, signs of a convergence between the health levels of the two populations are observed, as emerges from the international literature. In addition, duration of permanence has proved to be a factor of interaction with the individual characteristics linked to the socio-economic sphere in the host country. The association between time spent in the country and poor health proved stronger for those exposed to the most disadvantageous socio-economic conditions, for all three indicators (Loi, 2016).

Asylum-seekers and Refugees

Currently, there are no data for an in-depth study of health conditions, and, still less, for mortality, of asylum seekers and refugees, who certainly deserve special attention for at least two reasons. First, we may reasonably believe that asylum seekers and refugees are less selected at origin than the so-called 'economic' migrants. Secondly, it is clear that the reason for migration and, above all, the means used, often by sea in dangerous conditions, may constitute an important risk factor, both for health and mortality.

From the analyses carried out so far, three fundamental aspects emerge, closely connected with the recent Italian migration history and the different individual characteristics – demographic and migratory – of the foreign population. The first is the negative relation between health and poor working conditions for foreign men. The second is the need for public health assistance for foreign women in reproductive ages. The third is the need, which has emerged in recent years, to guarantee an emergency health service for the growing number of persons saved in the Mediterranean who have landed in the ports of Southern Italy.

A HIDDEN REALITY OR A REAL PHENOMENON: WHEN A NEGATIVE EVENT HIGHLIGHTS A PRIVILEGE

It is well-known that life expectancy is the mirror image of mortality, and so low levels of mortality correspond to high survival and vice versa. Italy, which has a life expectancy at birth in 2014 of 85 years for women and 80 years for men, can boast one of the highest survival levels in the world. These levels tend to grow, year by year, by effect of a constant decline in adult mortality and, above all, that of old people. It is, then, difficult to imagine that those arriving in Italy from Eastern Europe or the poorer countries of the world, which are strongly penalized by low or very low survival levels, may seem favored by a lower average adult mortality than the Italian level of mortality. Yet this result appears in all the analyses carried out so far.

Before analyzing levels and characteristics of mortality of the foreign population, we should emphasize that we cannot provide a summary indicator which links mortality to life expectancy at birth. Nor can we construct the risks of death for ages over 65, given the very few foreigners of this age in Italy (see the age pyramid in Figure 13.2). For now, the mortality histories of foreigners are therefore incomplete, and, even if we wanted to complete them with estimates, we cannot as there is no information, direct or indirect, we can refer to.

This is not the only obstacle. The construction of mortality indicators, age-specific or standardized, requires consistency between the figures for the numerator and the denominator. First, some of the deaths of foreigners registered as resident in Italy occur outside the country. The salmon bias is a highly significant phenomenon, particularly in some nationalities, and has become the object of discussion beyond individual episodes that have been highlighted by the national press. The tendency to re-enter one's country of origin when one has an incurable disease has been noted in other European countries too (Khlat and Courbage, 1995; Tribalat, 1996). This occurs for sentimental and cultural reasons, which drive the sick individuals to return to their family of origin to spend what may be the last period of their life (Tribalat, 1996). This may also occur for economic reasons, as the cost of funerals is very high in Italy and, equally, the cost of the repatriation of the corpse may be beyond the means of a family of foreign workers. In addition, given the large number of Muslims in Italy, the difference in funeral rites drives many in this community to return to the country of origin at the onset of a possibly fatal disease. At other times, the desire to return home at least when dead can lead to behaviors perceived as strange or illegal. The Chinese community, for example, is perceived in Italy as 'immortal', registering only very few deaths despite its growing numbers.

To estimate the mortality of foreigners the National Institute of Statistics (Istat, 2015) suggests referring merely to deaths of those resident legally and permanently in the country. In this way, we can calculate a mortality rate where both the events in the numerator and the individuals in the denominator refer only to the population resident in the country. No estimate of the error owing to the salmon bias is possible, as it is unlikely that an individual who leaves for serious reasons of health will proceed to cancel himself or herself from the register of the resident population. This means that some deaths coming from the population in the denominator of the mortality rate will not be in the numerator of the same rate.

To contain the so-called salmon bias, the National Report on Population Health (Osservatorio Nazionale sulla Salute, 2012, 2014), like other studies on the subject (Bruzzone and Mignolli, 2002; Maccheroni et al., 2007), presents the mortality rates for the age range 18–64 years. This extensive age range has mortality levels that are significantly consistent, and is also regarded by experts as where those who have spent a long period of time in Italy are concentrated and have a growing level of permanence, and hence are less likely to return to their country of origin for health reasons. In addition, as we have mentioned, the history of the mortality of foreigners after 65 years is still unwritten, while that for the younger ages has been little studied and, as is well known, presents low risks of death. Special mention, however, should be given to the analysis of infant mortality, which is treated separately in Chapter 14 in this volume.

Adult Mortality

The analysis that follows seeks to offer as complete a summary as possible of the recent development of the mortality of the foreign population with reference to the reconstruction of both the last two reports of Osservatorio Nazionale sulla Salute (2012, 2014) and in some publications (Bruzzone et al., 2000; Bruzzone and Mignolli, 2002, 2003, 2012, 2014). Thus, for adult mortality (18–64 years) we refer to the standardized mortality rates (SMR) calculated by gender, areas of nationality, and principal cause of death category. The standardization of rates was carried out by Istat with the direct method, known also as the population type, identified in the world standard population (Bruzzone and Mignolli, 2012, 2014).

Two aspects of the phenomenon appear very clearly in Table 13.4, which shows the development of rates from 2003 to 2012 for men and women, and for the four macro-areas of nationality indicated: the lower values of foreigners over Italians, irrespective of gender, and the lower mortality for women over men, irrespective of nationality, with values that are almost always half those of their peers. These results remind us that what makes any comparison with the Italian figures peculiar is tied to the particular selection of the foreign population – a selection that derives from an essentially good state of health. The relatively low mortality rates seem to be in line with the well-known theory of the so-called healthy immigrant effect (HIE), an effect that, at least for the population considered, might be enhanced if the population had average educational levels higher than those of the Italian population.

More recently, irrespective of corrections, comparing Italian adult mortality with that of foreigners in the CSMP group (96 percent of the total of foreigners) we note a clear contrast in the two trends. While the values of the former tend to decrease for men and remain substantially stable for women, for the latter, irrespective of gender, the trend is upwards. For Italian adult mortality, the figures have recently shown a reduction in the gender distance (the male/female mortality ratio goes down from 2.02 in 2003 to 1.82 in 2012), owing to a more marked decline in male mortality in these ages. This has been interpreted as indicating an improvement in male lifestyles in the more recent adult generations; as a result of greater primary and secondary prevention, they have managed to obtain important reductions in mortality levels for diseases in the circulatory system and, especially, lung cancer (Caselli, 2015).

To better understand the characteristics of mortality and the differences noted so far, we may usefully refer to mortality by cause. If we look at the levels for 2011 in Table 13.5 (Bruzzone and Mignolli, 2014, p. 317), the result is truly surprising. First, comparing the mortality of Italians with that of foreigners in the CSMP group, we note that only for causes of external and violent nature for women is the risk of death higher for foreigners (relative risk equal to 1.1). Again, for women, the relative risk of death by infectious diseases is equal to 1, while for all other causes it is less than 1. By contrast, when we compare the values for Italians with those for foreigners who entered the EU from 2007 on, the relative risks for mortality for all causes of death considered, apart from respiratory ones, show that

Table 13.4 *Mortality rates standardized with direct method of foreign population resident in Italy and Italians aged 18–64 by gender and area of citizenship, values per 10 000, 2003–12*

Areas of citizenship	2003	2004	2005	2006	2007	2008	2009	2010*	2011*	2012*
Males										
Highly developed countries – HDC	10.2	10.1	11.5	10.6	8.5	9.2	8.7	10.7	17.2	11.4
Countries with strong migratory pressure – CSMP	17.0	19.5	17.4	16.1	12.0	15.5	14.5	14.0	14.5	15.2
Of which: countries that have recently joined the EU		22.7	27.3	20.8	19.6	15.7	15	19.7	26.6	21.4
Italians	26.5	24.9	24.3	23.6	23.0	22.3	21.8	21.1	21.0	20.6
Females										
Highly developed countries – HDC	5.2	7.0	7.7	7.7	7.7	5.1	4.6	7.0	7.8	7.2
Countries with strong migratory pressure – CSMP	8.5	6.8	6.6	6.9	5.6	6.8	5.7	5.6	5.9	6.6
Of which: countries that have recently joined the EU	7.6	6.4	6.7	6.0	6.5	7.2	5.6	6.8	8.9	8.5
Italians	13.1	12.3	12.2	11.8	11.7	11.5	11.7	11.2	11.4	11.3

Note: * Until 2009 the denominators of the rates refer to the average resident population at 1 January year t and $t + 1$. From year 2010 to 2012 the population refers to 2011 census data.

Sources: Maccheroni et al. (2007); Bruzzone and Mignolli (2014); Bruzzone and Mignolli (2015).

Table 13.5 Mortality rate and relative risks of the foreign population resident in Italy and of Italians aged 18–64 years by gender, cause of death and area of citizenship, values per 10 000, 2011

Causes of death	SMR age 18–64 years		Relative risks	
	Men	Women	Men	Women
CSMP				
Infectious and parasitic diseases	0.51	0.25	0.8	1.0
Tumors	4.58	2.69	0.5	0.4
Diseases of the circulatory system	3.71	1.55	0.8	0.7
Diseases of the respiratory system	0.46	0.13	0.8	0.4
External or violent causes	3.25	0.83	1.0	1.1
Other diseases	1.99	0.94	0.6	0.5
Total rate	14.48	5.92	0.7	0.5
Countries who had recently joined the EU 2007				
Infectious and parasitic diseases	0.25	0.34	0.4	1.4
Tumors	10.60	4.30	1.2	0.6
Diseases of the circulatory system	5.93	1.34	1.3	0.8
Diseases of the respiratory system	0.51	0.06	0.9	0.2
External or violent causes	5.48	1.58	1.7	2.1
Other diseases	3.78	1.27	1.1	0.7
Total rate	26.55	8.89	1.3	0.8
Italy				
Infectious and parasitic diseases	0.61	0.25	1.0	1.0
Tumors	8.49	6.72	1.0	1.0
Diseases of the circulatory system	4.45	1.58	1.0	1.0
Diseases of the respiratory system	0.59	0.32	1.0	1.0
External or violent causes	3.26	0.76	1.0	1.0
Other diseases	3.58	1.81	1.0	1.0
Total rate	20.98	11.44	1.0	1.0

Notes:
The groups of causes of death are taken from the tenth revision of the International Classification of Diseases ICD 10: Infectious and parasitic diseases (A00-B99), Tumors (C00–D48), Diseases of the circulatory system (I00-I99); Diseases of the respiratory system (J00–J99); External causes of morbidity and mortality (V01–Y98); Other diseases (D50–H95; K00–K93; L00-Q99; R00–R99).
Population standard used is the world population.

Source: Bruzzone and Mignolli (2014).

the men from these countries are more penalized than Italians. These risks reach 1.7 in cases of causes of an external and violent nature. For women, the risk of death by these causes for foreigners is twice that for Italians (Vicarelli, 1994). Death by infections show a relationship above 1.0 too, while mortality for all others causes is relatively lower. For these foreign nationals, violent behaviors and work-related risks result in higher male mortality for violent or external causes, but, together with the unhealthy lifestyles – individual and collective – that these foreigners were exposed to even before their arrival in Italy, also result in higher mortality in adult age for tumors and diseases of the circulatory system (Vallin et al., 2001; Bruzzone and Mignolli, 2014). What we have seen in analyzing the health of these nationals is evident too in their risk of death, with the result of a higher mortality even though the estimates of deaths may be considered lower than the real value, for all the reasons previously described.

Although the information is incomplete and the period of study limited, the study of the mortality of foreigners clearly cannot be related to an average value, but needs to be examined with reference to the various nationalities, as these bring with them different social and cultural life histories, and, above all, different life styles and work histories, which have an important role in determining the various risks of disease and death.

Infant Mortality

Focusing on the infant mortality of the foreign population resident in Italy and comparing it with that of Italian children may give interesting indications on the different degree of well-being of the two groups. In particular, as mortality in the first year of life in the developed countries is concentrated mainly in the neonatal period (0–30 days), this information further helps us in formulating hypotheses that might explain the existing differences.

Istat calculates the rates of infant mortality by making the numerator of the relation the number of deaths in the first year (or first month) in a given period, and the denominator all the live births in the same period, expressing the rate of deaths per thousand live births. Istat has supplied some results for the periods 2006–08 and 2009–11 (Istat, 2014, pp. 10–12). First, the rate of mortality in the first year of life for foreign children resident in Italy is always higher than that for Italian children. In the first period, for the foreigners it is equal to 4.71 per thousand, while for the Italians it is 3.15 per thousand. In the second period, although the distance observed in the period 2006–08 is maintained, the numbers decrease for both groups to 4.55 per thousand and 3.01 per thousand, respectively.

Higher infant mortality among foreigners is certainly linked to their lower economic resources and the social hardship they often experience – the same factors that also penalize reproductive and maternal infant health, and that lead foreign women to make less use both of the health systems in the first months of pregnancy and of therapeutic abortion than Italian women (1.7 percent against 4.2 percent). These factors may create more difficult conditions of health and survival for a newborn child who is the result of a risky pregnancy. This consideration is supported by an analysis of infant mortality by cause of death. The risk of death, particularly for congenital malformations and morbid conditions in the prenatal period, as we have already seen in the case of perinatal health in the previous section, is higher for foreign children than for Italians: 1.25 per thousand against 0.69 per thousand for the pathologies of the first group, and 2.39 per thousand against 1.78 per thousand for those of the second. In confirmation of this, we may recall that, in the case of foreign children, there is less information on the pathological situation available to the doctor at the moment of certifying death (Osservatorio Nazionale sulla Salute, 2012; Di Fraia et al., 2015).

Some mortality differences from the countries of origin of foreign children were brought out in the 2012 Osservasalute Report (Osservatorio Nazionale sulla Salute, 2012). In this case, the rate of infant mortality was calculated using longitudinal data (deaths and births in the same generation), for the years 2005–09 (see Table 13.6). The foreigners of the CSMP countries showed the highest levels: those countries accounted for 80 percent of foreign deaths in the first year of life. Among these, the deaths of African children were in first place, owing to the high number of deaths of Moroccan children, a result that was in line with what has already been noted in perinatal health (Bruzzone and Mignolli, 2012, p. 246). Of the Europeans in 2005, the Romanian community had some of the highest values of infant mortality, though the values rapidly decreased, only to rise again (in the great immigration period following Romania's entrance into the EU) and then, in 2009, actually settle below the Italian values.

Table 13.6 *Infant mortality rates of the foreign population resident in Italy and of Italians by area of citizenship from 2005 to 2009, values per 1000 live births, 2011*

Areas of citizenship	2005	2006	2007	2008	2009
Foreigners from CSMP	5.0	4.4	3.9	3.8	4.0
Of which: *countries that joined the EU in 2007*	5.6	3.8	2.5	4.0	3.0
Romania	5.4	3.9	2.8	4.0	3.0
Africa	5.7	4.9	4.7	4.6	5.1
Italy	3.6	3.4	3.3	3.3	3.3

Source: Authors' elaboration on data of Bruzzone and Mignolli (2012).

In general, the trend of infant mortality in the period 2005–09 shows a gradual narrowing of the gap between Italian and foreign children, at least until 2008, even though the latter are still relatively at greater risk. The same change can be seen for the children, though with positions reversed, as for the adults, particularly the men: a tendency for the mortality levels to converge, perfectly in line with the reduction in the distances observed in analyzing health conditions.

CONCLUSION: WHAT WILL BE THE FUTURE OF THE HEALTH AND MORTALITY OF SUCH A HETEROGENEOUS POPULATION THAT IS CONSTANTLY DEVELOPING?

We have provided an overall picture of the characteristics of recent Italian immigration as it concerns some well-known and less well-known aspects of the health and mortality of the foreign population resident in Italy. We want to insist that this work analyzes for the first time the health of foreigners with reference to the data in the European EU-Silc survey on perceived health. The analysis of these figures – together with those from other sources – allows us to compare the health of foreigners with that of Italians, and to note that, though the former enjoy better conditions of health, the distance from the latter tends to converge as time of permanence increases. This leads to the conclusion that their living conditions – socio-economic, family and working – in the host country are unfavorable to maintaining the initial good conditions of health and their advantage over the Italians.

Given the more recent face of immigration in Italy, characterized by an increasing number of refugees and asylum seekers, in the future mental health problems may become more and more important. This is an aspect which requires the availability of specific data that until now have not been available. In order to overcome the lack of these data one possibility would be to undertake observational studies on new immigrant communities. Longitudinal designs would be even more useful in order to better comprehend how migrants' socio-economic and health conditions, both physical and mental, change over time in the host country.

As for health, for adult and infant mortality too, the distance between foreigners and Italians tends to reduce, showing a clear convergence – particularly for adult men – toward the same levels. This suggests that with the passage of time, when the migrant's previous life history plays a less important role than that lived in the country of arrival, mortality histories become more similar. Obviously, this is pure speculation, as there are insufficient data available, and they do not lend themselves to analyses requiring a longitudinal perspective in studying health and mortality.

Compared with the present picture, mortality differences in adult ages that are to be found among groups of different nationalities suggest that life experiences after migration, like the type of activity performed in Italy, play an important role in determining levels and characteristics by cause of death.

One of the limitations of the results presented is that they refer to more recent migration, which is more numerous but also has completely different characteristics by gender and origin from the first migration of the 1980s and 1990s. The greatest limitation, however, is that of not providing results on the health and mortality of the old (aged 65+) – that part of the population that in Italy in 2014 determines 85 percent of deaths and accounts for 70 percent of overall health expenditure. It is clear that the current numbers of adult foreigners and their growing weight on the total of the population constitute one of the most important problems that Italy will have to face in the near future – a future difficult to foresee as it could have two such different faces as to require the implementation of contrasting health policies. Indeed, if the present immigrants, on reaching retirement age, decided to return to their country of origin, they would not contribute to increasing the aged population, and hence health expenditure would be reduced by a deceleration in aging. However, if they decided to remain in Italy, the effect on the growing number of old people, at least as an absolute value, would be notable and entail a significant increase in the demand for health services and health expenditure. In this second perspective, the models of mortality in old age might change too. It is a question of understanding if the 'foreign' old person, as a result of a social and working life that was unfavorable to survival in the destination country, is destined to have a lower longevity than that of the Italian old person. If that happened, given the large number of foreigners, in a not too distant future the positive development of survival levels experienced so far in Italy would also be called into question.

Although studying the health and mortality of migrants in Italy is difficult, given the limitations mentioned and the fluid nature of the situation, it is even more difficult to foresee what the future will be for this share of the population, which is already so different in its characteristics of origin, and whose future retirement plans are completely unknown. To forecast, it is useful to think in a longitudinal perspective, on the basis of information concerning the development of health and mortality in the present generations of migrants, working with the hypothesis that those who continue to arrive will not be too different from the foreign adults of today. This is no easy task for the experts and the future is uncertain for implementing good health policies.

NOTE

1. Law 943/1986, accessed October 2015 at http://www.stranieriinitalia.it/briguglio/immigrazione-e-asilo/1992/luglio/legge-943-86.html.
2. The CSMP group includes all African countries, those of Central-Southern America, Asia (apart from Japan, Israel and South Korea), Oceania (apart from Australia and New Zealand); countries that have joined the EU since May 2004 and January 2007 (excluding Malta and Cyprus), i.e. Czech Republic, Estonia, Hungary, Latvia, Lithuania, Poland, Slovakia, Slovenia, Bulgaria and Romania; and all the remaining countries of Eastern Europe. Highly Developed Countries (HDC) include the countries of EU-15, Norway, Iceland, Switzerland, Liechtenstein, Monaco, Andorra, Cyprus, Malta, Japan, Israel, Australia, New Zealand, Canada, the United States and South Korea.

REFERENCES

Abella, M.I., Y. Park and W.R. Bohning (1995), 'Adjustments to labour shortages and foreign workers in the Republic of Korea', International Migration Papers No. 1, International Labour Office, Geneva.

Ambrosini, M. (2005), *Sociologia delle migrazioni*, Bologna: Il Mulino.

Barbagli, M., A. Colombo and G. Sciortino (eds) (2004), *I sommersi e i sanati. Le regolarizzazioni degli immigrati in Italia*, Bologna: Il Mulino.

Berkman, L.F., I. Kawachi and T. Theorell (2014), 'Working conditions and health', in L. Berkman, I. Kawachi, and M.M. Glymour (eds), *Social Epidemiology*, 2nd edn, Oxford: Oxford University Press, pp. 153–81.

Birindelli, A.M. (1989), 'Le migrazioni con l'estero. Chiusura di un ciclo e avvio di una nuova fase', in E. Sonnino (ed.), *Demografia e società in Italia*, Rome: Editori Riuniti, pp. 189223.

Blangiardo, G.C. and M.L. Tanturri (2006), 'How many and who? An up-date picture of the foreign migrants in Italy', paper presented at the European Population Conference 2006, Liverpool.

Bonifazi, C. (2013), *L' Italia delle migrazioni*, Bologna: Il Mulino.

Bruzzone, S., and N. Mignolli (2002), 'Lo studio della mortalità per causa della popolazione straniera in Italia: problematiche metodologiche e disponibilità dei dati', *Atti del Settimo Seminario Internazionale di Geografia Medica del 2001*, Perugia: RUX editrice, pp. 395–410.

Bruzzone, S. and N. Mignolli (2003), 'La mortalità per causa degli immigrati nell' Unione Europea e nei Paesi Candidati: documentazione e criteri di misura', in M. Natale and E. Moretti (eds), *Siamo pochi o siamo troppi? Alcuni aspetti delle relazioni tra evoluzione demografica e sviluppo economico e sociale*, Milan: Franco Angeli, pp. 412–33.

Bruzzone, S. and N. Mignolli (2012), 'Mortalità per causa tra gli stranieri in Italia', in 'Rapporto Osservasalute 2012: stato di salute e qualità dell'assistenza nelle regioni italiane', Milan, Università Cattolica del Sacro Cuore, pp. 242–6.

Bruzzone, S. and N. Mignolli (2014), 'Mortalità per causa tra gli stranieri in Italia', in 'Rapporto Osservasalute 2014: stato di salute e qualità dell'assistenza nelle regioni italiane', Università Cattolica del Sacro Cuore, Milan, pp. 310–18.

Bruzzone, S. and N. Mignolli (2015), 'Mortalità per causa tra gli stranieri in Italia',

in *Rapporto Osservasalute 2015: stato di salute e qualità dell'assistenza nelle regioni italiane*, Milan: Università Cattolica del Sacro Cuore, pp. 293–301.
Bruzzone, S., A. Carciotto, G. Cariani, N. Mignolli and A. Reale (2000), 'Studi differenziali sulla mortalità degli immigrati stranieri in Italia', *Atti XL Riunione Scientifica della Societa Italiana di Statistica (SIS)*, Rome: Istat, pp. 115–18.
Cacciani, L., G. Baglio and L. Rossi, E. Materia, M. Marceca, S. Geraci et al. (2006), 'Hospitalization among immigrants in Italy', *Emerging Themes in Epidemiology*, **3** (1), 1.
Cacciani, L., S. Asola and A. Polo, F. Franco, R. Lucchini, M. De Curtis et al. (2011), 'Perinatal outcomes among immigrant mothers over two periods in a region of central Italy', *BMC Public Health*, **11** (1), 1.
Caselli, G. (2015), 'Gender differences in longevity and health', paper presented to the conference on Socio-Demographic Impact of Longevity: Evolution and Emerging Characteristics in the Population at Advanced Ages, Madrid, 20 October.
Caselli, G. and V. Egidi (2011), 'Una vita più lunga e più sana. Riflessioni sul passato per immaginare il futuro', in A. Golini A. and A. Rosina (eds), *Il secolo degli anziani. Come cambierà la società italiana*, Bologna: Il Mulino – Prismi, pp. 29–45.
Cox, B., H. Van Oyen, E. Cambois, C. Jagger, S. Le Roy, J.M. Robine and I. Romieu (2009), 'The reliability of the minimum European health module', *International Journal of Public Health*, **54** (2), 55–60.
Dalla Zuanna, G., P. Farina and S. Strozza (2009), *Nuovi italiani. I giovani immigrati cambieranno il nostro paese?*, Bologna: Il Mulino.
Di Comite, L. (1986), 'L'immigration tunisienne en Italie: quelques données censitaires', *Studi Emigrazione*, **82–3**, 217–27.
Di Fraia, G., S. Simeoni, C. Orsi and L. Frova (2015), 'La mortalità infantile degli stranieri residenti in Italia', Giornate di Studio sulla popolazione, Associazione Italiana per lo Studio del Pancreas (AISP), Palermo.
Geraci, S., G. Baglio and A. Burgio (2014), 'Salute degli immigrati', in *Osservasalute 2014: stato di salute e qualità dell'assistenza nelle regioni italiane*, Milan: Università Cattolica del Sacro Cuore, pp. 263–309.
Golini, A. (1997), 'Le migrazioni nella storia dell'Europa', in AA.VV., *L'Europa dei popoli*, Rome: Istituto Poligrafico e Zecca dello Stato: Editalia.
Impicciatore, R. and S. Strozza (2015), 'Migrazioni internazionali e interne di italiani e stranieri', in A. De Rose and S. Strozza (eds), *Rapporto sulla popolazione. L'Italia nella crisi economica*, Bologna: Il Mulino, pp. 109–40.
Istat (2009a), 'IT-Silc, Italian Statistics on Income and Living Conditions', IT-SILC XUDB 2009 – second version, August 2013.
Istat (2009b), 'EU-Silc, Reddito e condizioni di vita delle famiglie con stranieri', UDB CVS2009 – January 2012 version.
Istat (2014), 'Anni 1887–2011. La mortalità dei bambini ieri e oggi in Italia', Statistiche Focus, accessed October 2015 at http://www.istat.it.
Istat (2015), 'Popolazione straniera residente al 1° gennaio per età e sesso', accessed October 2015 at www.demo.istat.it.
Khlat, M. and Y. Courbage (1995), 'La mortalité et les causes de décès des Marocains en France 1979 à 1991. II. Les causes de décès', *Population*, **50** (2), 447–71.
Loi, S. (2016), 'Social determinants of migrants' health in Italy: evidence from duration of stay and migration history', doctoral thesis, Sapienza University of Rome.

Maccheroni, C., S. Bruzzone and M. Mignolli (2007), *La mortalità degli stranieri in Italia: metodi di misura a confronto*, Collana Quaderni del Dipartimento per lo studio delle società del Mediterraneo, Bari: Cacucci Editore.

Mazziotta, M. (2014), 'L'indagine di copertura (PES) del 15° Censimento generale della popolazione e delle abitazioni. I risultati definitivi, Seminario su "La misurazione della qualità del 15° Censimento generale della popolazione e delle abitazioni: i risultati dell'indagine di copertura (PES)', 27 June, Rome, Istat.

Osservatorio Nazionale sulla Salute (2012), 'Rapporto Osservasalute 2012: Stato di salute e qualità dell'assistenza nelle regioni italiane', Università Cattolica del Sacro Cuore, Milan.

Osservatorio Nazionale sulla Salute (2014), 'Rapporto Osservasalute 2014: Stato di salute e qualità dell'assistenza nelle regioni italiane', Università Cattolica del Sacro Cuore, Milan.

Peixoto, J., J. Arango, C. Bonifazi, C. Finotelli, C. Sabino, S. Strozza and A. Triandafyllidou (2012), 'Immigrants, markets and policies in Southern Europe: the making of an immigration model?', in M. Okólski (ed.), *European Immigration. Trends, Structures and Policy Implications*, IMISCOE Research, Amsterdam: Amsterdam University Press pp. 107–47.

Rosano, A., E. Ronda and F.G. Benavides, L. Cacciani, G. Baglio and A. Spagnolo (2012), 'Work-related health problems among resident immigrant workers in Italy and Spain', *Italian Journal of Public Health*, **9** (3), 68–74.

Rossi, F. and S. Strozza (2007), 'Mobilità della popolazione, immigrazione e presenza straniera', in GCD-SIS, *Rapporto sulla popolazione. L'Italia all'inizio del XXI secolo*, Bologna: Il Mulino, pp. 111–37.

Salvatore, M. A., G. Baglio and L. Cacciani, A. Spagnolo and A. Rosano (2013), 'Work-related injuries among immigrant workers in Italy', *Journal of Immigrant and Minority Health*, **15** (1), 182–7.

Strozza, S. (2009), 'Le seconde generazioni in Italia: i numeri di un fenomeno in ascesa', in O. Casacchia, L. Natale, and A. Guarneri (eds), *Tra i banchi di scuola. Alunni stranieri e italiani a Roma e nel Lazio*, Milan: Franco Angeli, pp. 19–42.

Strozza, S. (2010), 'International migration in Europe in the first decade of the 21st century', *Rivista Italiana di Economia Demografia e Statistica*, **64** (3), 7–43.

Strozza, S. (2015), 'La presenza straniera in Italia', in AA.VV., *L'integrazione delle comunità immigrate e l'imprenditoria straniera*, Florence: Neodemos, pp. 9–30.

Strozza, S. and E. Zucchetti (eds) (2006), *Il Mezzogiorno dopo la grande regolarizzazione. Vecchi e nuovi volti della presenza migratoria*, vol. 2, Milan: Franco Angeli.

Tribalat, M. (1996), 'Cronique dell' immigration', *Population*, **51** (1), 141–94.

Vallin, J., F. Meslé and T. Valkonen (2001), *Trends in Mortality and Differential Mortality*. Strasbourg: Council of Europe.

Vicarelli, G. (ed.) (1994), *Le mani invisibili. La vita e il lavoro delle donne immigrate*, Rome. Ediesse.

Zanfrini, L. (2002), 'Politiche delle "quote" ed etnicizzazione del mercato del lavoro italiano', *Sociologia del lavoro*, **88**, 186–226.

14. Mortality and health of immigrants and their children in Belgium in the 2000s

Patrick Deboosere and Hadewijch Vandenheede

INTRODUCTION

The aim of this chapter is to unravel differences in (cause-specific) mortality, life expectancy and health by migrant background[1] in Belgium. Before going into detail about the health and mortality patterns of immigrants in Belgium, we briefly describe Belgium's migration history and elaborate upon theories on immigrants' health and mortality. After focusing on life expectancy and cause-specific mortality, we very briefly touch upon migrant health through the analysis of a case study: diabetes among populations of Moroccan and Turkish origin. Finally we illustrate the shift in mortality patterns occurring between generations.

BELGIUM'S MIGRATION HISTORY: A BRIEF OVERVIEW

Belgium, as many other European countries, has been an emigration country during most of the nineteenth century. After a very short and strong upsurge of emigration during and after the First World War, the migration balance of Belgium turned positive and the country became and remains an immigration country (Lesthaeghe, 2000; Deboosere, 2012). At the beginning of the twentieth century, 254000 persons were registered as migrants in a population total of 6.1 million persons. The large majority (86 per cent) came from the neighbouring countries and crossed a largely theoretical border sometimes only a few kilometres from their birthplace (Eggerickx et al., 1999). To palliate the shortage of workers in the mines and heavy industry, Belgian authorities started recruiting actively in Southern and Eastern Europe. In 1930, 18 per cent of miners were of migrant background, mostly from Poland and Italy, and already with a large Maghrebian presence (Eggerickx and Sanderson, 2004). From 1930 onwards, protectionist policies dominated the international scene with a sharp decline in international labour migration as a consequence.

In 1945, in the immediate aftermath of the Second World War, the Belgian government began recruiting again large contingents of foreign workers for the mining and metal industries. On 20 June 1946, an agreement was signed between Belgium and Italy stipulating the weekly arrival of 2000 Italian workers in exchange for the engagement of Belgium to sell a fixed amount of coal to Italy (Martens, 1985; Morelli, 1988). The mining disaster of le Bois du Cazier in Marcinelle (8 August 1956), with 262 miners killed, among whom 136 were of Italian origin, put an end to this agreement. The Italian migration slowed down, but recruitment was already extended to the whole northern part of the Mediterranean area with workers coming from Spain, Greece, Portugal and the former Yugoslavia. In the 1960s this recruitment area was enlarged to Morocco and Turkey. Increasingly more industrial sectors, the construction industry and the service sector, started recruiting foreign workers as well (Moulaert, 1985). The petroleum crisis of 1973 put an end to the organized labour migration and, similar to other European countries, Belgium installed a 'migration stop' in 1974. From 1974 onwards, family reunification became the main migration channel and migration lost its dominant male character. During the 1970s a Congolese community emerged from former students and migrants arriving often as political refugees or asylum seekers. By the census of 1991 the Congolese community living in Belgium reached 10 000 persons (Eggerickx et al., 1999).

The years between 1974 and the beginning of the 1990s remained a period of relatively low net migration. Belgium counted 878 000 persons of foreign origin in the census of 1981; this was 9 per cent of the total population. In 1996 it was still about 9 per cent and in absolute numbers not much higher at 909 769 according to the then recently introduced Central Population Register. The so-called 'law Gol' of 28 June 1984 granted Belgian nationality to each child born with one Belgian parent. Belgian nationality was automatically accorded to all children under the age of 18 born to a Belgian mother, reducing the foreign population by more than 75 000 individuals on 1 January 1985. The Wathelet legislation of 3 September 1991 extended Belgian nationality further to all children born in Belgium, adding principles of the *ius solis* to those of the *ius sanguinis*. Without changes in naturalization the total number of foreign inhabitants in the 1991 census should have been over 1.1 million persons instead of the 900 855 counted.

From the 1990s onwards immigration increasingly outnumbers emigration again. There is an important group of asylum seekers and refugees starting with the Yugoslavian wars and followed by those fleeing the wars in former Soviet republics. The Rwandan genocide and the successive Congolese wars strongly increased the sub-Saharan migration. However, it was the adoption of the European Treaty and especially the 2004 and 2007 enlargements of the European Union with Central and Eastern European countries that boosted net migration.

The important migration flows of the past quarter century rapidly altered the composition of the Belgian population. In the census of 2001, Belgium had a population of 10 295 724 with 846 903 persons of foreign nationality, and 557 602 Belgians born with a foreign nationality (Deboosere et al., 2007). On 1 January 2015 the Belgian Federal Migration Centre reported 1 605 776 immigrants. A person is considered an immigrant when he or she is not born in Belgium and moved from another country to become officially a Belgian resident, regardless of the current nationality. If current nationality is the criterion, 1 255 270 persons with a foreign nationality are living in Belgium of a total population of 11 209 259 inhabitants. Persons with a foreign nationality are not necessarily immigrants as they can be born in Belgium. However, if nationality at birth is the criterion, regardless of the current nationality and of the fact that a person is born in Belgium or abroad, then 2 206 259 residents of Belgium can be considered of foreign origin (Myria, 2016). Table 14.1 summarizes the main nationalities of persons of foreign origin living in Belgium based on nationality at birth. When we extend these combined criteria and include all persons with at least one parent of foreign origin, about three out of ten inhabitants of Belgium can be considered to be from recent migrant background.

As the 2001 Belgian census is the main data source for the analysis in this chapter, it is a good starting point for an overview of the main population groups in Belgium by year of birth and country of birth. The graphs in Figure 14.1 illustrate different populations living in Belgium according to the country of origin, distinguishing those born in the origin country and those born in Belgium. The populations of French and Dutch origin have a long history of transborder migration, mixed with more recent intra-European migration often linked to work or studies. The population of Italian origin has a migration history going back to the inter-bellum with the first labour migrations, but also with a strong contribution of political refugees fleeing the Mussolini regime. The populations of Moroccan and Turkish origin have a clear-cut starting point with the labour migration of the 1960s illustrated by the year when the second generation started to be born in Belgium.

Table 14.1 Persons with foreign nationality at birth living in Belgium (1 January 2015) by current nationality

Current foreign nationality		Current Belgian nationality	
France	159352	Morocco	224108
Italy	156977	Turkey	119011
Netherlands	149199	Italy	116206
Morocco	82009	France	50042
Poland	68403	DR Congo	37381
Romania	65768	Netherlands	31138
Spain	60386	Poland	23020
Portugal	42793	Ex-Yugoslavia	21998
Germany	39294	Algeria	17596
Turkey	36747	Germany	16325
Bulgaria	28721	Spain	13609
United Kingdom	23974	Russia	13417
DR Congo	20625	Tunisia	10932
Greece	16275	Romania	9586
Russia	12434	Rwanda	9541
Other	292313	Other	237079
Total	1255270	Total	950989

Source: Myria (2016, p. 60).

THEORETICAL PERSPECTIVES ON IMMIGRANTS' HEALTH AND MORTALITY

Migrant studies on all-cause mortality generally show a mortality advantage in first-generation (FG) immigrants, despite their oft-poorer socio-economic position (SEP) and living conditions (Courbage and Khlat, 1996; Kouris-Blazos, 2002; Deboosere and Gadeyne, 2005; Tarnutzer et al., 2012; Wallace and Kulu, 2014, 2015). This is often referred to as the 'adult migrant mortality paradox'. Among the theories to explain this is the 'healthy-migrant effect', which states that health selection takes place in the country of origin, with the healthiest individuals being selected into migration (Deboosere and Gadeyne, 2005; Nørredam et al., 2014). The 'salmon-bias hypothesis', on the other hand, predicts FG immigrants will return to their home countries when they become ill. Nevertheless, whether this holds for all FG immigrants is still debatable, since high-quality health services and the investment of settling in the host country could make a return less likely than suggested according to the theory (Deboosere and Gadeyne, 2005; Wallace and Kulu, 2014; Nørredam et al., 2014, 2015; Vandenheede et al., 2015).

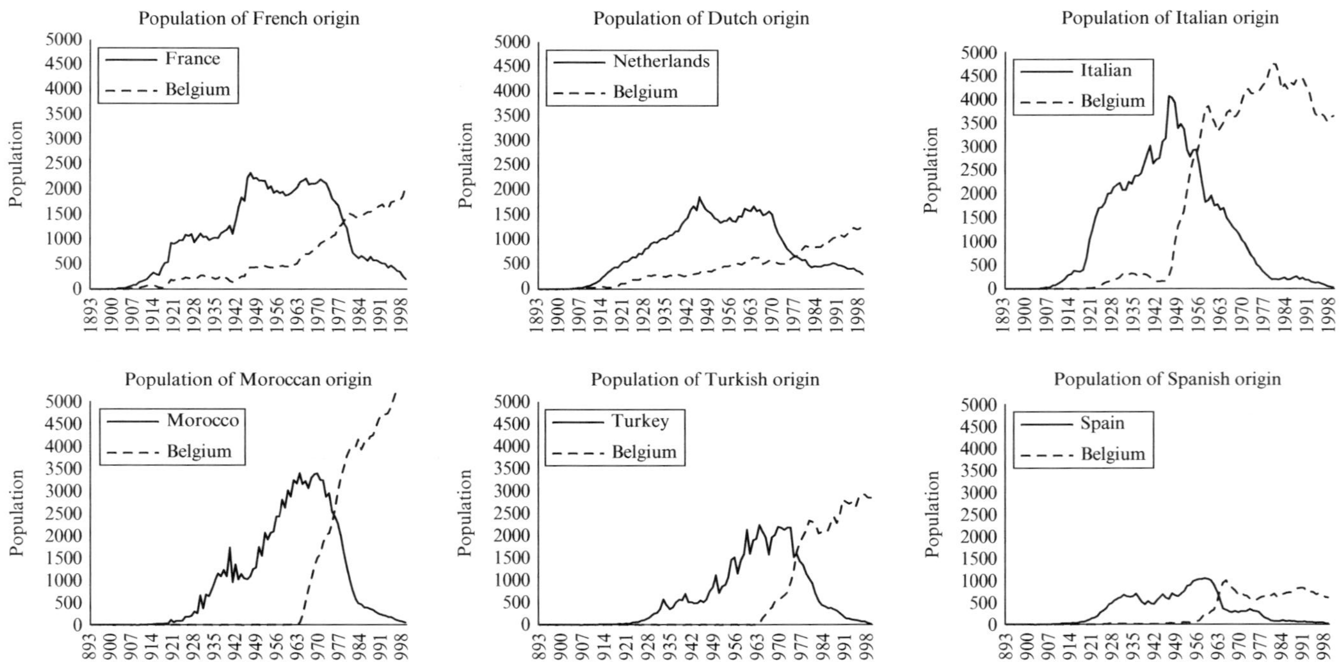

Figure 14.1 Selected population groups by nationality of origin and year of birth divided by births in the country of origin and births in Belgium, 2001 census

An explanation gaining momentum is the claim that FG immigrants from less industrialized countries moving to highly industrialized countries pass through the health transition – a shift in the cause-of-death profile from infectious to chronic diseases – at an accelerated pace (Razum and Twardella, 2002; Cappuccio, 2004; Spallek et al., 2011). As soon as FG immigrants from less industrialized countries arrive in the host country, they can benefit from more hygienic environmental conditions and high-quality medical care, leading to a fast decline in infectious-disease mortality. Simultaneously, upon arrival, FG immigrants are confronted with risk factors for chronic diseases. Yet these only result in chronic-disease mortality after a substantial lag period. In sum, this hypothesis assumes that the infectious-disease mortality (for example, tuberculosis) of FG immigrants from less industrialized countries will be high upon arrival and die out quickly after migration, whilst an increase in chronic-disease mortality (for example, cardiovascular mortality) does not follow immediately, entailing a migrant mortality advantage (Razum and Twardella, 2002; Cappuccio, 2004; Spallek et al., 2011). This hypothesis of 'migration as an unusually rapid health transition' has rarely been researched fully (Spallek et al., 2011; Wallace and Kulu, 2015). Yet the claims of this hypothesis are largely in line with observations from acculturation studies, showing that FG immigrants' health and mortality converge to host-country levels, with length of stay and over generations (Parkin and Khlat, 1996; Tarnutzer et al., 2012). However, small differences between these theories exist: while acculturation studies generally posit that acculturation is likely to occur sooner for some health outcomes than for others and that this process largely depends on the outcomes' webbing with culture and identity (Parkin and Khlat, 1996; Marsiglia et al., 2005; Harding et al., 2008; Kimbro, 2009; Nicolaou et al., 2009; Szaflarski et al., 2011), the focus of the migration-as-rapid-health-transition hypothesis is on differences in patterns of chronic versus infectious diseases (Razum and Twardella, 2002; Spallek et al., 2011). In the present study we look at this hypothesis by an analysis of differences in cause-specific mortality by migrant background in middle-aged adults, subdividing mortality into chronic and infectious types among other causes of death. We also probe into differences in life expectancy and health patterns. We discuss some of the mechanisms at play for the observed differences.

For the second generation a different health framework emerges. The prevalence of infectious diseases may be slightly higher than in the Belgian population because of the ongoing contact with the country of origin and the fact that the 'healthy-migrant effect' no longer plays a role. Rather, health and mortality patterns for this generation are largely determined by the socio-economic conditions of the parents and, later, by own socio-economic status. Still, lifestyle can be influenced by the specific cultural background of the country of origin and contribute to variations in health patterns. Finally, depending on the country of origin, discrimination and strong feelings of exclusion and non-acceptance by the host country can play an important role, especially in the case of mental health.

DATA

For the mortality and life expectancy analyses, the data are based on individual linked records from the Belgian 2001 census of population with the mortality register follow-up for the period 2001–11. Information on relevant covariates was available at baseline. Exposure and all-cause mortality were based on population register information, whereas the number of cause-specific deaths was derived from the mortality register.

LIFE EXPECTANCY BY NATIONALITY OF ORIGIN

Table 14.2 gives an overview of life expectancy at birth by nationality of origin including immigrants from a given country and their Belgian-born second generation descendants. Life expectancy has been calculated over a period of ten years (2001–11). Life expectancy over a ten-year period

Table 14.2 Life expectancy at birth by nationality of origin (own nationality or parents' nationality) based on the 2001 census population and mortality for the period 2001–11

Males		Females	
Nationality	Life expectancy at birth	Nationality	Life expectancy at birth
French	74.70	French	80.99
Eastern Europe	75.80	Other WE	81.56
Belgian	*76.49*	Turkish	81.74
Sub-Saharan	76.51	Eastern Europe	81.75
Turkish	76.88	*Belgian*	*82.11*
Italian	76.99	Sub-Saharan	82.20
Other SE	77.21	Italian	82.68
Other WE	77.53	Dutch	82.83
Dutch	78.27	Moroccan	83.89
Other	79.30	Other SE	83.98
Moroccan	79.73	Other	84.54

gives a mean that does not take the recent increases in life expectancy into account. Life expectancy of women and men in Belgium in 2015 was 83.5 and 78.6 respectively (Statistics Belgium, 2016).

Compared with Belgian men, most populations of migrant origin have higher life expectancy at birth. Only French and East-European men have a lower life expectancy. Moroccan men live three years longer than Belgian men and slightly longer than other non-European men. Dutch men have a life expectancy that is almost two years higher than Belgian men.

Life expectancy among women by nationality of origin basically follows the same order as for men, but even the best performing group among men has a life expectancy of minus two years versus the worst performing group among women, that is, French women. As with men, Moroccan and Dutch women have a higher life expectancy than Belgian women. Turkish women on the other hand end up with a lower life expectancy than Belgian women.

Differences in life expectancy between the population of Belgian origin and populations with a migrant background are the result of complex age-specific patterns with contributions that are not necessarily working in the same direction. Figure 14.2a gives the decomposition of the difference in life expectancy between Turkish and Belgian men for the 2001–11 period using the method of Arriaga (1984). The population of Turkish origin includes both the persons born in Turkey and their children (second generation) born in Belgium. The oldest age groups contain parents (or grandparents) who followed the labour migration of their children.

Men of Turkish origin have a slightly higher life expectancy than Belgian men by about a third of a year. The age-specific pattern reveals that adults between 20 and 64 years contribute to this higher life expectancy by almost one year and that another half-year comes from the oldest old. Negative contributions are divided between the older population (65–84 years) with a loss of half a year and the children with the remarkable high negative contribution of infant mortality. A similar pattern emerges among Turkish women (Figure 14.2b), although the adult mortality advantage compared with Belgian women is lower than among men and starts only at age 35. The net outcome of the age-specific contributions of Turkish women results also in a slightly lower life expectancy at birth than for Belgian women.

These results are influenced both by age-specific mortality patterns in the population of Turkish origin and in the Belgian population. Still it is remarkable how the decomposition gives a much more subtle image of the mortality differences, with lower adult mortality than the Belgian population and higher mortality among the elderly and children. For the oldest we have to take into account that the absolute numbers are relatively small and that a data artefact can more easily occur. However, a 'healthy migrant

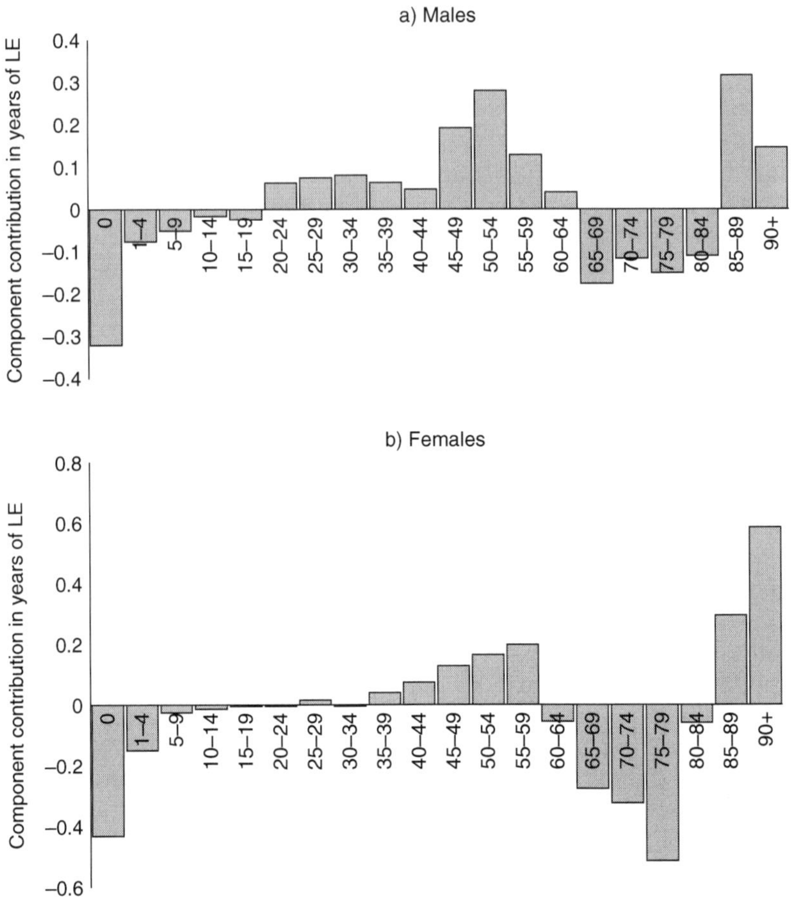

Figure 14.2 Age-specific contribution to differences in male and female life expectancy (LE) between the population of Turkish origin and the Belgian population

effect' cannot be excluded as it is probable that only the more healthy parents have followed their children who went to work overseas.

DECOMPOSITION BY AGE AND CAUSE

The decomposition of differences in life expectancy by age and cause are presented in Figures 14.3 to 14.5 for a selection of the most important populations by country of origin. Decomposition by age and cause

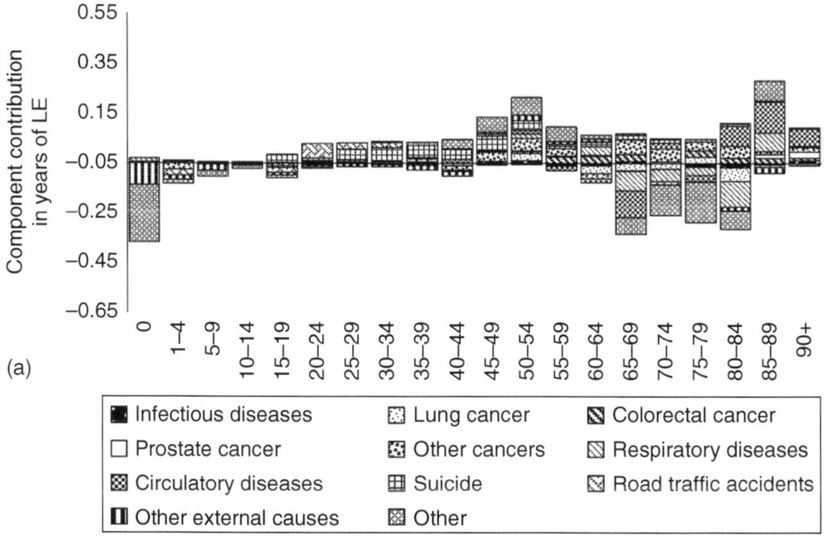

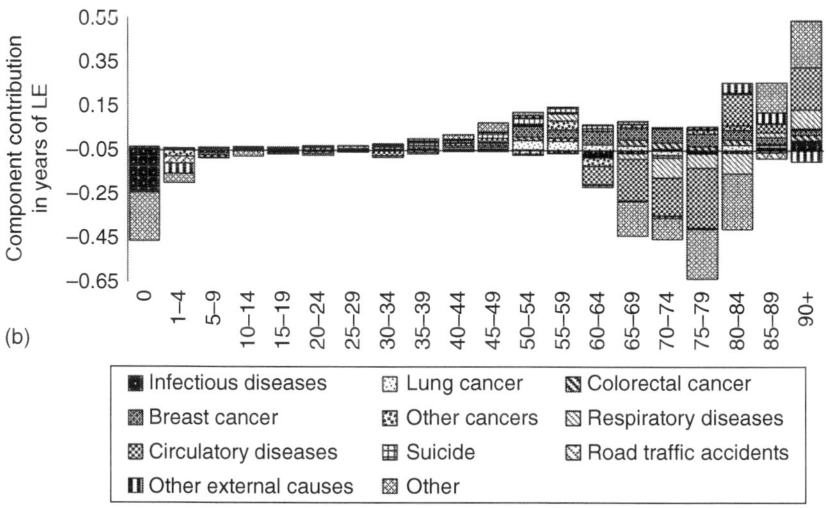

Figure 14.3 *Age-specific and cause-specific contribution to differences in male life expectancy (LE) between the population of Turkish origin males (a) and females (b) in relation to the Belgian population*

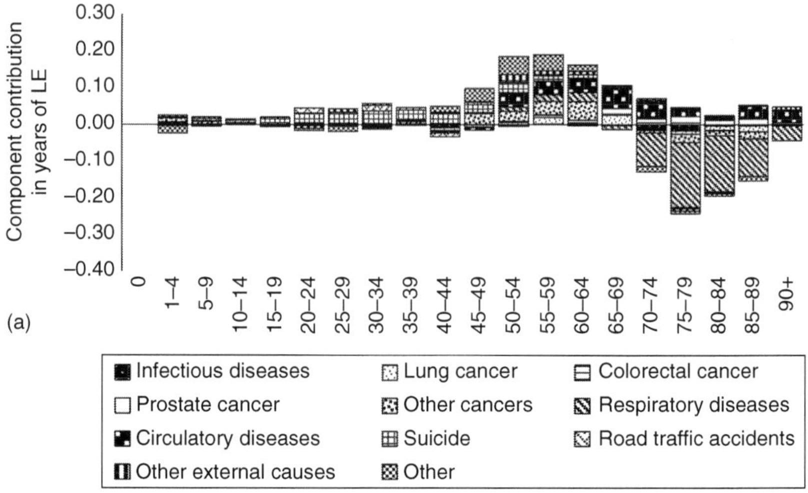

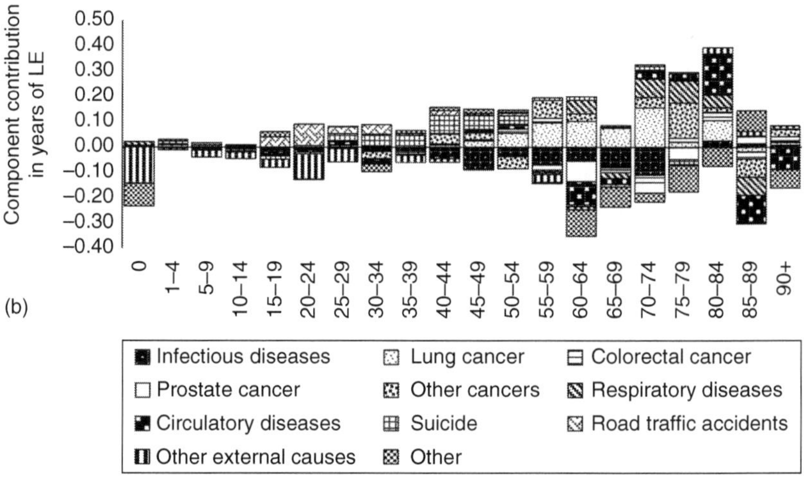

Figure 14.4 Age-specific and cause-specific contribution to differences in male life expectancy (LE) between the population of Italian males (a) and sub-Saharan males (b) in relation to the Belgian population

makes clear how a specific cause has contributed to the difference in life expectancy between Belgians as a reference population and the nationality of origin concerned. For each age group a specific cause can have a positive contribution, increasing life expectancy compared with the Belgian

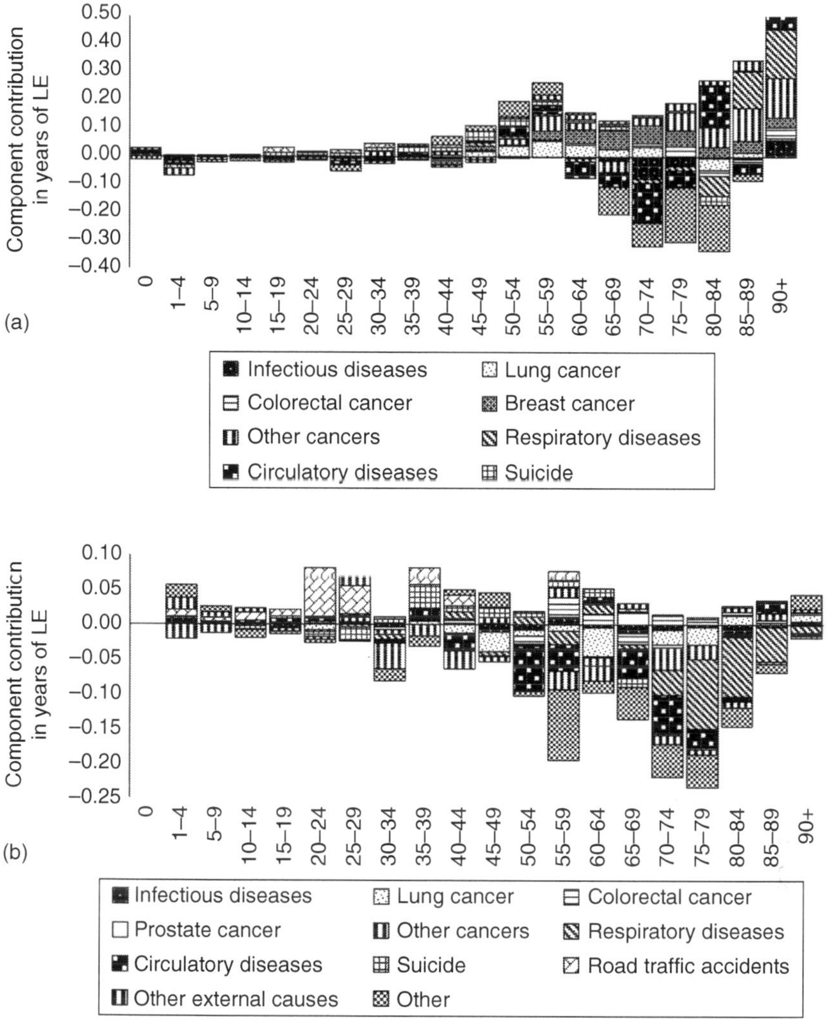

Figure 14.5 *Age-specific and cause-specific contribution to differences in life expectancy (LE) of Moroccan females (a) and East-European males (b) in relation to the Belgian population*

reference group, or a negative contribution, lowering life expectancy. For each age group these positive and negative contributions add up to the total contribution of the age group in life expectancy differences with the Belgian reference group. In Figure 14.3a, cause-specific mortality is added to the decomposition of life expectancy difference of Turkish men compared to Belgian men. The higher mortality among older Turkish men (65–84) is the result of counteracting causes. In the age group 65–69 there is a small contribution to higher mortality caused by lung cancer. Two more important negative contributors are the circulatory and the respiratory diseases. However, in the same age group we can discern a contribution to higher life expectancy owing to lower mortality for colorectal cancer, other cancers, suicide and road traffic accidents. A combination of residual causes (other), finally, has a negative impact on mortality.

For the whole age group 65–84 respiratory diseases, other diseases and to a lesser extent lung cancer have a negative contribution. Circulatory diseases show a more mixed result with a positive contribution among the 80–84 age group that persists in the oldest. This specific pattern hints towards a high tobacco consumption in the generations born after 1930 with even higher lung cancer mortality than among Belgian men maybe combined with lower exposure to air pollution over the life course for the oldest. Inversely the negative contribution of respiratory diseases in the age group 65–84 is probably influenced by the working conditions of these cohorts. Mineworkers have been heavily overrepresented in these age groups. From 1965 onwards there was an important recruitment of Turkish men for the Belgian coalmine industry. The Belgian coalmines have been progressively closed down, mostly towards the end of the 1980s.

Two causes dominate the contribution to lower mortality among Turkish adult men: lower road traffic accidents and lower suicide than among Belgian men. Both causes can also be related to marked lower alcohol consumption in the Turkish community, and explain the positive contribution of 'other' causes in this age group where excessive alcohol consumption is a killer among Belgian men.

Applying cause-specific information to the decomposition for Turkish women (Figure 14.3b) shows a large negative contribution of circulatory diseases in the age group 60–79 together with excess mortality for diabetes ('other') and some excess mortality for respiratory diseases. Contributing to higher life expectancy is the lower breast cancer mortality covering all age groups between 45 and 89 years.

In a similar vein decomposition of life expectancy differences by age and cause can be applied for men and women of all migrant communities. The most salient observations can be summarized as follows:

1. The heavy burden of the coalmine industry has left an imprint on the labour migration. Beginning immediately after the Second World War with the Italian migration and ending at the end of the 1980s with the closure of the Belgian coal industry, the male populations belonging to

the labour migration in 1945–73 all bear the traces of mine labour in their older cohorts. The mortality pattern of Italian men (Figure 14.4a) is very explicit in this regard with a clear-cut difference in the contribution of respiratory diseases to mortality between the younger and older adult population. Respiratory diseases above the age of 65 contribute to lower life expectancy than the Belgian population in a pattern that increases with age. Silicosis, pneumoconiosis, dust-related fibrosis and chronic obstructive pulmonary disease (COPD) testify how the oldest generation of Italian men were almost exclusively recruited to 'going down'. With the closure of the Belgian mines comes an end to the excess mortality in Italian men due to respiratory diseases. The lower mortality at younger ages reflects how the socio-economic status of the second generation gradually changes with increasing educational attainment. Also, newer migrants from Italy, attracted by the European institutions, are mostly highly educated, contributing to the changing composition of the population of Italian origin.

The mining industry has also left an impact on the mortality patterns of the population of East-European origin (Figure 14.5a) with the oldest generations coming predominantly from Poland, and on the other Mediterranean labour migrants (mainly Spain, Greece and Turkey) who have mainly been recruited in functions of the Belgian mining industry during the 1950s and 1960s.

2. Cardiovascular diseases in general contribute to a higher life expectancy in most migrant populations. It helps to explain how, notwithstanding the negative contribution of respiratory diseases, some nationalities end up with a higher life expectancy than the Belgian population. Lower tobacco consumption, a Mediterranean diet and growing up in less polluted regions during childhood are possible pathways explaining the lower mortality for cardiovascular diseases. Belgium belongs for many decades, and probably since the beginning of the industrial revolution, to the region in Europe with the highest air pollution (Nemery et al., 2001). Although air pollution has been continuously improving since the 1980s, the cumulative impact over a lifetime, and especially in younger ages, cannot be excluded and can explain differentials in health outcome between the Belgian population and migrants arriving at an adult age (Brook et al., 2004; Hoek et al., 2013).
3. Markedly lower suicide prevalence in populations of migrant origin, especially during the adult life under the age of 70, also contributes to higher life expectancy. Although small, the combined impact over all ages for the Italian male population (Figure 14.4a) results in a third of a year higher life expectancy. Populations of migrant origin form a mirror, revealing the high suicide prevalence in the Belgian population (Renard

et al., 2014), but the second generation already has higher suicide mortality, moving to an intermediate position between their parents and the Belgian population (Bauwelinck et al., 2016; Hjern and Allebeck, 2002).

4. Infectious diseases appear to have an important impact on life expectancy of some populations. In the male (Figure 14.4b) and female populations of sub-Saharan origin, infectious diseases have a negative impact in all adult age groups (for example, tuberculosis and other infectious diseases). A small negative impact of infectious diseases is also apparent among the older adults in the population of East-European origin (Figure 14.5b), as well as in other non-European populations.
5. Tobacco consumption plays an important role in the relatively lower life expectancy of the Belgian population compared with many populations of foreign origin. The contribution of lower lung cancer mortality to higher life expectancy among sub-Saharan African men (Figure 14.4b) is a clear illustration in this regard, contributing more than half a year of life expectancy. Tobacco consumption and especially cigarette smoking is known to contribute more than 80 per cent to lung cancer mortality. Again, the positive contribution of low lung cancer mortality among older adult sub-Saharan African (SSA) men has to be understood through the relative high tobacco consumption of Belgian men in the past decades. Lower tobacco consumption probably explains partially why many migrant communities have higher life expectancy than the Belgian population, even with a relatively low socio-economic status and worse working and living conditions. Lung cancer mortality is only an indicator of a much larger impact of smoking behaviour on many other causes, including circulatory conditions (Boyle, 1997; Van der Heyden et al., 2009). Figure 14.5a shows the positive contribution of lower lung cancer mortality among Moroccan women, notwithstanding the much lower lung cancer mortality in Belgian women than in Belgian men. Lung cancer mortality is extremely rare among Moroccan women.

   The situation is quite the opposite for men and women from East-European origin. As illustrated by Figure 14.5b for East-European men, tobacco consumption appears to be a major negative contributor to lower life expectancy, reflected in higher lung cancer mortality and higher mortality due to cardiovascular diseases.

Mortality differentials do not necessarily represent a full picture of health among migrant populations. For a more comprehensive understanding we should also take into account health differentials. Notwithstanding the fact that Belgian adults from migrant backgrounds often have a mortality advantage compared with the host population, their health, especially in those of non-western origin, is often worse. Below we examine the case of type 2 diabetes.

MIGRANT HEALTH: TYPE 2 DIABETES AS A CASE STUDY

Based on pooled data of the Belgian Health Interview Surveys of 1997, 2001 and 2004, persons of Turkish and Moroccan origin have a higher prevalence of diabetes than do Belgians. As shown below for men and women for the age groups of 35–74 years, the relative differences are particularly pronounced among women.

	Men (%)	Women (%)
Belgians	5.0	4.3
Turkish origin	5.8	18.7
Moroccan origin	6.5	11.9

Logistic regression confirms this pattern. Adjusted for age, the odds ratio of diabetes for Turkish versus Belgian men is 1.71; for Moroccan versus Belgian men 1.99 (Table 14.3, model 1). However, the odds for Turkish and Moroccan women is no fewer than 8.61 and 4.70 times greater than the odds for Belgian women (Table 14.3, model 1). If account is also taken of the differences in educational level, immigrant differences in diabetes' prevalence become smaller both for men and women (Table 14.3, model 2). In model 3 of Table 14.3, we included the lifestyle factors body mass index (BMI) and 'lack of physical activity' in the analyses. As expected both specific determinants show a positive association with diabetes. In 35- to 74-year-old men the ethnic differences in the prevalence of diabetes are no longer significant, if analyses are adjusted for these variables. In women the differences become smaller but the odds ratios remain very high, that is, 8.24 and 2.55 respectively for Turkish and Moroccan women. If level of education, BMI and lack of physical activity are all integrated in the analyses, immigrant differences in the prevalence of diabetes become even smaller (Table 14.3, model 4), but the odds ratios remain high. Thus, lifestyle and socioeconomic factors do not account for all immigrant differences in type 2 diabetes.

THE SHIFT IN MORTALITY PATTERN BETWEEN GENERATIONS

Results of direct standardization analyses with the Belgian population in 2001 as the standard are shown in Table 14.4. As for all-cause mortality, first-generation (FG) immigrants generally have a mortality advantage, while second-generation (SG) immigrants generally have a disadvantage relative to the host population. Particularly striking in this respect are

Table 14.3 Poisson regression odds ratios (OR) of diabetes according to age, ethnic origin, lifestyle factors, education and gender (ages 35–74)

		Model 1			Model 2			Model 3			Model 4		
		OR	se	Sign.	OR	se	Sign.	OR	se	Sign.	OR	se	Sign.
Males													
	Intercept	0.01	0.14	***	0.02	0.18	***	0.01	0.16	***	0.01	0.21	***
	Age – 35	1.07	0.01	***	1.07	0.01	***	1.07	0.01	***	1.07	0.01	***
Ethnic origin	Belgian (ref.)	1			1			1			1		
	Turkish	1.71	0.53		1.54	0.53		1.12	0.75		1.06	0.76	
	Moroccan	1.99	0.28	*	1.84	0.28	*	1.87	0.34		1.81	0.35	
BMI	> 25.77							1.1	0.01	***	1.09	0.01	***
Activity	Weekly physically active (ref.)							1			1		
	Sedentary							1.42	0.12	**	1.4	0.12	**
Education	No dipl./primary (ref.)				1						1		
	Lower secondary				1.06	0.15					1.02	0.16	
	Higher secondary				0.78	0.15					0.88	0.17	
	Higher education				0.72	1.16	*				0.81	0.17	
	−2 log-likelihood	2821			2812			2341			2339		
	Deviance[a]	200		***	209		***	244		***	247		***
	df	3			6			5			8		

Females													
	Intercept	0.01	0.15	***	0.02	0.18	***	0.01	0.18	***	0.01	0.23	***
	Age – 35	1.06	0.01	***	1.06	0.01	***	1.06	0.01	***	1.06	0.01	***
Ethnic origin	Belgian (ref.)	1			1						1		
	Turkish	8.61	0.32	***	6.01	0.33	***	8.24	0.39	***	6.87	0.4	***
	Moroccan	4.7	0.24	***	3.5	0.24	***	2.55	0.33	**	2.22	0.34	*
BMI	– 25.77							1.13	0.01	***	1.12		
Activity	Weekly physically active (ref.)							1			1		
	Sedentary							2.02	0.13	***	1.93		
Education	No dipl./primary (ref.)				1						1		
	Lower secondary				0.76	0.14	*				0.86	0.16	
	Higher secondary				0.66	0.15	**				0.83	0.17	
	Higher education				0.32	0.21	***				0.49	0.23	
	−2 log-likelihood	2748			2712			2073			2062		
	Deviance[a]; df	220/3		***	257/6		***	374/5		***	385/8		***

Notes:
se = standard error; ref. = reference group; [a] based on comparison of the respective intercept models.
Significance): *** p <0.001; ** p < 0.01; * p <0.05.

Table 14.4 All-cause age-standardized mortality rates (ASMR), number of deaths, and person-years by migrant background and sex, ages 25–54, 2001–11

	Males			Females		
Migrant background	ASMR per 100 000 [95% CI]	Deaths	Person-years	ASMR per 100 000 [95% CI]	Deaths	Person-years
Belgian	385.1 [382.2–387.9]	70 244	18 242 457	217.8 [215.6–219.9]	39 506	18 139 967
Western, FG, 0–9 yrs in Belgium	245.8 [228.0–263.6]	791	417 759	156.1 [141.5–170.7]	516	472 300
Western, FG, ≥10 yrs in Belgium	327.7 [314.8–340.6]	2 984	690 183	191.7 [182.1–201.3]	1 781	728 876
Western, SG	431.9 [416.4–447.5]	3 605	1 218 174	237.0 [224.7–249.3]	1 695	1 074 360
Non-western, FG, 0–9 yrs in Belgium	227.2 [192.9–261.6]	421	393 226	147.2 [125.5–168.9]	318	356 100
Non-western, FG, ≥10 yrs in Belgium	278.3 [264.0–292.6]	1 487	530 260	161.9 [150.6–173.2]	819	525 625
Non-western, SG	738.7 [639.2–838.2]	479	208 307	350.8 [266.7–434.9]	178	189 247
Italian, FG, 0–9 yrs in Belgium	226.0 [161.1–290.9]	54	33 491	145.3 [83.7–206.9]	24	24 472
Italian, FG, ≥10 yrs in Belgium	275.3 [255.4–295.3]	1 031	257 692	152.5 [136.3–168.7]	452	212 311
Italian, SG	362.8 [341.6–384.1]	1 488	566 263	202.4 [185.8–219.1]	739	519 940
French, FG, 0–9 yrs in Belgium	351.5 [298.8–404.3]	201	87 338	179.1 [140.1–218.1]	108	92 308
French, FG, ≥10 yrs in Belgium	479.3 [444.9–513.7]	838	139 036	262.5 [239.6–285.3]	557	174 303
French, SG	601.0 [549.1–652.9]	649	182 700	318.3 [280.0–356.6]	312	162 220
Dutch, FG, 0–9 yrs in Belgium	215.2 [185.7–244.7]	207	105 387	166.9 [138.3–195.5]	135	96 896
Dutch, FG, ≥10 yrs in Belgium	257.7 [224.3–291.1]	254	77 789	173.1 [147.6–198.5]	191	88 887
Dutch, SG	356.4 [317.2–395.7]	355	138 291	169.0 [136.9–201.0]	122	108 250

Moroccan, FG, 0–9 yrs in Belgium	225.6 [141.8–309.4]	127	167 320	153.7 [109.9–197.5]	80	102 308
Moroccan, FG, ≥10 yrs in Belgium	268.3 [246.3–290.3]	584	212 666	147.3 [130.4–164.3]	303	206 694
Moroccan, SG	832.1 [664.2–999.9]	251	108 977	351.2 [215.5–486.9]	85	101 482
Turkish, FG, 0–9 yrs in Belgium	310.3 [199.7–420.9]	79	72 967	119.0 [62.8–175.1]	31	51 806
Turkish, FG, ≥10 yrs in Belgium	269.1 [241.4–296.8]	377	148 719	149.3 [127.6–170.9]	197	145 176
Turkish, SG	705.4 [468.8–942.1]	90	48 403	418.6 [157.0–680.2]	36	41 813
Sub-Saharan African, FG, 0–9 yrs in Belgium	288.3 [213.2–363.5]	108	62 378	235.8 [177.7–294.0]	121	72 648
Sub-Saharan African, FG, ≥10 yrs in Belgium	344.4 [291.4–397.4]	170	49 359	261.2 [216.9–305.6]	139	55 865
Sub-Saharan African, SG	626.7 [358.1–895.3]	34	14 259	413.2 [177.3–649.1]	21	13 376

Note: FG = first generation; SG = second generation.

Source: Belgian 2001 census linked to National Register (2001–11).

Table 14.5 Cause-specific mortality rate ratios with 95 per cent confidence intervals by migrant background for men aged 25–54, 2001–11

Migrant background	Cardiovascular diseases		Cancer
	Model 1	Model 2	Model 1
Belgian	1.00 (ref.)	1.00 (ref.)	1.00 (ref.)
Western, FG, 0–9 yrs	0.63 [0.53–0.74]	0.50 [0.42–0.59]	0.58 [0.50–0.66]
Western, FG, ≥ 10 yrs	0.83 [0.77–0.90]	0.72 [0.66–0.78]	0.88 [0.83–0.94]
Western, SG	1.06 [0.97–1.15]	0.95 [0.87–1.03]	1.04 [0.98–1.12]
Non-western, FG, 0–9 yrs	0.57 [0.45–0.73]	0.36 [0.28–0.46]	0.45 [0.36–0.56]
Non-western, FG, ≥ 10 yrs	0.79 [0.71–0.88]	0.59 [0.53–0.66]	0.71 [0.65–0.78]
Non-western, SG	1.34 [0.98–1.83]	1.01 [0.74–1.39]	1.06 [0.78–1.44]
Italian, FG, 0–9 yrs	0.81 [0.47–1.40]	0.53 [0.31–0.91]	0.52 [0.30–0.90]
Italian, FG, ≥ 10 yrs	0.83 [0.74–0.95]	0.71 [0.63–0.81]	0.80 [0.73–0.88]
Italian, SG	0.93 [0.82–1.06]	0.85 [0.75–0.97]	0.91 [0.82–1.01]
French, FG, 0–9 yrs	0.78 [0.55–1.11]	0.57 [0.40–0.81]	0.68 [0.50–0.92]
French, FG, ≥ 10 yrs	1.06 [0.90–1.24]	0.85 [0.72–1.00]	1.24 [1.10–1.39]
French, SG	1.27 [1.03–1.56]	1.04 [0.85–1.28]	1.40 [1.20–1.64]
Dutch, FG, 0–9 yrs	0.62 [0.44–0.84]	0.63 [0.47–0.84]	0.58 [0.46–0.74]
Dutch, FG, ≥ 10 yrs	0.62 [0.47–0.82]	0.64 [0.48–0.85]	0.80 [0.66–0.97]
Dutch, SG	0.74 [0.56–0.96]	0.70 [0.54–0.92]	0.92 [0.76–1.12]
Moroccan, FG, 0–9 yrs	0.28 [0.16–0.49]	0.15 [0.09–0.27]	0.55 [0.39–0.78]
Moroccan, FG, ≥ 10 yrs	0.65 [0.54–0.79]	0.45 [0.37–0.54]	0.80 [0.70–0.91]
Moroccan, SG	1.46 [0.92–2.33]	0.99 [0.62–1.59]	0.95 [0.57–1.57]
Turkish, FG, 0–9 yrs	0.89 [0.54–1.48]	0.55 [0.33–0.91]	0.68 [0.42–1.11]
Turkish, FG, ≥ 10 yrs	0.80 [0.65–1.00]	0.59 [0.47–0.73]	0.68 [0.57–0.82]
Turkish, SG	1.11 [0.50–2.47]	0.86 [0.38–1.92]	0.72 [0.30–1.73]
Sub-Saharan African, FG, 0–9 yrs	0.74 [0.46–1.17]	0.50 [0.31–0.80]	0.39 [0.23–0.66]
Sub-Saharan African, FG, ≥ 10 yrs	1.05 [0.77–1.44]	0.93 [0.68–1.27]	0.79 [0.60–1.05]
Sub-Saharan African, SG	1.62 [0.15–2.46]	0.55 [0.14–2.21]	0.86 [0.32–2.29]

Notes:
FG = first generation; SG = second generation.
Model 1: controlled for age; Model 2: controlled for age, urbanicity and socio-economic position (education, housing status, and employment status).

Source: Belgian 2001 census linked to National Register and Mortality Register (2001–11).

the high mortality rates in non-western immigrants of the SG. The age standardized mortality rate (ASMR) in men of this background amounts to 738.7 per 100 000 (95% CI 639.2–838.2), compared with 385.1 (95% CI 382.2–387.9) in Belgian men.

If we look into the mortality pattern of specific immigrant groups, a more heterogeneous picture emerges. However, most immigrant groups follow the general pattern and thus experience a mortality advantage in the FG and a disadvantage in the SG relative to the host population. Notable

Cancer	Infectious diseases		Lung cancer	
Model 2	Model 1	Model 2	Model 1	Model 2
1.00 (ref.)	1.00 (ref.)	1.00 (ref.)	1.00 (ref.)	1.00 (ref.)
0.49 [0.43–0.57]	0.63 [0.48–0.81]	0.45 [0.35–0.59]	0.50 [0.39–0.65]	0.43 [0.33–0.55]
0.78 [0.73–0.83]	1.03 [0.92–1.16]	0.85 [0.75–0.96]	0.99 [0.90–1.10]	0.84 [0.76–0.93]
0.95 [0.89–1.02]	1.13 [0.99–1.28]	0.97 [0.86–1.10]	1.06 [0.94–1.19]	0.94 [0.84–1.06]
0.31 [0.25–0.39]	1.29 [1.01–1.65]	0.68 [0.53–0.87]	0.43 [0.28–0.67]	0.28 [0.18–0.43]
0.56 [0.51–0.61]	1.11 [0.95–1.29]	0.73 [0.62–0.85]	0.75 [0.65–0.88]	0.56 [0.48–0.65]
0.85 [0.63–1.16]	2.45 [1.75–3.43]	1.63 [1.16–2.27]	1.69 [0.97–2.92]	1.34 [0.77–2.31]
0.37 [0.22–0.64]	1.10 [0.52–2.30]	0.62 [0.30–1.31]	0.64 [0.27–1.55]	0.43 [0.18–1.02]
0.70 [0.63–0.77]	1.01 [0.83–1.21]	0.82 [0.68–0.99]	0.94 [0.80–1.09]	0.77 [0.66–0.90]
0.84 [0.76–0.93]	1.03 [0.85–1.24]	0.90 [0.75–1.09]	0.96 [0.80–1.14]	0.86 [0.72–1.03]
0.54 [0.40–0.73]	0.82 [0.47–1.41]	0.53 [0.31–0.92]	0.68 [0.39–1.17]	0.53 [0.31–0.91]
1.04 [0.93–1.17]	1.39 [1.11–1.75]	1.09 [0.87–1.37]	1.45 [1.21–1.74]	1.16 [0.83–1.48]
1.20 [1.02–1.40]	1.54 [1.14–2.06]	1.22 [0.91–1.64]	1.37 [1.02–1.83]	1.11 [0.95–1.64]
0.60 [0.47–0.76]	0.39 [0.22–0.71]	0.40 [0.22–0.72]	0.34 [0.20–0.58]	0.35 [0.20–0.61]
0.82 [0.68–1.00]	0.44 [0.26–0.77]	0.47 [0.27–0.81]	0.79 [0.57–1.10]	0.82 [0.59–1.14]
0.88 [0.73–1.07]	0.60 [0.37–0.96]	0.57 [0.35–0.91]	0.89 [0.63–1.26]	0.84 [0.59–1.18]
0.34 [0.24–0.49]	1.12 [0.73–1.72]	0.53 [0.34–0.81]	0.73 [0.40–1.32]	0.40 [0.22–0.72]
0.58 [0.51–0.67]	1.04 [0.82–1.33]	0.61 [0.48–0.78]	0.98 [0.79–1.21]	0.65 [0.53–0.81]
0.70 [0.42–1.16]	2.49 [1.51–4.10]	1.45 [0.88–2.39]	2.13 [0.88–5.17]	1.48 [0.61–3.60]
0.45 [0.28–0.74]	0.27 [0.07–1.07]	0.14 [0.04–0.58]	1.02 [0.46–2.26]	0.59 [0.27–1.32]
0.52 [0.43–0.63]	0.79 [0.56–1.12]	0.53 [0.37–0.75]	0.82 [0.61–1.10]	0.56 [0.42–0.76]
0.58 [0.24–1.41]	2.46 [1.17–5.19]	1.74 [0.83–3.68]	No deaths	No deaths
0.29 [0.17–0.50]	2.71 [1.86–3.96]	1.52 [1.04–2.22]	0.19 [0.05–0.76]	0.15 [0.04–0.58]
0.74 [0.56–0.99]	2.27 [1.61–3.19]	1.72 [1.22–2.43]	0.44 [0.23–0.84]	0.44 [0.23–0.84]
0.81 [0.30–2.15]	1.39 [0.35–5.57]	1.12 [0.28–4.47]	No deaths	No deaths

exceptions to this pattern are FG French men and women experiencing either comparable mortality to the host population or a disadvantage, and SG Dutch women having an advantage. As for FG SSA, the picture is diversified. FG SSA men residing for up to nine years in Belgium have a mortality advantage, while all other FG SSA have mortality rates that are comparable to those of the Belgian host population. Yet, confidence intervals are large owing to relatively small population numbers and few deaths, and, hence, should be interpreted cautiously.

In Tables 14.5 and 14.6, the results on mortality for four major causes of death (cardiovascular disease, cancer, infectious diseases, lung cancer) are based on Poisson regression, using person-years as the offset. Model 1 only controls for age, whereas model 2 controls also for socio-economic variables (compare below). The Belgian host population is used as the reference category.

Table 14.6 Cause-specific mortality rate ratios with 95 per cent confidence intervals by migrant background for women aged 25–54, 2001–11

Migrant background	Cardiovascular diseases		Cancer
	Model 1	Model 2	Model 1
Belgian	1.00 (ref.)	1.00 (ref.)	1.00 (ref.)
Western, FG, 0–9 yrs	0.60 [0.47–0.78]	0.44 [0.34–0.57]	0.64 [0.55–0.73]
Western, FG, ≥ 10 yrs	0.82 [0.72–0.92]	0.65 [0.58–0.74]	0.89 [0.83–0.96]
Western, SG	1.02 [0.89–1.17]	0.88 [0.77–1.01]	1.02 [0.95–1.10]
Non-western, FG, 0–9 yrs	0.76 [0.56–1.03]	0.41 [0.30–0.56]	0.50 [0.41–0.62]
Non-western, FG, ≥ 10 yrs	0.76 [0.63–0.91]	0.48 [0.40–0.57]	0.70 [0.63–0.78]
Non-western, SG	0.99 [0.58–1.68]	0.68 [0.40–1.16]	0.84 [0.61–1.16]
Italian, FG, 0–9 yrs	0.79 [0.30–2.11]	0.48 [0.18–1.27]	0.38 [0.17–0.85]
Italian, FG, ≥ 10 yrs	0.80 [0.64–1.00]	0.62 [0.50–0.78]	0.74 [0.65–0.84]
Italian, SG	0.87 [0.72–1.07]	0.75 [0.61–0.91]	0.97 [0.87–1.08]
French, FG, 0–9 yrs	0.73 [0.41–1.28]	0.51 [0.29–0.91]	0.64 [0.45–0.90]
French, FG, ≥ 10 yrs	1.00 [0.79–1.27]	0.76 [0.60–0.96]	1.13 [0.99–1.28]
French, SG	1.36 [1.00–1.85]	1.09 [0.80–1.48]	1.24 [1.03–1.48]
Dutch, FG, 0–9 yrs	0.68 [0.43–1.08]	0.68 [0.43–1.08]	0.79 [0.62–1.00]
Dutch, FG, ≥ 10 yrs	0.94 [0.66–1.32]	0.93 [0.66–1.30]	0.90 [0.74–1.10]
Dutch, SG	0.84 [0.54–1.32]	0.80 [0.51–1.25]	0.66 [0.50–0.88]
Moroccan, FG, 0–9 yrs	0.61 [0.32–1.17]	0.27 [0.14–0.53]	0.59 [0.40–0.85]
Moroccan, FG, ≥ 10 yrs	0.58 [0.42–0.80]	0.32 [0.23–0.44]	0.74 [0.63–0.87]
Moroccan, SG	1.07 [0.51–2.27]	0.66 [0.31–1.40]	0.72 [0.44–1.20]
Turkish, FG, 0–9 yrs	0.60 [0.22–1.60]	0.30 [0.11–0.80]	0.48 [0.26–0.89]
Turkish, FG, ≥ 10 yrs	0.86 [0.62–1.20]	0.52 [0.37–0.72]	0.61 [0.49–0.76]
Turkish, SG	1.53 [0.57–4.10]	1.03 [0.38–2.75]	0.48 [0.18–1.29]
Sub-Saharan African, FG, 0–9 yrs	1.23 [0.74–2.04]	0.69 [0.42–1.15]	0.55 [0.36–0.84]
Sub-Saharan African, FG, ≥ 10 yrs	1.59 [1.10–2.31]	1.17 [0.81–1.70]	0.82 [0.61–1.09]
Sub-Saharan African, SG	0.65 [0.09–4.62]	0.56 [0.08–3.96]	1.04 [0.43–2.50]

Notes:
FG = first generation; SG = second generation.
Model 1: controlled for age; Model 2: controlled for age, urbanicity and socio-economic position (education, housing status, and employment status).

Source: Belgian 2001 census linked to National Register and Mortality Register (2001–11).

Chronic-disease mortality is generally low in all recent FG western and non-western immigrants, and this advantage diminishes with length of stay. In the SG, chronic-disease mortality in immigrants often reaches a comparable level of that of Belgians. For example, cardiovascular mortality rate ratios (MRRs) in SG Moroccan women is 1.07 (95% CI 0.51–2.27) (Table 14.6, model 1).

Infectious-disease mortality is high in FG SSA, whereas it is low in all

Cancer	Infectious diseases		Lung cancer	
Model 2	Model 1	Model 2	Model 1	Model 2
1.00 (ref.)	1.00 (ref.)	1.00 (ref.)	1.00 (ref.)	1.00 (ref.)
0.55 [0.48–0.64]	0.59 [0.42–0.83]	0.41 [0.29–0.57]	0.79 [0.59–1.07]	0.62 [0.46–0.83]
0.81 [0.75–0.86]	0.98 [0.84–1.15]	0.78 [0.67–0.92]	0.81 [0.69–0.95]	0.65 [0.56–0.77]
0.95 [0.88–1.03]	1.11 [0.94–1.41]	0.94 [0.80–1.11]	1.18 [1.00–1.39]	1.01 [0.86–1.20]
0.37 [0.30–0.46]	1.86 [1.45–2.39]	0.96 [0.75–1.24]	0.31 [0.16–0.60]	0.18 [0.09–0.34]
0.56 [0.50–0.62]	1.10 [0.91–1.34]	0.68 [0.56–0.83]	0.34 [0.24–0.48]	0.22 [0.15–0.30]
0.71 [0.51–0.98]	1.85 [1.15–2.95]	1.19 [0.74–1.91]	0.62 [0.20–1.93]	0.45 [0.14–1.40]
0.30 [0.13–0.67]	1.33 [0.50–3.55]	0.76 [0.28–2.02]	No deaths	No deaths
0.65 [0.57–0.74]	0.94 [0.71–1.23]	0.73 [0.55–0.96]	0.43 [0.29–0.62]	0.33 [0.23–0.48]
0.90 [0.81–1.00]	0.92 [0.72–1.19]	0.78 [0.60–1.00]	0.98 [0.76–1.25]	0.83 [0.65–1.07]
0.55 [0.39–0.77]	0.80 [0.40–1.61]	0.54 [0.27–1.08]	0.44 [0.17–1.18]	0.34 [0.13–0.90]
1.00 [0.88–1.13]	1.37 [1.05–1.79]	1.05 [0.80–1.37]	1.13 [0.85–1.49]	0.88 [0.67–1.17]
1.12 [0.93–1.35]	1.92 [1.38–2.69]	1.54 [1.10–2.15]	1.86 [1.31–2.65]	1.51 [1.06–2.15]
0.79 [0.62–1.00]	0.52 [0.26–1.04]	0.51 [0.26–1.03]	1.20 [0.76–1.88]	1.23 [0.78–1.93]
0.89 [0.73–1.09]	0.50 [0.27–0.93]	0.50 [0.27–0.92]	1.34 [0.93–1.92]	1.31 [0.91–1.87]
0.65 [0.48–0.86]	0.52 [0.25–1.09]	0.49 [0.23–1.03]	1.09 [0.65–1.84]	1.01 [0.60–1.71]
0.39 [0.27–0.57]	0.99 [0.51–1.90]	0.43 [0.22–0.82]	0.13 [0.02–0.96]	0.06 [0.01–0.43]
0.55 [0.47–0.65]	0.83 [0.58–1.18]	0.44 [0.31–0.64]	0.29 [0.17–0.52]	0.16 [0.09–0.28]
0.58 [0.35–0.96]	1.49 [0.70–3.14]	0.85 [0.40–1.80]	1.11 [0.27–4.46]	0.70 [0.17–2.83]
0.34 [0.18–0.64]	No deaths	No deaths	0.61 [0.15–2.45]	0.32 [0.08–1.26]
0.48 [0.38–0.60]	0.76 [0.48–1.21]	0.47 [0.29–0.74]	0.24 [0.11–0.54]	0.15 [0.07–0.33]
0.41 [0.15–1.08]	2.12 [0.79–5.67]	1.38 [0.51–3.70]	No deaths	No deaths
0.42 [0.27–0.64]	6.08 [4.52–8.16]	3.20 [2.37–4.31]	0.31 [0.08–1.23]	0.18 [0.05–0.72]
0.71 [0.53–0.95]	2.97 [2.00–4.26]	2.07 [1.44–2.97]	0.82 [0.43–1.57]	0.61 [0.32–1.18]
0.96 [0.40–2.31]	3.06 [0.98–9.50]	2.44 [0.79–7.58]	No deaths	No deaths

other migrant groups. For illustration, the MRR for SSA women residing fewer than ten years in Belgium amounts to 6.08 (95% CI 4.52–8.16), whereas in their Moroccan counterparts it amounts to 0.99 (95% CI 0.51–1.90) (Table 14.6, model 1). As for SG immigrants, a pattern of convergence towards the host population is generally observed. Yet, in both SG non-western immigrant men and women, mortality from infectious diseases remains rather high (Tables 14.5 and 14.6, model 1).

For most migrant groups mortality improves after control for socio-economic status. For FG migrants this means even lower mortality. For SG migrants with higher mortality than the Belgian reference group, their mortality tends to become comparable after controlling for the impact of socio-economic factors. Dutch migrants are a notable exception as their socio-economic status is comparable to the host population.

CONCLUSION

The analysis of mortality by age and cause allows for a better understanding of the pathways explaining the differentials in life expectancy for populations with a foreign background. The observed pattern by age and by cause strongly underscores the need to move behind mono-causal explanations of differentials in mortality. There is not a single factor explaining a migrant or ethnic mortality advantage. There are arguments in favour of a migrant health effect. The fact that the labour migration was composed of healthy men has certainly contributed to lower mortality in adult migrant populations in the past and currently. Working conditions did, however, work in an opposite direction. Much of this negative impact of lower socio-economic status and hence of bad working conditions only emerged after several decades. The respiratory diseases among older men of foreign origin are a clear testimony of these long-term effects.

A number of other causes of death are related to food and alcohol consumption and smoking behaviour, and demonstrate how the negative impact of bad socio-economic conditions on health can be largely compensated by better dietary habits. Cultural background (and religion as part of the culture of origin) also plays an obvious role in containing the negative impact of some causes as demonstrated by the low mortality due to alcohol-related diseases and the very low suicide figures. Detailed analysis of cause-specific mortality, however, indicates that food can also have a negative impact on mortality as illustrated by the higher stomach cancer mortality among several migrant groups. Observing the shift in food consumption among the second and third generations of migrant background and especially the growing importance of fast food, we can expect in the future the emergence of a different pattern of cause-specific mortality among the younger generations.

NOTE

1. In the remainder of this chapter, we use the terms 'migrant background' or 'immigrants' when both migrants (first-generation immigrants) and their descendants (second-generation immigrants) are implied.

REFERENCES

Arriaga, E. (1984), 'Measuring and explaining the change in life expectancies', *Demography*, **21** (1), 83–96.

Bauwelinck, M., P. Deboosere, D. Willaert and H. Vandenheede (2016), 'Suicide mortality in Belgium at the beginning of the 21st century: differences according to migrant background', *European Journal of Public Health*, **27** (1), 111–16, doi:10.1093/eurpub/ckw159.

Boyle, P. (1997), 'Cancer, cigarette smoking and premature death in Europe: a review including the Recommendations of European Cancer Experts Consensus Meeting, Helsinki, October 1996', *Lung Cancer*, **17** (1), 1–60.

Brook, R.D., B. Franklin, W. Cascio, Y. Hong, G. Howard, M. Lipsett et al. (2004), 'Air pollution and cardiovascular disease: a statement for healthcare professionals from the Expert Panel on Population and Prevention Science of the American Heart Association', *Circulation*, **109** (21), 2655–71.

Cappuccio, F.P. (2004), 'Commentary: epidemiological transition, migration, and cardiovascular disease', *International Journal of Epidemiology*, **33** (2),387–8.

Courbage, Y. and M. Khlat (1996), 'Mortality and causes of death of Moroccans in France, 1979–91', *Population*, **8** (English selection), 59–94.

Deboosere, P. (2012), 'De stad van aankomst: de stedeling als migrant', in D. Holemans (ed.), *Mensen maken de Stad*, Berchem: EPO, pp.48–67.

Deboosere, P. and S. Gadeyne (2005), 'Adult migrant mortality advantage in Belgium: using census and register data to document different explanatory hypotheses', *Population*, **60** (4), 765–812.

Deboosere, P., R. Lesthaeghe, J. Surkeyn, D.Willaert, P.-M. Boulanger, A. Lambert and L. Lohlé-Tart (2007), *Huishoudens en gezinnen, Algemene socio-economische enquête 2001*, monograph, Brussels: FOD Economie.

Eggerickx, T. and J.-P. Sanderson (2004), 'Les migrations internationales. Observations, analyse et perspectives', conference paper, Budapest, 20–24 September.

Eggerickx, T., C. Kesteloot, M. Poulain, K. Peleman, T. Roesems and H. Vandenbroecke (1999), *De allochtone bevolking in België*, Monograph no. 3, Algemene Volks- en Woningtelling op 1 maart 1991, N.I.S.-D.W.T.C.

Harding, S., A. Teyhan, M.J. Maynard and J.K. Cruickshank (2008), 'Ethnic differences in overweight and obesity in early adolescence in the MRC DASH study: the role of adolescent and parental lifestyle', *International Journal of Epidemiology*, **37** (1), 162–72.

Hjern, A. and P. Allebeck (2002), 'Suicide in first- and second-generation immigrants in Sweden. A comparative study', *Social Psychiatry and Psychiatric Epidemiology*, **37** (9), 423–9.

Hoek, G., R.M. Krishnan, R. Beelen, A. Peters, B. Ostra, B. Brunekreef and J.D. Kaufman (2013), 'Long-term air pollution exposure and cardio-respiratory mortality: a review', *Environment and Health*, **12** (43), 15.

Kimbro, R.T. (2009), 'Acculturation in context: gender, age at migration, neighborhood ethnicity, and health behaviors', *Social Science Quarterly*, **90** (5), 1145–66.

Kouris-Blazos, A. (2002), 'Morbidity mortality paradox of 1st generation Greek Australians', *Asia Pacific Journal of Clinical Nutrition*, **11** (Supplement 3), S569–S575.

Lesthaeghe, R. (ed.) (2000), *Communities and Generations: Turkish and Moroccan Populations in Belgium*, Brussels: NIDI-CBGS Publications.

Marsiglia, F.F., S. Kulis, T. Nieri and M. Parsai (2005), 'God forbid! Substance use among religious and nonreligious youth', *American Journal of Orthopsychiatry*, **75** (4), 585–98.

Martens, A. (1985), Het na-oorlogse immigratiebeleid', in A. Martens and F. Moulaert (eds), *Buitenlandse minderheden in Vlaanderen en België*, Antwerp: Uitgeverij De Nederlandsche Boekhandel, pp. 169–81.

Morelli, A. (1988), 'L'Appel à la main d'oeuvre italienne pour les charbonnages et sa prise en charge à son arrivée en Belgique dans l'immédiat après-guerre', *BTNG–RBHC*, **19** (1–2), 83–130.

Moulaert, F. (1985), 'Vreemde werknemers, werkgelegenheid en sociale zekerheid', in A. Martens and F. Moulaert (eds), *Buitenlandse minderheden in Vlaanderen en België*, Antwerp: Uitgeverij de Nederlandsche Boekhandel, pp. 61–74.

Myria (2016), *Migratie in cijfers en in rechten*, Brussels: Federal Migration Centre, p. 249.

Nemery, B., P.H.M. Hoet and A. Nemmar (2001), 'The Meuse Valley fog of 1930: an air pollution disaster', *Lancet*, **357** (9257), 704–8.

Nicolaou, M., C.M. Doak R.M. van Dam, J. Brug, K. Stronks and J.C. Seidell (2009), 'Cultural and social influences on food consumption in Dutch residents of Turkish and Moroccan origin: a qualitative study', *Journal of Nutrition Education and Behavior*, **41** (4), 232–41.

Nørredam, M., C. Agyemang, O.K. Hoejbjerg Hansen, J.H Petersen, S. Byberg, A. Krasnik and A.E. Kunst (2014), 'Duration of residence and disease occurrence among refugees and family reunited immigrants: test of the "healthy migrant effect" hypothesis', *Tropical Medicine & International Health*, **19** (8), 958–67.

Nørredam, M., O.H. Hansen, J.H. Petersen and C. Agyemang (2015), 'Remigration of migrants with severe disease: myth or reality? A register-based cohort study', *European Journal of Public Health*, **25** (1), 84–9.

Parkin, D.M. and M. Khlat (1996), 'Studies of cancer in migrants: rationale and methodology', *European Journal of Cancer*, **32** (5), 761–71.

Razum, O. and D. Twardella (2002), 'Time travel with Oliver Twist – towards an explanation for a paradoxically low mortality among recent immigrants', *Tropical Medicine & International Health*, **7** (1), 4–10.

Renard, F., J. Tafforeau and P. Deboosere (2014), 'Premature mortality in Belgium in 1993–2009: leading causes, regional disparities and 15 years change', *Archives of Public Health*, **72** (1), 34.

Spallek, J., H. Zeeb and O. Razum (2011), 'What do we have to know from migrants' past exposures to understand their health status? A life course approach', *Emerging Themes in Epidemiology*, **8** (1), 6.

Statistics Belgium (2016), 'FOD Economie – Algemene Directie Statistiek en Economische Informatie', accessed 27 August 2016 at http://statbel.fgov.be.

Szaflarski, M., L.A. Cubbins and J. Ying (2011), 'Epidemiology of alcohol abuse among US immigrant populations', *Journal of Immigrant and Minority Health*, **13** (4), 647–58.

Tarnutzer, S., M. Bopp and the SNC study group (2012), 'Healthy migrants but unhealthy offspring? A retrospective cohort study among Italians in Switzerland', *BMC Public Health*, **12**, 1104, doi:10.1186%2F1471-2458-12-1104.

Vandenheede, H., D. Willaert, H. De Grande, S. Simoens and C. Vanroelen (2015), 'Mortality in adult immigrants in the 2000s in Belgium: a test of the "healthy migrant" and the "migration-as-rapid-health-transition" hypotheses', *Tropical Medicine & International Health*, **20** (12), 1832–45.

Van der Heyden, J.H.A., M.M. Schaap, A.E. Kunst, S. Esnaola, C. Borrell, B. Cox B. et al. (2009), 'Socioeconomic inequalities in lung cancer mortality in 16 European populations', *Lung Cancer*, **63** (3), 322–30.
Wallace, M. and H. Kulu (2014), 'Low immigrant mortality in England and Wales: a data artefact?', *Social Science & Medicine*, **120** (November), 100–109.
Wallace, M. and H. Kulu (2015), 'Mortality among immigrants in England and Wales by major causes of death, 1971–2012: a longitudinal analysis of register-based data', *Social Science & Medicine*, **147** (December), 209–21.

15. Reflections toward an organizing framework for the study of immigrant mortality

Frank Trovato

INTRODUCTION

As shown in this book, various hypotheses have been advanced in the migrant studies literature concerning health and mortality variations among immigrant populations, from the healthy migrant effect and negative acculturation explanations to the 'salmon bias', and accelerated health transition perspectives, among others. Our understanding of the complex dynamics and determinants of migrant health is certainly enhanced by this literature. At the same time, there is growing recognition that these explanatory frameworks do not fully capture the immigrant experience with respect to health and mortality. For instance, in some contexts immigrants do not uniformly exhibit characteristically low death rates as dictated by the healthy migrant thesis. Some immigrant groups may actually be more representative of vulnerable populations with unusually high morbidity and mortality rates (see for example Khlat and Guillot in this volume). Analyses of multiple groups often yield findings that are difficult to reconcile with the established explanations (Landrine and Klonoff, 2004). As described by Deboosere and Vandenheede in this volume, in actuality the causes of health and mortality variations among immigrants entail many interacting positive and negative factors that are often difficult to measure let alone conceptualize.

Currently, an all-encompassing theory of the causes of immigrant health and mortality change may not be possible. Therefore it may be useful to rely on delimited conceptual frameworks to help organize and interpret empirical observations. Figure 15.1 proposes one such framework that can suitably accommodate a wide range of possible analyses. Outcome variables include all-cause and cause-specific mortality for the major segments of the life course (infancy, childhood, teen years, young adulthood, and old age). It can accommodate a life-course approach to study

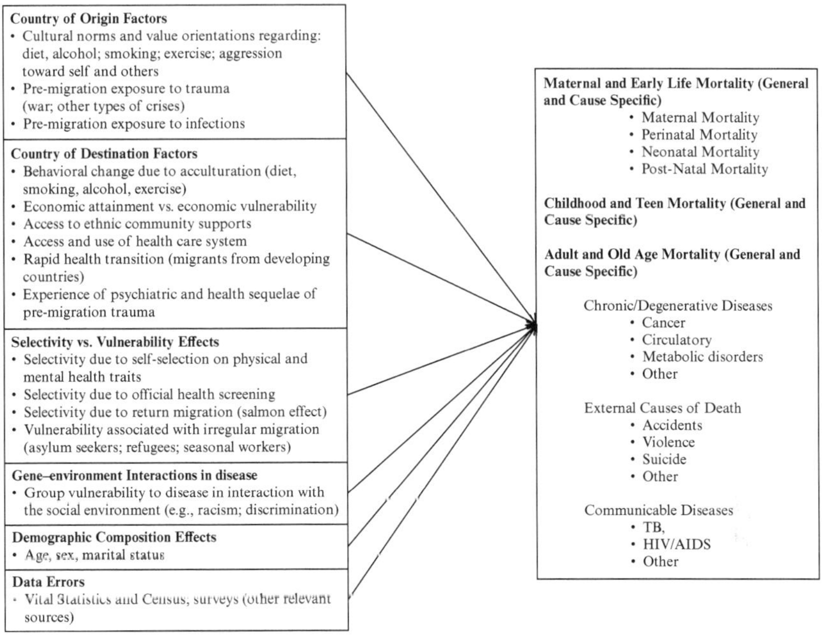

Figure 15.1 An organizing framework for the study of immigrant mortality

first generation migrants and their descendants. Pre-migration factors would be especially relevant in regard to the first generation. Different immigrant arrival cohorts could be studied and observed over age and time with this framework to allow for a more in-depth understanding of health change over time in the new environment. New arrivals bring with them better health due to the selectivity effect. More established migrants, on the other hand, have moved close to the epidemiological profile of the host population. In this dynamical context, the new arrivals help raise the overall health profile of the immigrant population while the more established segments of the migrant population experience health erosion. This type of ongoing process involving new and established migrant cohorts accounts for a large part of the immigrant health advantage observed in cross-sectional studies.

The proposed schema could be extended to study health and mortality variations among refugees and asylum seekers. Short- and long-term effects of pre-migration exposure to traumatic conditions could be researched and monitored. Old world (that is, European) and new wave (that is, from non-European origins) migrants may be compared in terms of differential mortality from infectious, chronic, and external types of mortality.

COUNTRY OF ORIGIN (PRE-MIGRATION) FACTORS

Immigrants' health and mortality patterns are closely linked to pre-migration factors (Kliewer, 1992). For example, many immigrants carry with them to the new country latent tuberculosis that becomes manifest later in the new country. Stomach cancer may arise from a combination of early infections (for example, *Helicobacter pylori*) pre-migration and dietary change. The experience of psychological trauma among refugees can result in additional physical and psychiatric problems post-migration. Background culture determines to a large extent the health behaviors of migrants, particularly in regard to smoking, alcohol use, and diet. Culture may be a factor in the extent to which individuals directed frustration and other forms of psychic conflict inwardly (for example, suicide) as opposed to outwardly (for example, homicide) (Durkheim, 1897 [1951]; Wolfgang and Ferracuti, 1967).

COUNTRY OF DESTINATION FACTORS

In the new country, migrants face conditions that can enhance or erode health and survival probabilities. Socioeconomic improvements would be expected to improve health and well-being. As members of a new society migrants must also confront and reconcile elements of their own culture with that of the host society. In this sense acculturation may be closely associated with health and mortality convergence with the host population (Berry, 1997). Certain features of the adopted society can operate in the opposite way, to improve health and survival, as for example having access to health care or belonging to a cohesive ethnic community (Trovato and Jarvis, 1986; Wolf and Bruhn, 1998).

SELECTIVITY VERSUS VULNERABILITY

Health selection underlies a good portion of the often observed migrant survival advantage (Razum et al., 2000; Wallace and Kulu, 2014a). However, this explanation may not apply to irregular migrants, particularly asylum seekers, refugees and seasonal workers. These groups may be more representative of vulnerable populations.

GENE–ENVIRONMENT INTERACTIONS

In epidemiology, migrant populations provide a natural experiment for the study of the effect of environmental change on disease (Mascie-Taylor and Lasker, 2009). Some migrant groups may share with their home population common genetic predisposition to certain diseases. For instance, some populations are more prone than others to single-gene related disorders responsible for ailments such as thalassemia, cystic fibrosis, sickle-cell anemia, non-insulin dependent diabetes (adult onset) mellitus, and certain cancers (Polednak, 1989). Genetic predispositions may be amplified by conditions in the social environment, as illustrated by Cooper et al. (1999), in the case of African Americans, a group with high levels of hypertension. Although black people do carry genes that make them more susceptible to hypertensive disease, this alone does not fully explain the very high prevalence of this disease among African Americans. Rather, it is the genetic predisposition in interaction with the experience of racism and discrimination that produces the racial disparity in hypertensive disease in the United States. Depending on the national context, some immigrant populations may experience a similar situation to African Americans. The idea of a possible interaction between genetic predisposition to disease and the quality of the social environment for immigrants is worthy of further exploration.

DEMOGRAPHIC COMPOSITION

Variations in demographic composition can confound statistical comparisons. Older populations may have high death rates from aging-related diseases, as compared to younger populations. Populations with a preponderance of unmarried persons might experience higher incidence of morbidity and mortality from external types of death in relation to those with a more balanced marital composition. Highly skewed sex ratios may account for unusual health and mortality patterns within immigrant populations.

DATA ERRORS

Problems are frequently found in vital statistics and census data, specifically with respect to under-registration of deaths and in some cases overestimation of the immigrant population (Weitoft et al., 1999; Wallace and Kulu, 2014b). A common problem is the presence of missing information on the death certificates.

CONCLUSION

Currently, given the state of the literature, an overarching theory of the causes of variations in immigrant mortality in host countries does not seem possible. Organizing conceptual frameworks delimited to a specific study context or setting (that is, national, subnational, group specific, multi-group, and so on) can help researchers interpret empirical observations.

REFERENCES

Berry, J.W. (1997), 'Immigration, acculturation, and adaptation', *Applied Psychology*, **46** (1), 5–34.

Cooper, R.S., C.N. Rotimi and R. Ward (1999), 'The puzzle of hypertension in African-Americans', *Scientific American*, **280** (1), 56–63.

Durkheim, E. (1897), *Suicide*, J.A. Spaulding and G. Simpson (trans.) 1951, Glencoe, IL: Free Press.

Kliewer, E. (1992), 'Epidemiology of diseases among migrants', *International Migration*, **30** (supplement 1), 141–65.

Landrine, H. and E.A. Klonoff (2004), 'Culture change and ethnic-minority health behavior: an operant theory of acculturation', *Journal of Behavioral Medicine*, **27** (6), 527–55.

Mascie-Taylor, N.C.G. and G.W. Lasker (eds) (2009), *Biological Aspects of Human Migration*, Cambridge: Cambridge University Press.

Polednak, A.P. (1989), *Racial and Ethnic Differences in Disease*, New York: Oxford University Press.

Razum, O., H. Zeeb and S. Rohrmann (2000), 'The "healthy immigrant effect" – not merely a fallacy of inaccurate denominator figures (letter to the editor)', *International Journal of Epidemiology*, **29** (1), 191–2.

Trovato, F. and G. Jarvis (1986), 'Immigrant suicide in Canada', *Social Forces*, **65** (2), 433–57.

Wallace, M. and H. Kulu (2014a), 'Migration and health in England and Scotland: a study of migrant selectivity and salmon bias', *Population, Space and Place*, **20** (8), 694–708.

Wallace, M. and H. Kulu (2014b), 'Low immigrant mortality in England and Wales: a data artefact?', *Social Science & Medicine*, **120** (November), 100–109.

Weitoft, G.R., A Gullberg, A. Hjern and M. Rosen (1999), 'Mortality statics in immigrant research: Method for adjusting underestimation of mortality', *International Journal of Epidemiology*, **28** (4), 756–63.

Wolf, S. and J.G. Bruhn (1998), *The Power of Clan: A 25-Year Prospective Study of Roseto, Pennsylvania*, New Brunswick, NJ: Transaction.

Wolfgang, M. and F. Ferracuti (1967), *The Subculture of Violence*, London: Tavistock.

Index